MARY PUTNAM JACOBI *&* THE POLITICS OF

MEDICINE IN NINETEENTH-CENTURY AMERICA

✦

Studies in Social Medicine

ALLAN M. BRANDT AND LARRY R. CHURCHILL, *editors*

CARLA BITTEL

✦

Mary Putnam Jacobi

& THE POLITICS OF MEDICINE IN

NINETEENTH-CENTURY AMERICA

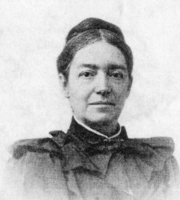

THE UNIVERSITY OF NORTH CAROLINA PRESS *Chapel Hill*

This volume was published with the assistance of the Greensboro Women's Fund of the University of North Carolina Press. Founding Contributors: Linda Arnold Carlisle, Sally Schindel Cone, Anne Faircloth, Bonnie McElveen Hunter, Linda Bullard Jennings, Janice J. Kerley (in honor of Margaret Supplee Smith), Nancy Rouzer May, and Betty Hughes Nichols.

Designed by Courtney Leigh Baker Set in Arno Pro by Rebecca Evans

The paper in this book meets the guidelines for permanence and durability of the Committee on Production Guidelines for Book Longevity of the Council on Library Resources.

The University of North Carolina Press has been a member of the Green Press Initiative since 2003.

Library of Congress Cataloging-in-Publication Data
Bittel, Carla Jean.
Mary Putnam Jacobi and the politics of medicine in nineteenth-century America / Carla Bittel.
p. ; cm. — (Studies in social medicine)
Includes bibliographical references and index.
ISBN 978-0-8078-3283-7 (cloth: alk. paper)
1. Jacobi, Mary Putnam, 1842-1906.
2. Women physicians—New York (State)—Biography.
3. Women's rights—United States—History—19th century. 4. Sex differences—History—19th century.
I. Title. II. Series: Studies in social medicine.
[DNLM: 1. Jacobi, Mary Putnam, 1842-1906.
2. Physicians, Women—United States—Biography.
3. History, 19th Century—United States. 4. Women's Rights—United States—Biography. 5. Women's Rights—history—United States. WZ 100 J1596b 2009]
R692.J33B58 2009
610.82092—dc22
[B]
2009011531

Portions of this work appeared previously in somewhat different form in Carla Bittel, "Science, Suffrage, and Experimentation: Mary Putnam Jacobi and the Controversy over Vivisection in Late Nineteenth-Century America," *Bulletin of the History of Medicine* 79:4 (2005): 664–94; and "Mary Putnam Jacobi and the Nineteenth-Century Politics of Women's Health Research," in *Women Physicians and the Cultures of Medicine*, edited by Ellen S. More, Elizabeth Fee, and Manon Parry (Baltimore: Johns Hopkins University Press, 2009), 23–51; both © Johns Hopkins University Press, and reprinted with permission of Johns Hopkins University Press.

CLOTH   13 12 11 10 09   5 4 3 2 1

To my mother,

JEANNE MARGARET BITTEL,

and in memory of my father,

GREGORY CARL BITTEL (1940–2004),

who gave me history

✴

Contents

Acknowledgments xi   *Introduction* 1

1 · CONVERSIONS OF YOUTH 15

2 · ON THE BORDERLAND 50
A Medical and Political Education in Paris

3 · SCIENCE AND SOCIAL EMANCIPATION 86

4 · FIGHTING SCIENCE WITH SCIENCE 116

5 · A MEDICAL MARRIAGE 154

6 · HIGHLY EVOLVED ORGANISMS 194

EPILOGUE · A GAUZE VEIL 226

Notes 235   *Bibliography* 281   *Index* 313

Illustrations

George Palmer Putnam 18

Page one of Mary Putnam's
    medical thesis, "Theorae ad
    lienis officium" 40

Mary Corinna Putnam, c. 1866 52

École de Médecine, Paris 64

Élisée Reclus, c. 1870 70

Reclus family circle 70

The New York Infirmary for
    Women and Children 102

Sphygmograph on a woman's
    arm 131

Illustration from Mary
    Putnam Jacobi's "Studies in
    Endometritis," 1885 134

Sphygmographic tracings 140

The Butler Health Lift 140

Illustration from Mary Putnam
    Jacobi's "Case of Absent Uterus,"
    1895 147

Abraham Jacobi, c. 1869 160

Hiawatha Island, Lake George,
    N.Y. 165

Ernst Jacobi 168

Marjorie Jacobi 168

Ernst Jacobi Memorial, Hiawatha
    Island, Lake George, N.Y. 171

Calling card from Mary Putnam
    Jacobi to Fanny Garrison Villard,
    1890 172

Jacobi and Schurz families, Lake
    George, N.Y. 191

Abraham Jacobi with grandchildren,
    c. 1917 192

Jacobi gravesite, Green-Wood
    Cemetery, Brooklyn, N.Y. 193

Acknowledgments

Writing a biographical study has been a constant reminder of how a life is never solitary, and neither is a book project. As was Mary Putnam Jacobi, this book was shaped by a large network of influence and many incredible minds; I just now hope the book can do them some justice.

I begin by expressing my deepest appreciation to my mentor and dear friend, Joan Jacobs Brumberg. From the first day I arrived at Cornell, she pushed me to think harder, dig deeper, and keep writing. Her encouragement and support continues today; I am extremely grateful for her many years of advice and inspiration.

Several other scholars inspired me in my early years of historical work and introduced me to the practice of history. It all began in a "Women and Medicine" course with Deborah Harkness and continued with the guidance of Paula Findlen, Karen Halttunen, Catherine Kudlick, and the late Roland Marchand. When I moved on to Cornell, I had the great pleasure of working with Mary Beth Norton, Peter Dear, Ronald R. Kline, and R. Laurence Moore. I also truly benefited from the Cornell Science Studies Reading Group during the earliest stages of this research.

I am extremely grateful to the many librarians, archivists, and historians who helped me gather materials for the book. In New York, I am thankful for the assistance of Arlene Shaner at the New York Academy of Medicine Library; Tara C. Craig at Columbia University Rare Book and Manuscript Library; Jeffrey I. Richman at Green-Wood Cemetery, Brooklyn; and Donald Glassman at the Barnard College Archives. I am also grateful for the assistance I received at the Mount Sinai School of Medicine Archives, the Museum of the City of New York, the New York Public Library, the New-York Historical Society, the

Columbia University Augustus C. Long Health Science Library, the New York City Municipal Archives, the Weill Cornell Medical College Archive, and the New York Downtown Hospital. At Lake George, New York, I received assistance from Pat Babé at the Historical Society of the Town of Bolton, Bolton Historical Museum. I thank Jack Eckert at the Francis A. Countway Library of Medicine at Harvard Medical School in Boston, and the staffs of Houghton Library and the Schlesinger Library, Harvard University, in Cambridge, Massachusetts. I appreciate the ongoing assistance of Barbara Williams and Joanne Grossman at the Archives and Special Collections on Women in Medicine and Homeopathy, Drexel College of Medicine in Philadelphia. I thank the staff of the Library of Congress, and am particularly grateful to Kristi Finefield in the Prints and Photographs Division. Several people made it possible for me to carry on my research in Los Angeles: Alan Jutzi and the staff at the Huntington Library; the staff of the UCLA Louise M. Darling Biomedical Library, History and Special Collections; and Cynthia Becht, Rhonda Rosen, Glenn Johnson-Grau, Erik Osuna, Orlando Penetrante, and Molly Parks at the Von der Ahe Library, Loyola Marymount University (LMU).

I was overjoyed to meet descendants of the Jacobi family, who were equally enthusiastic to learn more about Mary and Abraham. Thanks to Susan Boyd Joyce, Katharine Jacobi Boyd, Katharine Ciganovic, and Wendy McAneny Bradburn for their suggestions, correspondence, phone calls, and willingness to share what they know. At Lake George, Susan kindly showed me Jacobi Point, Abraham Jacobi and Carl Schurz Park, and the shores where the Jacobis spent their summers. In addition, I am grateful to Mary Martialay and Judy Martialay for allowing me to visit and photograph Hiawatha Island.

Several institutions provided invaluable funding so that I could continue and complete this project. I am extremely grateful to the National Science Foundation for the Scholars Award, grant no. 0724513, that allowed me to finish the book, and I thank Frederick Kronz for his assistance through the grant process. The Gilder Lehrman Institute of American History provided me a research fellowship so I could return to New York. I am grateful to the Huntington Library for the Mayers and Helen Bing Fellowships, and to Roy Ritchie for welcoming me again and again to the library, my second (academic) home in southern California. Finally, the College Fellowship and Summer Research Grants from Loyola Marymount University offered me vital assistance during crucial points of revision; I give special thanks to Dean Michael Engh for supporting and encouraging research at LMU. Any opinions, findings, and conclusions or recommendations expressed in this book are solely mine, and do not necessarily reflect the views of the National Science Foundation or any of the above institutions.

Several audiences heard different versions of this research and offered feedback. Thanks to the UCLA U.S. History Colloquium; members of the Loyola Marymount History Department at the Julia Stearns Dockweiler Tuesday Conversations on Scholarship; the UC Berkeley/UCSF Colloquium in the History of Science, Technology, and Medicine; the National Library of Medicine Symposium "Women Physicians, Women's Politics, and Women's Health: Emerging Narratives"; the Northwestern University Science and Human Culture Program; the Berkshire Conference on the History of Women; and members of the American Association for the History of Medicine and the History of Science Society. I am especially grateful to Nancy Cott and the Schlesinger Library Summer Seminar as well as to the Huntington-USC Institute on California and the West, Medicine/Public Health Working Group, who read my work and offered many suggestions.

A distinctive group of scholars provided me with a range of assistance over the years. For sharing their invaluable insights and knowledge on women physicians, I wish to sincerely thank Arleen M. Tuchman, Ellen S. More, and Regina Morantz-Sanchez. Janet Golden, Heather Munro Prescott, and Barbara Sicherman also provided vital feedback. Other colleagues in the history of medicine offered important suggestions: Toby Appel, Lynne Getz, Steven J. Peitzman, Naomi Rogers, David Sloane, Elizabeth Siegal Watkins, and Susan Wells. Over the years, Joan Jacobs Brumberg, G. David Brumberg, Faye Dudden, and Carol Groneman shared scholarly advice and their hospitality during my trips back to New York. Lisa Forman Cody and Cheryl Koos read and commented on sections, just when I needed their help the most. Jane Dabel and Diana Selig always offered sage advice. Last, but definitely not least, I am indebted to my wonderful writing group, who endured and seemed to enjoy my drafts: Emily K. Abel, Janet Farrell Brodie, Sharla Fett, Devra Weber, and Alice Wexler.

At Loyola Marymount University, a network of support kept me going through this project. I am lucky to have such wonderful colleagues in the history department, who each offered particular bits of help and words of encouragement. Special thanks to Anthony Perron and Nigel Raab, who gave translation advice, and to John Grever, who, as chair, supported my research in numerous ways. Teresa Hackett is our administrative assistant and the department's center of gravity. In the Office of Sponsored Projects, Joseph McNicholas and Yolanda Uzzell assisted me with grant applications and helped me to laugh in the grave final hours of submission. Several student research assistants provided great support at different stages of the project; I wish to thank Jennifer Allan Goldman, Romina Samplina, Christine Morrison, Ashley Balducci, and most importantly, Andrea Ryken, who inspired me as she did her own research.

I am extremely grateful to the staff at the University of North Carolina Press for all of their efforts and assistance. I was especially lucky to work with Sian Hunter, my trusted editor, who always gave smart advice, astute comments, and just the right words of encouragement. I also thank Dino Battista, Paul Betz, Ellen Bush, Mary Caviness, Beth Lassiter, and Heidi Perov. Finally, it is a privilege to be part of the Studies in Social Medicine Series, and I truly appreciate the support of the editors, Allan M. Brandt and Larry R. Churchill.

I have many friends and/or fellow scholars to thank who have touched both my life and this project. Diane Meyer used her photographic talent to assist me with images; she and Anna Muraco kept my spirits up in our shared Santa Monica neighborhood. Jodi Finkel restored my optimism and faith in myself, and humanity, over chicken dinners. Kristina Malsberger, friend and writer extraordinaire, gave editorial advice while reminding me to live. I am grateful for my Pasadena family, which originated at the Huntington Library and has helped me greatly over the years: John Herron, Joshua Piker, Charles Romney, Susanah Romney, Francesca Sawaya, Mark Wild, the late Clark Davis, and especially Cheryl Koos and Jackson Davis. My closest friends from graduate school remain dear: Laura E. Free, Kate Haulman, and Shobita Parthasarathy. Shobita read drafts, asked hard questions, offered strong insights, and shared unforgettable times in urban adventures. Daniel Martinico has been a gift to me; he saw me through the end of this project and made me immensely happy.

Family and friends in the Bay Area gave me their infinite love and support: Joanie and Larry Jones, Ryan Jones, Adam Jones, Clara Bianchi, Janice and Bob Graves, and Joe and Maureen Volpi. Unfortunately, three important people in my life are no longer around to see this book in print. My great uncle Orlando Petroni (1922–2006) was a surrogate grandfather and one of my biggest fans. My grandmother Margaret Petroni (1920–2008) taught me so much and showed me how to be a "wonder woman." My father, Gregory Bittel (1940–2004), was the family's original historian, whose daily lessons encouraged my love and appreciation for the past.

My mother, Jeanne Bittel, remains my rock of support. Her tireless listening, endless encouragement, and sound advice mean the world to me; she has sustained me through this project. She also offered her research assistance, as we followed the Jacobis around Lake George and lost our way in Brooklyn. My mother and father gave me history, not just through birth, but through their love, sacrifices, faith, and unconditional support, which enabled me to pursue what I loved. It is to them that I dedicate this book.

MARY PUTNAM JACOBI & THE POLITICS OF

MEDICINE IN NINETEENTH-CENTURY AMERICA

✳

Introduction

In 1873, in the United States and across the Atlantic, Victorians began talking about a controversial new book: *Sex in Education; or, A Fair Chance for the Girls*. Written by the now-infamous Edward H. Clarke, a physician at Harvard University, the book cautioned middle-class families that their daughters were seriously at risk for illness, with catastrophic consequences. The author warned that young women had unique and fragile constitutions and that they could become physically depleted or sterile when taxed by the rigors of coeducational studies, especially during menstruation.[1] As more and more young women sought higher education, Clarke's work set off a firestorm of debate, as women's rights activists rejected his alarming predictions.

Spearheading the fight against Clarke was Mary Putnam Jacobi, a physician from New York, who provided scientific ammunition to refute his claims. Her own study showed the opposite to be true: women were healthy when they *were* educated, mentally engaged, and physically active.[2] Women were not perpetually ill during menstruation, nor were they hindered by their biology, she insisted. Social limitations, not biology, constrained women and threatened their health.[3]

Edward Clarke has come to represent an effort by Victorian-era medicine to use biology as reinforcement for female subordination. Today, it seems obvious that Clarke's reactionary study was not based on pure science, but it was also a reflection of his gender politics. But so was Mary Putnam Jacobi's. Her version of the "truth" about women's bodies was also deeply connected to her own notions of gender and her hopes for female equality. She used the tools of scientific medicine, especially the laboratory, to prove that women were biologically capable of being equal players in the public sphere. She tried to depathologize and normalize the female body to show that women were capable of higher education, professional careers, and political participation. Most radically, she argued that men and women were not so different, and had the majority of human physiological and mental traits in common.

In the late nineteenth century, the body occupied a central position in battles over "the woman question." Many observers looked to the biology of sex differences to justify the social and symbolic separation of men and women. At a critical moment of professionalization, a number of orthodox physicians defined themselves as experts on women's nature and reinforced a model of sex differences that portrayed men and women as physical opposites. Some medical men claimed that female uniqueness was tantamount to women's physical weakness and mental inferiority.

Scholars have shown how Victorian gender ideology shaped knowledge on female health, focusing on medicine's masculine bias.[4] While many scientists and physicians were intent on using biological knowledge to demonstrate female fragility, they did not go unchallenged. A dialogue on differences between the sexes contained many voices and interpretations, both male and female. Women physicians played a large part in this debate, and Jacobi's was one of the loudest voices. A leading expert for feminist causes, she was called on by women's organizations, journals, and the women's rights leadership to set the record straight and provide medical evidence to support female vitality.[5] Reflecting their own views on female nature, women defined members of their sex in ways that reflected their own politics. They, too, were medical activists who could not separate their social values from their "sexual science."[6]

This book is the first scholarly treatment of Jacobi that focuses on the interrelationship of her social activism and her scientific inquiry, arguing that her science and politics were one and the same. Although it is a biographical study of an atypical woman, its significance goes beyond an individual life to the heart of American social, cultural, and political life. Her story serves as a vehicle for the analysis of the politics of gender and medical knowledge in late-nineteenth-century America. It also provides an open window into the contested world of nineteenth-century medicine and provides historical perspective on heated debates about the nature of gender that continue today.

✦ MARY PUTNAM JACOBI is now considered one of the most important figures in the history of American medicine. In her own time, leading medical practitioners — men and women — agreed that she was at the forefront of the profession. She has been called a "pathfinder" in medicine for her accomplishments and extensive education, standing out among both women and men for earning three degrees.[7] She first studied at the New York College of Pharmacy and received a degree in 1863; she then attended the Female (later Woman's) Medical College of Pennsylvania in Philadelphia, where she received her first M.D. in 1864. Dissatisfied with her education in America, she traveled to France and became the first woman admitted to the École de Médecine in Paris, receiving her second M.D. in 1871 and graduating with high honors. Her two medical school theses, the first in Latin and the second in French, reveal a conscious, early effort to define herself as a woman of science.[8] In the course of her career, she accessed a medical world dominated by men and won admission to several American medical societies that had historically been unfriendly to women. Combining therapeutics, research, and activism, she was also a prolific author who published several books and over 120 articles. Within her own lifetime, and also in historical memory, she represented a model of medicine based on scientific rigor and has become symbolic of women physicians who valued science over sentiment.

And yet, up until now, she has not been the subject of a full-scale study. Certainly, Jacobi is a central figure in Regina Morantz-Sanchez's groundbreaking work on women physicians, *Sympathy and Science: Women Physicians in American Medicine*.[9] Morantz-Sanchez was the first to describe Jacobi's scientific sensibility in contrast to the "sympathetic" approaches of other women physicians who emphasized maternalism, spirituality, and female nurture over rationalism and experimentalism. Other scholars have documented certain elements of Jacobi's life, including her education, Paris experience, writing, and relationship with her husband, Abraham Jacobi, who has been called the "father of pediatrics."[10] And still, historians have yet to fully examine her as a political activist and medical scientist, in tandem, as this book does.

Jacobi's background has been of great interest to historians because the Putnam family had deep roots in American culture. Mary Corinna Putnam was the first daughter and eldest child of George Palmer Putnam, one of New York's leading publishers, and his wife, Victorine Haven Putnam. From Protestant New England stock, her father's family first arrived in America in 1642 and settled in Salem, Massachusetts. In 1692, Putnam family members were, now famously, the most active accusers in the Salem witch crisis. Mary descended from other famous Putnams, including heroes of the American Revolution, Generals Israel Putnam and Rufus Putnam.[11] But by the mid-nineteenth century, the Putnam family name had become synonymous with publishing.

Mary Putnam was born into the world of literature, arriving in 1842 while her parents were living abroad in London and her father was employed in the transatlantic book trade. She returned to the United States at age five, with younger brother, Haven, and sister, Edith. The family eventually grew to include eleven children, with Mary as the eldest. Her siblings are historically significant in their own right, becoming active writers and key figures in the publishing industry.[12] A learned middle-class family, the Putnams encouraged their eldest daughter's education. At a young age, Mary began to establish herself as an essay and fiction writer, using her father's connections to get her pieces in print. But then she had a scientific "awakening" and began to pursue a medical education.

In an unpublished autobiography, penned in convalescence during her final years of life, she tried to explain her unconventional choice to pursue science and medicine, citing an almost uncontrollable desire as a young girl to carry out her own "anatomical experiment." After finding a dead rat in the barn of her family's Staten Island home, she wanted to cut it open to look at its insides. While most girls would have screamed in disgust at the dead rodent, Putnam recalled thinking, "If I had the courage I could cut that rat open and find his heart which I greatly longed to see." Her mother put a stop to her plans, and she noted, "I was secretly . . . relieved at the forcible delay of my anatomical studies."[13] Like many women doctors who wrote memoirs, she tried to explain her unusual life choices, and described animal experimentation as an early instinct. Looking back on years of dealing with disease and death, and spending more time in the hospital than the home, she returned to events of her childhood to claim that her study of science was a natural inclination.

But Putnam's career was not predestined. Rather, she pursued science as an antidote for spiritual confusion and gender conflicts. Her childhood years were plagued by her struggles with religion, particularly fending off pressure from her grandmother, an evangelical who expected a youthful conversion experience. While the evangelical tradition has been shown to be a source of social capital and power for many young women, particularly during the Second Great Awakening, Putnam wanted to be liberated from religious doctrine and rejected women's secondary status in churches and society.[14] In the volatile Civil War era, she desired more concrete, pragmatic, immediate solutions to social crises, as well as a way out of the gender role expectations of her class. She found an escape through the study of science.

Putnam's story illustrates the route traveled by women who reconfigured religion into a scientific faith. As she dramatically shifted her worldview, Putnam found new sources of devotion in medical scripture and in hospitals as temples of health. Her life story foreshadows the "spiritual crisis of the Gilded Age," that is, the process by which many members of the middle class participated in the secularization and medicalization of American society in the post–Civil War period. Many Americans found ways to harmonize science and religion; they would continue to worship, but they also placed their faith in numbers, knowledge, and practices produced within academic and political institutions. Middle-class women, through their work both at home and in public, as hygienic homemakers or health professionals, played an integral part in disseminating new scientific principles. Their ideas and activities would be critical for the making of twentieth-century America, a society that, increasingly, followed a "gospel of germs," pursued "magic bullets," and observed the authority of scientific knowledge.[15]

Putnam's years as a student in Paris solidified her scientific faith. Crossing the Atlantic in 1866, she spent almost five years in France, returning to New York at the end of 1871, degree in hand and personally transformed. She had acquired an unprecedented medical education for an American woman, studying in the halls of the École de Médecine, observing patients in the Paris clinics, and moreover, learning histology and cellular pathology in the city's microbiology laboratories. Putnam was inspired by French radical politics, associating with socialists and liberal reformers who mentored her personally and intellectually. She lived through the bombardment of Paris during the Franco-Prussian War and then witnessed the Paris Commune of 1871. In the next three decades, she integrated science and medicine, and blended science and politics, becoming, arguably, the most significant woman physician of her time.

In New York, she quickly built her reputation on her extensive education and numerous articles in leading medical journals. As a professor and a practitioner, she soon took on leadership roles and affiliations at numerous medical institutions in the city. She was most famously a lecturer and then professor of materia medica and therapeutics at the Woman's Medical College of the New York Infirmary, her home base from 1871 to 1889, and worked until 1897 as an attending physician at the affiliated New York Infirmary for Women and Children, founded by Elizabeth Blackwell. She also taught at the New York Post-Graduate Medical School, served as a visiting physician at St. Mark's Hospital, and helped establish the Pediatric Clinic at Mount Sinai. Jacobi gained prominence as a physician in an era when female practitioners struggled for acceptance in orthodox medicine.

Inside and outside of medicine, there was great opposition to women physicians because they betrayed middle-class gender norms and challenged the notion that men and women occupied "separate spheres" of influence.[16] Moralists claimed it was improper for women to obtain intimate knowledge of the body. By touching patients and performing dissections, many critics argued, women violated natural law and rules of propriety. Some medical men, anxious to elevate their status, worried that female physicians would degrade the profession with their poor training and frail constitutions. Echoing Clarke, opponents of women in medicine argued that strenuous medical work threatened not only feminine character but women's health; it could also "unsex" women and destroy their ability to reproduce. For the white, Victorian middle class, so committed to fixed gender boundaries and binaries, the prospect of becoming genderless was both a biological and a social disaster. Despite opposition, the number of women physicians grew to approximately 7,000 in the United States by 1900, representing about 5 percent of the profession.[17]

In the post–Civil War era, physicians cultivated their influence and authority by expanding teaching and research institutions, improving inadequate education programs, regulating practice, and shrinking the marketplace of lay healers.[18] At the same time, a debate emerged among physicians about the role of science in medicine and the value of the laboratory for clinical practice. While some physicians clung to the idea that empirical observation should direct treatment, others turned to testing, measurement, and experimentation for answers.[19] They disagreed whether and to what extent the laboratory should shape therapeutics. Some medical men tried to define medicine as a masculine domain and rejuvenate an old alliance in the Western tradition between science and masculinity. As physicians debated the meaning and worth of "science" in medicine, many of them saw it as a way to establish certain types of expertise and assign them to men. Jacobi actively inserted herself in this debate and supported the expansion of science in medicine, while criticizing men who did not agree. With the profession in transition, she and other women took advantage of its fluidity to pursue science in different forms. Jacobi ultimately did not persuade the medical profession to open all of its doors to women, but her moments of protest and activity at the center of orthodox medicine demonstrate that associations between manhood and medical practice were neither stable nor set in stone in the late nineteenth century.[20]

Jacobi associated most with the school of physiological therapeutics that argued scientific medicine, particularly experimentalism, should directly inform clinical care.[21] She focused heavily on "nutrition," applying histological and physiological knowledge to her studies on women's health and prescriptions for treatment. Influenced by the chemical and metabolic studies of European experimental science and concepts of cellular generation and pathology, Jacobi understood most female diseases as a result of failed nutrition.[22] Although extremely knowledgeable about gynecology and obstetrics, she grounded most of her work, especially mental health therapeutics and research, in physiology and neurology. In the latter half of her career, she explored the physiology of memory, perception, and cognition, but the majority of her studies focused on somatic manifestations of disease.[23]

For Jacobi, science, as both knowledge and practice, was the main pathway for political action. The scientific project, she believed, could wipe away the gender barriers that divided society. As a physician and researcher, she prided herself on being a generalist with a broad knowledge of medicine. Although she did not want to be narrowly defined as a woman practitioner who only knew obstetrics and pediatrics, she devoted her career to studying and treating the diseases of women and children. Serving the city's most marginalized and vulnerable populations, she realized that good health care could shift some measure of power to her struggling patients. Her husband understood this too.

Science was a very personal matter for Mary Putnam, particularly when she met Abraham Jacobi, a German-Jewish physician and exile from the 1848 revolutions in Prussia.[24] Jacobi was a widower who had been married twice before. Although the couple had very different backgrounds, and some serious disagreements, Mary and Abraham found that they shared an uncompromising passion for medicine and politics. They met soon after she returned from Paris and married in 1873. Together, they had three children, but only two survived infancy. The first was a female infant who lived only one day.[25] They then had a son, Ernst, and a daughter, Marjorie (or "Grete," as Abraham called her).[26] In an age when some women physicians chose not to marry and have children, Mary Putnam Jacobi stands out for combining, even merging, professional and family life. In fact, pediatrics and childhood illness were personal, professional, and political priorities for the couple, who saw protecting child health as a way to rectify social inequalities. Publicly, Abraham Jacobi fought to control infectious diseases and improve infant diets. In his own life, he had experienced enormous losses; in 1883, when Ernst died of diphtheria, the "father of pediatrics" had actually lost his seventh child.[27]

The merging of medicine and feminist activism remained a constant in Mary Putnam Jacobi's life, but the nature and focus of that activism evolved over time. In the 1870s and 1880s, she concentrated on women's health issues in coordination with campaigning on behalf of medical education, higher education, and participation in the professions. This was the era of her famous study and rebuttal to Edward Clarke, *The Question of Rest for Women during Menstruation* (1877), which won Harvard's Boylston Prize, as well as her neurological work on hysteria and brain tumors.[28] This first phase of activism was inspired by her experience as a medical student in Paris, steeped in socialism in the "age of positivism." Becoming a committed disciple of August Comte, she believed that knowledge was social power and interpreted Comte to meet the needs of educated women, arguing women could best improve their social positions through learning and disseminating information, especially in the sciences. Although often resigned to working in women's institutions due to gender barriers, Jacobi idealistically hoped gender equality could be achieved through the combined energies of men and women.

In the late 1880s and 1890s, Jacobi's politics shifted, as she became involved in reform movements and began to identify herself more with the collective action of women. Her activism was now more "Progressive" in character, as she geared her science toward institutions for social improvement; it was also grounded in metaphors of evolution, applied to a women's rights agenda as well as labor and political reform. Most strikingly, she had a change of heart about woman suffrage. Although she once believed that health, science, and education were far more important than voting rights for women, she now became a leader in the New York City and State campaigns. Along with many other feminist activists, Jacobi cited women's growing achievements to argue not only that white, middle-class women deserved to vote but that society needed them to vote.[29]

Like many thinkers of her time, Jacobi interpreted social relations through the lens of evolution, applying variations of Darwinism to her own political agenda. Rejecting the views of other theorists, she argued that males and females had evolved in a parallel fashion, not in opposition. But as she downplayed sex differences, she often reinforced class and race differences by privileging the expertise and leadership of the middle class over the working class, immigrants, and nonwhite citizens. Although Jacobi tried to create greater social unity, she accepted an uneven social hierarchy as a natural stage of evolution. She stood with many reformers of the period who called for freedom and social justice and worked to improve health and labor conditions but often did not treat all classes and races as inherently equal.

From today's vantage point, Jacobi's life was full of apparent contradictions that made her a complex character. For example, she had both strong alliances and contentious disagreements with other women activists; she dedicated her career to teaching women while remaining highly critical of them as students. She worked tirelessly to alter views of women's bodies and yet condoned the removal of female body parts through risky gynecological surgery. She sought to create a united social body but treated human and animal bodies as objects of investigation. She was an advocate for women as a class but denied the uniqueness of her sex. Though Jacobi was not a "model" feminist, her ideas reveal the different notions of womanhood and feminism that coexisted in the late nineteenth century. Her views and practices need to be understood within the social, cultural, and intellectual context of her time, as well as the power dynamics of her profession and political position.

Focusing on women in medicine, this study examines the fundamental interaction between private and public life, sometimes a difficult task with Mary Putnam Jacobi.[30] For a woman of her stature and education, a relatively small amount of personal correspondence survives.[31] We have only a few photos of her because, as her daughter joked, "she never would have her picture taken except at the point of a pistol."[32] Only one letter remains between her and her husband. This may be due, in part, to the fire that consumed the family cabin at Lake George, New York, in 1918 and destroyed Abraham Jacobi's personal papers, one year before his death, just as he prepared to write his memoirs. Accessing both the personal and the political in Mary Putnam Jacobi's life requires reading carefully into her published work and public worlds, linking her intellectual biography and her more personal relationships. It also demands that we listen to the voices of her contemporaries.

With a national and international reputation, and status as a medical "celebrity," Jacobi drew great admiration from her colleagues. Women physicians revered her as a brave foremother, one of the "feminine trail blazers in a nineteenth-century masculine wilderness."[33] They were awed by her intelligence, calling her a genius and a savant who was fearless and brilliant.[34] Despite her small size — "a little figure in a black shawl and bonnet"—she reportedly had a powerful disposition and a remarkable presence when she entered a room.[35] While younger women colleagues marveled at her, they also withstood her judgment, criticisms, and impatience with inadequate medicine; "[this] did not always add to her popularity," explained Emily Blackwell.[36] Medical men held her in high regard, seeing her as an exceptional woman of talent and genius who was also a trusted friend. "We, [men], all liked Dr. Jacobi very much as a woman and as a woman physician," said physician Charles L. Dana.[37] But they also recognized her personal intensity, that she was "tenacious in her opinions" and even combative.[38] Although she was widely admired, colleagues saw her as a force to be reckoned with.

Family, friends, and political comrades also knew her as a strong and dynamic personality. Although she shied away from the camera, she did not avoid social engagements and public discourse. In fact, her daughter remembered how her mother loved parties but that she took very little time off from work, leaving medicine behind only on Sunday afternoons. Some found Jacobi extremely "talkative," at times, to a fault.[39] She was dynamic and witty but could also be austere, brusque, and somewhat stern.[40] Underneath a tough exterior, she had deep affection for her family and a highly developed concern for human welfare. Her husband sometimes saw her strength as stubbornness and her commitment to work as neglectful of familial duties, but he was married to an unconventional woman who challenged Victorian femininity to the core.

Rejecting social codes of gender behavior, Jacobi crafted a scientific identity and embodied the idea that scientific knowledge and medical skills were not exclusively masculine. She rejected the nurturing and sympathetic model of medicine invoked by many of her female peers in medicine, most famously Elizabeth Blackwell. Instead, she presented herself as a woman of science, who actively engaged with experimentation.[41] While several women physicians in the late nineteenth century combined elements of these two models, or created "balance," Jacobi held firmly to her scientific identity.[42] But within this scientific model, she maintained her feminine exterior, not through fashion, delicacy, or sentimentality, but with a femininity based on composure, competence, and womanly character.

Jacobi did not advocate that women act and behave like men, nor that they deny their femininity, but that men and women should exhibit similar qualities. She believed that scientific practice belonged to both genders, in pursuit of knowledge about the natural world.[43] Women physicians needed to become more scientific as practitioners, she insisted, but so did men. She urged both male and female colleagues to treat therapeutics like a science and envisioned a medical world in which men and women worked together, side by side as equals, in the pursuit of "truths" about the human body. In these ways, Jacobi made science itself a political act.

Mary Putnam Jacobi enhances our understanding of how medical women not only crafted their identities but also engaged in gender "performance" in the context of medical practice.[44] Jacobi aimed not to act masculine but to act more scientific as a woman, by performing her expertise. In conversation or debate with medical men, she made overt efforts to demonstrate her superior knowledge and skills, advertising her own scientific rigor and accuracy.[45] When Jacobi debated medical men about the nature of menstruation, hysteria, and various "female maladies," she defined her own work as scientific and their work as biased and tainted. In the midst of gender conflict, she engaged in "boundary work," constructing lines between science and non-science, legitimate and illegitimate knowledge.[46] She promoted her own technical credentials and denied those of her ideological opponents. She also performed neutrality and detachment, pursuing the nineteenth century's definition and formulation of objectivity, through data collection, diagnostic technologies, and representations of cells and tissues.[47] By sustaining herself as an authority, she hoped that her research could help improve the health of women and, more fundamentally, that knowledge could reconstitute gender and power relations. Jacobi's work reminds us not only that science and culture intersect but also that science is embedded with politics, even feminist politics.[48]

Jacobi's story also undermines the assumption that science is, and was, essentially a "masculine project" because of the ways she used science to advance women's place in American society. Her story turns us further away from narratives that equate medical science with female subordination. Instead, a close reading of her work and career shows us how women utilized science, as theory, as practice, and as a source of identity and power. Historians once focused on how men of medicine pathologized the female body to stop the growth of women's participation in education and the public sphere. Labeled as hysterics and subjected to invasive, undesirable procedures, women endured manipulation and subordination by the masculine project of medicine. While some medical men pathologized women and employed science to exclude them from their ranks, some women physicians and reformers also used scientific discourse and sources of inquiry as tools for female advancement.[49] In addition, some men earnestly supported women physicians, promoted active womanhood, and shared reservations about popular medical explanations for female invalidism.[50]

This book is part of a larger scholarly movement to study women who pursued various models of science and medicine.[51] In the 1970s, historians of women, as part of a broader critique of orthodox medicine, tended to show greater interest in women physicians who identified with a "sympathetic" model of medicine and were more separatist in orientation. Since then, scholars have more closely examined women who combined characteristics of "sympathy and science."[52] Historians are also looking at women physicians, like Jacobi, Marie Zakrzewska, and Mary Dixon Jones, who denied that science had a masculine character, to understand how women physicians took "feminist" political stances while rejecting the notion of "feminized" medicine.[53]

Mary Putnam Jacobi presents another opportunity to rethink early research in feminist science studies that condemned "androcentric science." While some scholars critiqued masculine modes of inquiry and notions of objectivity, others suggested women scientists could provide unique and better perspectives on the natural world by conducting a feminine style of science, one that balanced emotionality with reason and was based on a reverence and kinship with nature.[54] To avoid essentialism, scholars are now more interested in how scientific knowledge is "situated" in particular contexts.[55] Within this analytical frame, readers will see how Jacobi produced medical knowledge from a complex gender position that reflected her class and racial status, her own interrelated notions of gender and nature, as well as her scientific training, professional standing, and networks in the medical community. She pursued a particular version of "objective" science, one shaped by positivism and experimentalism that was inseparable from her political ideologies.[56] She had her own version of "biological determinism," in which nature demanded an active female body and mind.

Jacobi's work also highlights the role of gender in the making of scientific medicine and the ways in which medical science and gender were "co-produced."[57] The "idiom of co-production," as Sheila Jasanoff calls it, is useful for understanding how the "woman question" and the debate over science in medicine overlapped and converged, illuminating how science and the social order are created and sustained together. In Jacobi's time, scientific knowledge legitimized gender codes; these gender codes then, in return, reified the authority of science. Science was used to separate the sexes and define men as rational; notions of masculine rationality then served to reinforce scientific authority. While many physicians tried to construct science and sex to the advantage of men and the exclusion of women, Jacobi resisted and defined both medicine as scientific and women as scientific, in an effort to simultaneously reform medicine and revise gender relationships. These intersections remind us how science and social order are deeply embedded and mutually reinforcing in the past, as they are today.

This book moves chronologically through Jacobi's life but does not follow her day to day or word by word. Instead, I use her life as an assay to unlock selected themes in late-nineteenth-century life, including religion and secularization, transatlantic intellectual exchange, professionalization, gender relations, and debates over medical knowledge. Chapter 1, "Conversions of Youth," follows her spiritual, familial, and intellectual struggles, including her rebellion against genteel girlhood. This chapter illuminates her scientific awakening, explaining the appeal of science as a philosophy, practice, and faith in itself. Chapter 2, "On the Borderland," takes the reader across the Atlantic, where Putnam and other "foreign" women negotiated their way into French medical schools. It shows how Putnam experienced medicine and politics as one, and how her transnational experience was part of a broader pattern of intellectual exchange between the United States and Europe in the late nineteenth century.[58]

Chapter 3, "Science and Social Emancipation," examines Jacobi's medical work in New York in the 1870s and 1880s to show how she enrolled science and positivism in the struggle for gender equality. As a practitioner, professor, and experimenter, she simultaneously promoted science in medicine and women in medicine, trying to elevate women's place in the profession and beyond. Chapter 4, "Fighting Science with Science," revisits nineteenth-century medical and cultural debates over sex differences and female maladies from the perspective of a woman physician determined to normalize female biology through positivist means. Jacobi tried to downplay the physiological differences between men and women and "prove" that women would be healthier if they had expanded roles and rights. Chapter 5, "A Medical Marriage," examines the medical and political union of Mary Putnam and Abraham Jacobi. It compares them personally and professionally and demonstrates their centrality in different medical debates of the time, particularly over the value of bacteriology and the meaning of scientific medicine. Beyond the Jacobi/ Blackwell comparison, this chapter analyzes a man and a woman on a spectrum of healing. Chapter 6, "Highly Evolved Organisms," looks at Jacobi's collective political and medical activism in New York in the late 1880s and 1890s, which combined science, suffrage, and reform, grounded in evolutionary biology. With the coming of Progressivism, Jacobi played a key role in integrating science into women's reform movements at the turn of the century.

Jacobi's story brings us into the streets of late-nineteenth-century New York, traversing immigrant neighborhoods and uptown brownstones, infirmaries for the poor and private offices for the middle class. It follows Jacobi into crowded hospitals and teeming children's wards as well as dissecting rooms and vivisection laboratories. It bridges the closed communities of medical men with the small havens for medical women, showing the tensions and unexpected overlap between these "separate spheres" of the profession. Finally, it views the nineteenth century through the lens of a woman who sought to promote scientific practices, redefine womanhood, and ultimately, redesign the gender blueprint of her times.

Throughout her life, Jacobi knew full well that ideas about the body had serious cultural power to shape how Americans understood women's professional abilities. This still holds sway, as the most recent debates about biology and sex differences have shown. In the early twenty-first century, biological determinism is again in vogue, and Americans look to science to explain differences and inequalities. To fully understand this national debate and questions about women in science today, we need historical perspective to remind us that the biology of sex differences always carries political weight. In the work of Mary Putnam Jacobi, we find continuities with our own time, through historical conflicts that help put into perspective our own political battles over what it means to be male or female.

CONVERSIONS OF YOUTH

"Unknown things want *science* to make them known," wrote Mary Putnam in 1864 in the first line of her medical thesis, submitted to the faculty of the Female Medical College of Pennsylvania. In her opening statement, Putnam professed that only science could unlock truths about the physical world and the physical body. In this sixty-page, handwritten, Latin thesis, "Theorae ad lienis officium," Putnam illustrated her claim by focusing on a somewhat obscure, baffling body part: the spleen. Anatomists had been puzzled by the spleen for centuries, trying to understand its purpose and function. Once considered the source of emotions or the capsule of the soul, it had been, what Putnam called, "an organ shrouded in mystery."[1] Determined to put metaphysical explanations to rest, she insisted that only rational science could uncover the true significance of the spleen. While she produced this thesis to graduate, she also used it to prove her medical competence and demonstrate that the spleen was not a spiritual or mystical force but a purely physical entity with a significant role in controlling the interior body. Her thesis reveals how, as a young woman, she rejected religion in favor of scientific "ways of knowing."[2]

Putnam arrived at this stance two years prior, when at the age of twenty, she had a conversion experience. Hers was not the typical evangelical rebirth associated with so many young women of the nineteenth century, but a scientific awakening. After struggling for years with uncertainties about salvation, Mary Putnam turned away from her family's religious affiliations in favor of a new faith: science. Thereafter, scientific thinking became the cornerstone of Putnam's personal identity, and soon her political life.

In the early 1860s, dramatic change swept through New York and the nation at large. During this volatile time of intense urbanization and industrialization, and the coming of the Civil War, religion was an empowering source for many Americans, particularly young evangelical women.[3] Faith and domesticity provided some women comfort, security, and a sense of value in their communities. But for other women, religion was confining and limiting, especially when they struggled with the notion of conversion.[4]

For Mary Putnam, several factors converged to draw her away from religion and toward a life of science. As she reached adulthood, she experienced a series of family crises and personal tragedies that forced her to reexamine her principles. She also began to address theological problems that she could not resolve. Just when her mind was confounded by religious questions, she found answers through the study of science, as she began informal medical training in 1860; her ideas then solidified as she moved on to the New York College of Pharmacy and the Female Medical College of Pennsylvania.

By questioning her Christian faith, Putnam also challenged what it meant to be a woman in nineteenth-century America. She was not alone. Interested in social reform and feminist causes, other women began to challenge the traditional authority of the church and express disagreement with women's place in the social hierarchy.[5] Elizabeth Cady Stanton, leader of the American women's movement at midcentury, most famously critiqued the failures of religion to promote an equal and just society.[6] When confronting the vast change and social problems of the nineteenth century, many women reformers began to place greater faith in scientific intervention. Putnam went further than most, making medicine and science her core values, much like a religion.

Science did not squarely displace religion in Putnam's life. Rather, science was a new faith that provided an alternative lens for understanding society and interpreting the natural world. Though based on different skills, discourse, and forms of knowledge, science had its own sacred texts, institutions, and rituals. But unlike the structure of Christian churches, science and medicine could, potentially, allow for the equal participation of men and women, or so Putnam believed. Traditionally, women had been healers as mothers and midwives; she hoped they could now reclaim this role and gain new legitimacy in the public sphere through knowledge of science.

Of course, women who pursued medicine, including Putnam, faced great resistance. Still, she held onto the belief that science could help produce a just society. But long before Putnam ever learned cell theory, she had trouble with religious ways of knowing the world, and the social expectations placed on young women. Her long-term crisis of faith, and its gender components, had roots in the personal and familial challenges of her youth. It is in her childhood, then, that we begin to learn how and why she ultimately pursued a life of science.

Faith: A Family Matter

In the late 1850s, the Putnam family experienced a period of misfortune that was linked to growing instability in the nation at large. The financial crisis that swept America in 1857 abruptly ended Mary's comfortable, leisured girlhood rooted in her father's world of literature. It also tested the family's faith.

At the side of George Palmer Putnam, Mary had witnessed the birth of the modern American publishing industry. Although her father's career had humble beginnings, he became a man of letters and a primary leader in establishing New York as the capital of American print culture.[7] George Putnam started as an assistant in the bookstores of George W. Bleecker and Jonathan Leavitt in Manhattan. He eventually joined the publishing house of Wiley and Long and traveled to London in 1836 as the firm's junior partner. In England, he promoted the company's overseas markets and arranged for the firm to sell and reprint foreign books to an American audience. He soon became a partner in the business and made his company a leader in the transatlantic book trade. Putnam effectively used his social networks to increase the company's publication list, develop a periodical market, and promote American writers in Britain. After working for seven years in London, his firm was at the forefront of the publishing business and Putnam was a leader in a growing industry.[8]

In June of 1847, George Putnam moved his wife, Victorine, and family back to New York and started his own business. He settled his family on Staten Island and opened a Manhattan office on Broadway where as "G. P. Putnam" he sold retail books and courted some of the biggest authors in American literature. George Putnam won the allegiance of Washington Irving, his first major client, most famous for his stories "The Legend of Sleepy Hollow" and "Rip Van Winkle." He also focused his business on the publication of belles lettres, poetry, fiction, and criticism, many penned by female writers.[9] With the launching of his magazine, *Putnam's Monthly*, in 1853, he focused on publishing more political and reform-minded writers who addressed distinctly American topics.[10] This strategy helped him become one of the leading publishers in New York by midcentury.

But in the economic crisis of 1857, George Putnam's publishing house encountered deep financial trouble. That year he expanded his business with a longer list and new types of publications, including books on travel, the sci-

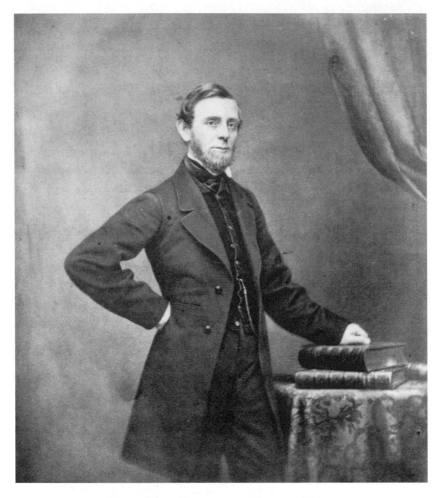

George Palmer Putnam, c. 1860. Courtesy of Prints
and Photographs Division, Library of Congress.

·✦· ·✦· ·✦·

ences, and contemporary fiction.[11] Although he knew his business and many
others in New York were overextended, Putnam optimistically watched as
American industry grew at an unprecedented rate. This economic boom,
fueled by the extension of the railroad system and land speculation, promised
great fortune, but it delivered a national financial crisis instead. Banks that had
once offered easy credit now began to call in their loans as interest rates rose
and stock prices fell. Although the financial damage stretched to the West, busi-
nesses in the urban Northeast were most severely paralyzed.[12] The publishing

industry was no exception as sales declined and many houses were forced to close their doors.

The country's financial disaster came at a particularly unfortunate time for George Putnam. External economic pressure combined with internal problems within his own firm, bringing Putnam's to the edge of bankruptcy. His partner, John Leslie, who handled their accounts, had not only extended the company's credit too far, but he had also used company funds for personal investments.[13] On 4 July 1857, the Putnam family learned that Leslie had drowned during a boat outing, possibly in an act of suicide, as his embezzlement schemes failed and the company's debt came to light. Years later, Mary speculated, "Whether knowing that he was to blame for this disaster, he determined to commit suicide, or whether it was really an accident, I don't think anyone knows."[14] One thing was certain; Mary knew that this disaster was "the great misfortune of [her] father's life." It was also a serious loss for the family who shared George Putnam's disappointment and financial hardships.[15]

Heretofore, the Putnams were a moderately religious couple, taking their children to an Episcopal church. While George Putnam's mother had always been a religious enthusiast, historically, his own family had devoted more of their energy to literary, political, and cultural interests than religion. But this all changed when the economy plummeted and revivalism offered the promise of spiritual renewal.

Nearing bankruptcy in 1857, Mary's characteristically secular father sought consolation in religion. Along with numerous other businessmen burdened with financial debt, George Putnam's despair drove him to seek solace in the evangelical movements in Manhattan, many of them located downtown in the city's financial center. The 1857 revivals — portrayed as a "masculine millennium"— attracted a number of businessmen eager to experience rebirth and reassurance in a time of uncertainty.[16]

The revivals of lower Manhattan were also popular because of their youthful, charismatic leadership. Abner Kingman Nott, the young pastor of the First Baptist Church on Broome Street ushered the entire Putnam family into the revivals. Nott had just finished his training at the Baptist Theological Seminary in Rochester, New York, when he arrived at the home church of Catherine Putnam, Mary's grandmother. Only twenty-three when he started at Broome Street, he was an overnight success, attracting large crowds to hear his sermons and converting at least two hundred people during his two-year tenure. It was in November 1857 that George Putnam first heard Nott sermonize, and he remembered later: "His mode of elucidating religious truth was to me peculiarly interesting, even as an intellectual exercise; for I could but admire his ever-ready, fluent, earnest eloquence — his dignified bearing and self-posses- sion — his happy choice of language — and the winning, sympathetic tones of his voice; and above all, the manly sincerity and truly Christian spirit that breathed through all he said. If ever my own inmost consciousness has been touched and enlightened by divine truths, it has been through the words which fell from his lips."[17] Nott's "intellectual exercise" moved the literary-minded Putnam, who appreciated the way Nott combined sympathy and manliness at a time when he needed both strength and understanding. In an unexpected shift from Episcopalian to Baptist, George Putnam and his family began to travel on Sundays from their home, then in the Bronx, to the southern end of Manhattan to attend Nott's church.

Besides the elder Putnam, Nott successfully drew all of the older members of the Putnam family into the church, counting Victorine, Haven, and Mary among his many converts. As George Putnam recalled, Nott "baptized my wife and daughter in May, and myself in August of that year."[18] Haven remembered, Nott's leadership "proved to be sufficient to bring me also into the Baptist communion, and what was, under the circumstances, much more surprising, stirred in the same direction my active-minded sister Minnie."[19] Haven was surprised that Mary, or "Minnie," as they nicknamed her, would be so easily swept up by the revivals, for she had spent most of her childhood confounded by questions of faith.

As a small child, Mary had followed the spiritual lead of her parents, at- tending church with her family and sessions of Episcopal Sunday school. She was primarily occupied with reading, lessons, playing music, and even going to the gymnasium, but like many Victorian girls, she made evaluating her per- formance as a Christian a high priority. At age eleven, she was extremely self- aware and reflective about conduct and character. Putnam monitored her own behavior, making a list of "virtues and vices" in the back her mother's ledger book. She noted when she had been "guilty" of being unkind to her mother and "disagreeable" to her siblings. To her younger sister Edith, she was "self- ish," "hasty," and ". . . silly. Burst[ing] into tears at a disappointment." She also marked down when she was careless or, even worse, "dawdling," for not being industrious. Putnam also took note of her virtues, including her "generosity . . . To a poor woman," her kindness, and her obedience.[20] In this mode of self- evaluation, very common in the nineteenth century, she tried to decipher her moral worth, and, ultimately, the destiny of her soul.

But Mary Putnam's spiritual troubles began the next year. On her twelfth birthday, she turned to her paternal grandmother for help. The family matriarch, a Sunday school teacher and devout Baptist herself, Catherine Putnam was eager to offer Mary guidance. She tried to comfort her granddaughter, becoming her religious counselor and confidante, and committed herself to leading her down the road to evangelical conversion. This was easier said than done; Mary often stirred up trouble in Sunday school with her "inquiring mind" and posed questions that fundamentally challenged what it meant to be a true believer.[21] She was not sure about her ability to "love Christ"—an evangelical requirement — and she questioned the presence of God in the lives of human beings.

A portend of the future, Putnam explained her confusion with allusions to scientific method. She claimed to spend three years conducting what she called "*experiments* upon the power of God," asking for divine intervention during times of family illness and waiting for results and evidence of divine power. She then decided to "apply the *proofs* of salvation" to herself to test whether she was worthy of or ready for conversion. Finally, after some serious contemplation, she came to a realization: "I do love to pray to God, and . . . nothing but salvation will satisfy me," and looked forward to being saved one day.[22]

Putnam may have temporarily soothed her own anxieties, but she then redirected her fears about salvation to her brother, Haven. Giving him an evangelical volume on "the eternal welfare of an immortal soul," Mary begged him, in an impassioned letter, to fear God and prepare to face his judgment. By expressing such pressing concern for her brother, Mary showed great unease about her own sins and chances at salvation.[23]

Still confused and conflicted, Mary sought relief on the eve of her sixteenth birthday. In 1858, she followed her father and her entire family into the Baptist faith and officially became a member of her grandmother's church on Broome Street. Catherine Putnam could not take credit for resolving her granddaughter's spiritual doubts. Rather, it was Abner Kingman Nott, the young charismatic preacher, who temporarily relieved Mary of her spiritual troubles.

At twenty-five, Nott made a devout, pious life accessible and attractive to Mary and many of her peers.[24] Though popular among elder parishioners, Nott was most deeply involved in counseling youth, or his "little band of converts," as he called them.[25] Preaching about the parallels between rebirth through conversion and Christ's resurrection, Nott tried to resolve the religious dilemmas that Mary faced in her younger years.[26] And because of his intellect and dynamic personality, Mary became enamored of the young preacher. Quite infatuated with him, she told a friend that they were "constantly associated together" during his visits, that they read together and engaged intellectually over theological topics. She recalled that Nott was "the only visitor we had constantly that I cared anything about."[27] Considered "one of the family," he visited the Putnams frequently and accompanied them on recreational excursions.[28] As George Putnam remembered, "His coming was always hailed with delight by the *little* children as well as the oldest," a reference to Nott's close relationship with Mary.[29] Although she was easily swept into the church by her fondness for Nott, her faith was short-lived.

In addition to their financial problems in the late 1850s, the Putnams suffered a series of personal losses. First, the family faced the death of George Putnam's four-year-old nephew, Duncan Smith, the son of his sister Elizabeth and her husband Isaac Smith. Next, the family's nurse, Isabella Cole, who moved with them from England to New York, died of a "failing heart."[30] The third loss, probably the most shocking, was the death of Abner Kingman Nott at age twenty-five. In early July, he drowned while swimming with friends near Perth Amboy in the waters between New Jersey and Staten Island. Unfortunately for the Putnams, drowning had become an all-too-frequent tragedy in their family. As a child, Mary had a near fatal swimming accident herself. After the loss of John Leslie and then Nott, the waters surrounding New York began to have dangerous associations.

According to his brother, Nott drowned because he was physically and emotionally exhausted from a rigorous preaching and traveling schedule. He died peacefully, the brother said, while floating on his back, as "God had called him home."[31] Nott's death was regarded as the climactic ending to his short but noble life and dynamic career as an apostle to the people. His memoir, reprinted several times in the late nineteenth century, was a didactic evangelical biography that presented Nott as the ultimate model for Christian youth.

Members of Nott's congregation were devastated by his death, especially George Putnam and his family. Mary described her father's response to the loss: "A strong man trembling almost under a shock that blasted a long pleasant path of life, leading to the very innermost depths of the soul."[32] Not long after Nott's drowning, George Putnam's "orthodoxy as a Calvinist was brought into question" and he left the First Baptist Church.[33] While Nott became a martyr whose story drew in young converts, his death was an important turning point away from religion for Mary Putnam. Though devastated by the loss, she refused at first to grieve over his death, accepting it as God's will. She reminded friend Mary Swift that, "according to the prevailing ideas nominally accepted on the subject," they should not be sad about Nott's passing because he entered an "eternity of irreversible happiness."[34] But Mary did not feel the full impact of Nott's death until months later, when the next pastor at the First Baptist Church failed to provide her with the same sense of comfort. For it was in 1859, the year of Nott's death, that she began the final phase of questioning her faith which lead to her final break with the church in 1863.

A House of Letters

Mary Putnam's spiritual journey was mirrored in her growth as a writer and the evolution of her commentaries on matters of gender and faith. Born into the publishing world, she grew up surrounded by men and women with great literary ambitions, and, at a very young age, the intellectually precocious Putnam saw a future for herself in writing. Following in the footsteps of many "literary domestics," she realized that publications could provide a solid income, particularly for middle-class women with few options for independent earnings.[35] It also provided women with a public voice. And while many women used this voice to extol the virtues of domesticity, and express Christian devotion, Putnam learned that it could also serve as an outlet for expressing dissatisfaction with religion and gender conventions. While young women used reading and writing to cultivate the inner self, words provided a much-desired mode of self-expression and independent thinking.[36] As Putnam matured, surrounded by the printed word, putting pen to paper was more than an intellectual exercise; it was an act of defiance.

During her childhood, Putnam's family encouraged her education and, in fact, facilitated her accelerated training. She and her siblings were educated primarily at home, where they learned to read and write from their mother or family nurse. Putnam began to study Latin at age twelve, and then continued lessons with private tutors. She joined many other young women in this period who took advantage of the expansion of educational opportunities for girls in the urban Northeast.

At fifteen, upon the suggestion of her paternal grandmother, a veteran teacher herself, Putnam enrolled in the newly established public and progressive Twelfth Street School in Manhattan. The school fostered confidence and independence in girls, so, as one supporter quipped, they could avoid the "prison-house" of domesticity. It prepared girls to pursue careers in the newly feminized professions, particularly teaching. Putnam received encouragement from principal Lydia F. Wadleigh, who took "especial interest . . . in the medical education of women from the beginning" and was a "life-long advocate of the higher education of women."[37] The school also facilitated her writing and literary pursuits, offering the intellectual space to question and comment on prescribed gender roles.[38] She benefited from studying outside the home, with other young women as a peer group, rather than just her siblings. As historian Jane Hunter has shown, high schools like Wadleigh's allowed girls to bond and in the process "challenged maternal domesticity" and undermined girls' subordination at home and in public, paving the way for the "new girl" and New Woman, icons of female autonomy at the end of the century.[39]

But on the surface, the Putnam family subscribed to Victorian ideologies with regard to gender. George Putnam and his wife viewed the public world as a masculine domain and the home as a sanctuary.[40] Putnam built his publishing empire in the competitive business world of Manhattan, while Victorine managed the home, preparing for her husband's business dinners and social gatherings as well as raising and educating their children. But the line between public and private life was actually quite blurry because George Putnam's world of letters carried over into his home, where the business of literature, social reform, and family life merged into one. To the family's house on Staten Island he brought the latest novels and periodicals, both American and European. Reading manuscripts, reviewing proofs, and discussing potential publications was a family affair. George Putnam brought both writers and the writing process into the domestic circle, inviting clients for social calls and for extended visits. While Mary's mother and grandmother oversaw her daily lessons, it was the lessons learned from her father's literary world that sparked her interest in books and ideas, and planted the notion that she, too, could become a writer.

The family belonged to a culture that was learned and middle class. Shortly after they returned from Britain, the Putnams lived a comfortable existence with private carriages and servants, and the financial means to welcome numerous guests and attend musical performances. The family spent their Sundays in church but otherwise amused themselves with games, the piano, and, above all, books, reading aloud in English and French. They also carried on traditions they had learned in England, particularly afternoon teas. While the Putnams were characteristically middle class, their income and stability did vary during difficult economic times. But the family valued ideas over materialism, and were more socially conscious than individualistic. More like the Beecher family than the Astors, they were literary-minded and made the printed word not only a source of income but a central part of daily life.[41]

Leading members of New York's literary and artistic communities visited the Putnam home throughout the 1850s. Women writers, especially, not only socialized and did business with George Putnam, but they became integrated into Putnam family life. Catharine Maria Sedgwick, a client from Putnam's London years, became a friend of the family and one of his first important female clients.[42] Two other women in particular, Fredrika Bremer, a Swedish writer, and Susan Warner, author of the best-selling novel *The Wide, Wide World*, were other influential visitors at the Putnam home.[43] Mary Putnam developed an admiration for both of these women who frequently visited the family and encouraged her early penchant for writing.

Warner, in particular, had a strong presence in the family circle. Mary's father decided to publish her book after receiving some encouragement from his mother, who reportedly said to her son: "If you never publish another book, publish this."[44] Warner's manuscript had been rejected by other publishers, but George Putnam recognized its potential in an expanding genre of didactic novels. But even he was surprised when it sold 40,000 copies in one year, and was published in thirteen editions over two years. George Putnam regularly supported the endeavors of female authors like Warner who needed to support their families by offering them an entrée into the literary world.[45] Many years later, in a eulogy to him, Mary recalled her father's sympathy toward "poor and solitary women struggling to maintain themselves by the uncertain profits of the pen."[46] His inclination to help "literary domestics" was also good business since a growing audience of literate middle-class women provided sound profits.

Susan Warner became a role model for Mary Putnam, demonstrating how Victorian women could apply their literary talents and earn an income. Warner spent several weeks in the Putnam's Staten Island home in 1850 reviewing her manuscript for *The Wide, Wide World*.[47] The socially active Putnams must have seemed overbearing to Warner, considering that she saw writing as a private matter and hid her true identity behind the pseudonym Elizabeth Wetherell.[48] Warner's novel was a religious allegory about a young woman left alone in the world. Ellen, the main character, has her faith tested, but she ultimately is dutiful and self-sacrificial, demonstrating her piety, evangelical temperament, personal fortitude, and faith in divine will. The themes in Warner's novel attracted the attention of many young women who were struggling to find their places in the world; it certainly left an impression on young Mary, who was only eight years old at the time of Warner's first visit. Mary was fascinated with the story after hearing a section read out loud in their home, finding meaning in it for her own life. To the surprise of Warner, Mary asked her mother when they could next hear "the story of Ellen." Warner spent time with her in conversation and also reading stories as she worked on her manuscript. "She is a very intelligent child," Warner told her sister. "She says people say she will be an author."[49]

Unlike Warner, Fredrika Bremer openly promoted herself as a writer and even became the center of a public commercial battle, as George Putnam and Harpers publishing vied for the rights to her work. Bremer captured the attention of American readers with her novels that focused on intimate matters of faith, the home, and womanhood. Bremer spent less time at the Putnam's than Warner, only briefly visiting in 1849, but her writings recounted the state of American domestic life and the vital role of women as keepers of a nation's moral fortitude. Putnam reprinted two of her works, *The Neighbors* and *Homes of the New World*, hoping to sell more elegant editions of her popular writings to American audiences.[50] While these books did not produce profits, they did further solidify Putnam's reputation with women writers, who continued to seek his association in the 1850s. Warner, Bremer, and others, all arbiters of religious culture and domesticity, may have reinforced the traditional values of American middle-class life, but in the Putnam home, they modeled for Mary a different future: one where she could become a writer, earn her own money, and even have an influential voice in society.

The Putnams enjoyed the company of even more writers when the family relocated to Manhattan in 1852, and their home became a center of New York cultural life. Now in a more fashionable abode, on East Sixteenth Street near Stuyvesant Square, the Putnams held social gatherings that attracted the literary icons of the city. The site of lively exchanges about social and political matters of the day, their home attracted academic, literary, and artistic types from the city and beyond. Susan Warner remembered how during one of the family's gatherings, Mary posted a sign on the door that read, "Nobody admitted who cannot talk."[51] With growing numbers of female socialites in the city, young Mary declared the importance of substantive verbal discourse in her home, and showed impatience for anyone not willing or able to perform intellectually.

Their eighteen months in Manhattan were critical for the expansion of George Putnam's publishing business and coincided with the launching of *Putnam's Monthly*. Putnam had a nationalistic vision for his new magazine and a political agenda that was antislavery and reform-minded.[52] With contributions from some of the most popular American writers, including Henry Wadsworth Longfellow, Henry David Thoreau, and Horace Greeley, *Putnam's* attracted an educated middle-class readership.[53]

The Putnam home continued to be a meeting place for literary figures of the age when the family moved to Yonkers in 1854.[54] Putnam helped organize a town library where he developed a series of lectures that drew preacher and reformer Henry Ward Beecher, author George Bethune, abolitionist Wendell Phillips, writer and lecturer George William Curtis, author and clergyman Edward Everett Hale, and many others, most of whom stayed in his home. During the 1856 election, George Palmer Putnam's antislavery stance led him to support John C. Fremont in the founding of the new Republican Party. His political activism inspired his children to engage with the social and political issues of the adult world.[55] In the spirit of her father's lyceum series, Mary started a debating society of her own and invited her peers, both boys and girls. Mirroring the adult discussions, the juvenile debating society of Yonkers addressed questions of slavery and black emancipation, the treatment of Native Americans, and women's rights. The group also produced a "local paper," edited and written largely by Mary.[56] At a relatively young age, she formulated political opinions and engaged other young women in the examination of social problems. As the parade of New York's literati continued through the Putnam home, and she found a voice in debate, Mary seriously began to envision a future for herself as a writer.

As early as age nine, Mary Putnam began to compose short essays and think pieces that imitated the didactic writings of the celebrated women authors she met in her own home. Her writings taught moral lessons by questioning and then affirming the definition of righteous living. Her message: material items and public acclaim may temporarily satisfy the individual, but they will not, in the long run, satisfy the needs of the soul. Although confused about religion, Putnam's writings suggested that one must answer to God, and they maintained that compassion, honesty, and sacrifice constituted life's great aims, carried out for the good of all. Ultimately, greed, idleness, and frivolity amounted to an empty life. For example, in "Three Paths of Life," three elderly men discuss how they spent their time on earth. A money-driven merchant and an aimless poet confront their shallow existence and selfishness, while a clergymen rejoices as he looks back on his fruitful course: "My purpose was gained. I have devoted my life to aiding my fellow men, and now I lay down not to die, but to live again."[57] In these pieces, there is a sense of searching and longing for purpose, a theme common to evangelical writing, and one central to Warner's *Wide, Wide World*.

In other writings of her youth, Putnam mimicked the style of the belles lettres published by her father.[58] These pieces continued to address moral questions but related them to a particular historical, philosophical, or literary theme. Describing an idyllic rural setting in "Life in the Country," for example, Putnam wrote a thick description contrasting "a perfect picture of rural felicity" to city life. She contemplated strength and leadership, particularly the reach of power (in France), in essays "Queen Marie Antoinette" and "Napoleon Bonaparte," and defended the people's right to demand liberty in "Revolutions." While most educated, middle-class girls wrote as an act of self-culture, Putnam composed from a unique vantage point, from inside the publishing world, knowing that it was possible and even likely to see her own words in print.

At the same time, Putnam's earliest writings express fierce resistance to the gender norms of her middle-class upbringing. As early as her twelfth birthday, she began to write about her struggle with Victorian codes of femininity. As she approached womanhood, Putnam saw no reason to celebrate, and instead complained: "Oh! The frivolous trivialities of decorum, the wearisomeness of propriety! . . . I am expected to cut off my childish things, to become a woman, while my heart is yet young, and why?" This outburst, penned in the aftermath of a confrontation with her mother, captured her need to "mourn" the loss of her childhood and resist the social expectations placed on her as a young woman of refinement. "To have one's least action pulled to pieces and criticized, the more so for its being trifling," she continued, "what do I care? Let the people talk, it hurts me not."[59] Intellectually precocious, inquisitive, and vocal in her opinions, Putnam came into conflict with her mother's observance of the "cult of true womanhood." Acting and playing as a child with no regard to gender, she experienced anxiety over accommodating to the codes of behavior observed by women in her social class.

Putnam even wrote from the voice of a young man in an essay called "Aims and Ends." It was not unusual for women writers at midcentury to disguise their gender, as Putnam would often do, and either sign their initials or use pseudonyms. In this unpublished piece, she instructed young men to choose careers that would reward them personally and, ultimately, spiritually. Speaking as one of them, she wrote, "We have our destinies to work out, and the time to begin is *now*."[60] In "Truth," she spoke to the need for honesty, specifically in boys, equating it with bravery, strength, and leading a moral life.[61] Overall, Putnam was concerned with moral fortitude, but in her writings she was also learning how to speak in a style and tone that did not suggest she was a woman.[62]

Over the years, some of Putnam's essays became increasingly and more explicitly critical of the expectations and constraints placed on women. For example, "Hair Chains" is a mythical tale set in the ancient world that expressed Mary Putnam's desire for education and her growing frustrations with the expectations of her society.[63] A young woman, Haguna, wants to study with a famous philosopher. The philosopher refuses because he believes she will distract the male pupils with her long golden hair, the symbol of her beauty. Frustrated with this rejection, Haguna complains, "Is it my fault that I am a girl? I come to you to learn, to satisfy the insatiable thirst for knowledge which you have awakened, — and you reproach me with my ignorance! I have just discovered that the one thing that I have secretly needed always was to learn to exercise my mind cramped with inaction, to share with you labor and toil."[64] To be taken seriously as a student, and to be welcomed into the philosopher's lessons, Haguna willingly cuts off all of her hair, sacrificing her beauty and the symbol of her womanhood. Now, unshackled from her golden locks, Haguna and a former suitor can engage in philosophical discussions on an equal footing. In this allegory, a young woman privileges learning over beauty, wisdom over attracting suitors; she also shows a degree of annoyance at being a "girl." Like Putnam, the character Haguna is frustrated by the ways femininity interfered with education, and she desires an egalitarian model of marriage and gender relations.

Putnam also wrote short nonfiction essays in which she confronted cultural understandings of physicality and femininity. In an essay titled "Effeminacy," she critiqued the preoccupation of her social class with illness and its repugnance for the body and its functions.[65] While it was fashionable to have contempt for "corporeal existence," she charged, people spent their time "fretting away" over pain and physical discomfort. She lamented, "What a vast amount of energy is expended in securing that trifling article, individual comfort." Putnam, still in her teen years, already seemed to understand the tensions around the body in nineteenth-century culture, as middle-class Americans tried to reconcile their physical and spiritual selves. She saw how anxiety about the body, especially feminine bodies, made the invalid a symbol of sentimental culture and an emblem of modern life. She also engaged with the debate surrounding the positive and negative effects of "civilization," pondering whether life in the nineteenth century constituted progress over the past, or whether luxury and comforts had weakened Americans, especially women.[66]

Beyond her own individual protests against prescribed gender roles, Putnam became more conscious about the broader status of women while a student at the progressive Twelfth Street School. In her essay on William the

Conqueror, completed just before graduation, Putnam overtly condemned female passivity. She called upon girls to be strong and powerful so that they might proudly and independently face the world, and the divine. She critiqued young women for their meekness and idleness: "Too lazy or too weak to *manfully* grapple with our own responsibilities, we gracefully throw them upon somebody else's shoulders, and delicately [*sic*] ourselves about some bolder and stronger minds. . . . A strong, powerful, and consequently honourable life, cannot [exist] with this shirking, this dependence."[67] That her class and culture had become "effeminate" bothered her; that women subjected themselves to the will of others was even more worrisome.

Immediately following her graduation from the Twelfth Street School, Putnam worked as an instructor at a local girls' school and took over her mother's role at home, tutoring her younger brothers and sisters. She also received private lessons in Greek.[68] Teaching school could provide her much-needed pecuniary supplements and serve as a viable occupation. Once a profession dominated by men, teaching was well on its way to becoming feminized by the 1860s and was regarded as an appropriate way for an unmarried, middle-class woman to spend her youthful years.[69] However, Putnam believed it was an occupation with serious limitations, for "the most honorable and lucrative posts of teaching [were] withheld from women," who were "underpaid" and subjected to "the dryest and most fatiguing duties of instruction." She lost interest because it had become "a mere traditionary employment for women; and if traditionary, then overcrowded and indiscriminate."[70] Moreover, it did not fully satisfy her growing thirst for knowledge or alleviate her ongoing feelings of spiritual isolation.

George Putnam foresaw an appropriate career for his daughter in writing, knowing that Mary was intellectually advanced beyond her years and that she deserved a formal education. He also recognized that advancing Mary's education would transform his oldest daughter into a family "breadwinner." During a rocky period in the publishing business, George Putnam welcomed his eldest child's small contributions to the family income. In the late 1850s she began to write pieces of short fiction with the hope of seeing them in print. With her father's assistance, she published her first story, "Found and Lost," in the *Atlantic Monthly* in April 1860 at the age of seventeen, receiving eighty dollars for her contribution.[71] The story opens on a stormy winter night, at a sickbed, with a physician sitting next to his recently deceased patient. The doctor decides to stay and read his patient's manuscript, which tells the story of a man's struggle to find a spiritual source, a fable that mimics Mary's own spiritual quest. Mixing a medical character with religious themes, it foretold the author's own search for faith. The work seemed to indicate that she was on her way to having a career in writing, as not just a witness but an active participant in her father's world.

Although Putnam had a genuine interest in literature, writing alone did not provide a constant or stable income, particularly during hard economic times. Writing and teaching were valuable occupations, but they limited her to working in the home or the now-feminized schoolroom. Unlike Ellen in *The Wide, Wide World*, and other young women of evangelical temperament, Putnam decided not to accept her position in life as God's will but eagerly sought to change it.[72] In April of 1860, just as she published "Found and Lost," she turned to medicine and mapped out a new course in life.

Reborn a Scientist

As in the case of many nineteenth-century religious conversions, Putnam documented her scientific conversion as a tale of her spiritual journey. Her notebook, recording her meetings with Dr. Thomas D. Anderson, the director of the First Baptist Church on Broome Street in lower Manhattan, serves as an alternative "conversion narrative."[73] Her meetings with Anderson in 1862 were designed as counseling sessions to comfort her and reinforce her faith, but instead she used these conversations to move away from the church. Putnam began her narrative skeptically: "I have now come to have doubts, very serious doubts, on the four [sic] points of the Calvinistic system: The doctrines of the Trinity, atonement, future punishment, and inspiration of the Bible."[74] She proclaimed a desire to reconcile with the church, but her narrative indicates little intent to do so. At the end of their sessions, the cleric concluded that Putnam was "on most dangerous ground."[75]

Less than one year after their conversations, in April of 1863, Putnam wrote a letter of resignation to the First Baptist Church, officially ending her membership. After trying to suppress her growing dissatisfaction, she finally made her formal break. She recalled the process: "I began [my] investigation in full faith and expectation that my doubts would speedily be settled, and my faith grounded anew, but today finds me a total disbeliever in the distinctive tenets of the technically called orthodox system of divinity."[76] With this statement, she voiced her "insuperable objections" to Calvinistic theology.[77] Unable to submit to the strict authority of the church, and accept the idea of eternal punishment, Putnam stepped away because "there is a point," she said, "where doctrines shrivel."[78]

Among several points of contention was Putnam's inability to reconcile spirituality and rationality. First, she rejected the utility of kneeling and carrying out conscious and verbal prayer. She confessed, "There seems to me an absurdity of stopping and saying actual words to God." If she prayed, she preferred to have her thoughts "flow back to him naturally from everything." This inclination led her to value the intellectual self over the emotional self. "The intellect," she said, "certainly builds the framework in which the rest of the nature lives, and lays its boundaries by means of ideas." Dr. Anderson lamented that Putnam had "too much cold intellectual activity and too little emotion."[79]

Putnam was also frustrated with notions of "true womanhood" and the patriarchal structure of her church. Gendered tensions run throughout her discussions with Dr. Anderson, as she openly challenged the elder pastor and commented on the false logic of his statements. Dr. Anderson found fault with her entire demeanor, which he perceived as unwomanly. He tried not only to restore her faith but also to put her in her place as an abiding female member of his congregation. Putnam resisted, often exaggerating or extending her opinions to provoke him. She pointed out the "weak point[s]" in his thinking and found flaws in his theories, making their meetings more of a theoretical debate than a counseling session.[80]

Putnam's narrative addressed many theological facets, but its most radical and innovative element involved employing science to overturn religious doctrine. She used cell theory and the concept of "reparative growth" as a metaphor to dispute notions of original sin and human damnation. New cells, she explained, were produced in the body not as exact copies of old cells. New cells "imitated" the characteristics of tissues but could diverge in character. This could be seen in embryonic cells, "where perfectly novel tissues are developed from neutral precedents." The same was true for people who inherited sin and past evils but who could be molded into better souls as well.[81]

Not coincidentally, Putnam's religious retreat overlapped with the start of her medical education. Her early training was informal, since there were few options for learning "regular" medicine in New York. She began by attending lectures and performing dissections, possibly her first, under the guidance of Dr. Samuel Percy at the New York Medical College. Though only open from 1850 to 1864, the New York Medical College was a respected institution; it adopted several American Medical Association reforms and employed some of New York's top medical men as instructors.[82] She also spent some time with Elizabeth Blackwell at the New York Infirmary on Second Avenue. In April 1860, Blackwell wrote about "two young ladies who will spend the coming year with us." One of the "students" was "a daughter of Putnam publisher" and "a very talented girl, only 17 however."[83] Blackwell had not yet opened the Woman's Medical College, but the infirmary offered opportunities for individual instruction: "The students from their first entrances are employed in the work — putting up medicines, examining patients, visiting the sick and gradually as knowledge increases, assuming more and more of the responsibility of practice, though still under the supervision of the senior physician."[84] Blackwell envisioned a four-year course of study for Putnam starting that November, but Putnam did not stay and moved on to the New York College of Pharmacy, where she could receive more formal instruction and earn an official degree.

In her first courses at the New York College of Pharmacy, she studied materia medica and the fabrication of medicine. It was a practical curriculum that covered the "history, composition, properties, preparations, impurities, and adulterations of all the officinal and the most important unofficinal drugs, employed [in the United States] and in Europe." She learned organic and inorganic chemistry and received "practical" training in science through "experiments, diagrams, specimens, and processes."[85] Most importantly, it was at pharmacy school that she most likely became knowledgeable about cell theory through her introductory courses in biology and that she began to use science to deconstruct tenets of Christian faith.

Cell theory argued that the cell was the basic form of human life and that cells generated from preexisting cells. The latter idea is associated with Rudolf Virchow, the German physician and pathologist who famously promoted the aphorism "*omnis cellula e cellula*" (each cell stems from another cell). Putnam applied these principles to dismantle the notion of inherited sinfulness, arguing that new cells are not exact copies of old cells, that they evolve and mature over time.[86] Virchow's positivist and materialist stance may also have contributed to her spiritual transition, convincing her that science could identify and address the ills of both the physical body and the social body.

The challenges faced by pharmacy schools at midcentury provided an opening for Mary Putnam. She became the first woman to attend the New York College of Pharmacy, taking advantage of the fact that pharmacy schools struggled with financial and organizational problems and desperately needed to maintain and graduate students. At the time she entered the college, lectures were held at a New York University building on Waverly Place.[87] A discipline on the periphery of the medical profession, pharmacy provided Putnam with the first phase of her training in the sciences as well as an unconventional path into medicine.

In the 1860s, pharmacy was a field transforming itself from a family business into a profession allied with the medical world. In New York, the production and distribution of medicines was part of the urban, antebellum commercial culture. Once trained in apprenticeships, pharmacists now strove to formalize education and create some type of authority for the practice. Aiming to professionalize their craft, they struggled to convince potential students, young apprentices, or sons of pharmacists that they needed institutional training.[88]

Putnam's decision to study at the College of Pharmacy caused a stir within the Putnam family. Although the family supported her work as a teacher and writer, they resisted her venturing outside the comforts of home and their community, and into the foreign world of scientific studies. Mary's father preferred that she stay home during these years and assist her mother with the care and teaching of her younger siblings while continuing her teaching at the nearby girls' school. In 1861, he wrote to her and asked, "What possible evil can result from your *suspending* those medical studies, entirely, except general reading at home, for the space of two years?" Her father even offered to pay his daughter to stay home, promising to reward her the $250 sum he had intended to spend on her medical education.[89] Mary temporarily gave in to his pleas but soon after proceeded with her plans, thereby overruling her father, who repeatedly expressed reservations about her study of medicine.

Upon the completion of her studies, she graduated from the college in March of 1863 with six other students, taking part in the college's first public commencement and becoming the first woman to graduate from the institution. She completed a thesis titled "Dialysis," which represented her studies in chemistry, and, according to the college president, it "compare[d] favorably with the productions of the other graduates."[90] But she did not receive her diploma until August; the institution's rules required that students be twenty-one years of age to officially receive the degree.[91]

The window of opportunity for female students was actually quite small. Thereafter, the college found no need to admit other women for revenue because enrollment had increased; Putnam was the only woman to graduate for the next twenty-five years.[92] It was not until the latter part of the nineteenth century that pharmacy became a popular and viable profession for American women interested in medicine and science.[93]

Putnam's early training in pharmacy had long-term consequences for her own identity as a practitioner. She was inspired by biological theories and chemical reactions, unlike many of her female peers, who were more interested in caring for and assisting patients. Although the first phase of her medical education was largely scientific and theoretical, Putnam soon learned how her new knowledge could have social and political significance and could be of use to the nation at large.

Medicine for the Union

In 1863, at the height of the Civil War, Mary Putnam traveled alone to the front lines. Refusing to sit passively in New York, she decided to use her new degree for the good of the Union. After learning that her brother Haven, a soldier stationed in Louisiana, had fallen ill with malaria, she journeyed south on a government steamship to New Orleans, determined to locate him and attend to his health. It was an opportunity not only to help her brother but to possibly doctor an entire regiment of Union soldiers struck with "swamp fever." With more than a touch of hubris, Putnam headed to Louisiana to help win the war.

Ultimately, Putnam's actual contributions to the cause were less significant than her experience during wartime, which had enormous long-term impact on her as a woman, physician, and activist. She served as a healer to her wounded brother and possibly to other fallen men in soldiers' hospitals.[94] She also worked briefly as a volunteer for the Freedmen's Bureau. From these experiences, Putnam witnessed the human suffering of the war, which cemented her interest in social improvement and reform and reaffirmed her feelings that women needed to be active citizens contributing in public rather than passive observers. Finally, she was easily convinced that the material and human losses of the war required new forms of organization to manage masses of bodies, dead and alive.

Like many Americans, Mary Putnam's Civil War experience began years before the fighting started. She grew up in a household that was ardently Republican and antislavery. In her father's social networks of reform-minded, middle-class people, the expansion of slavery presented a great threat to democracy and the social order. As the war loomed closer, the sectional conflict that dominated American politics in the 1850s was the leading subject of discussion and debate in the family home. The politics of the war drew almost the entire family into the conflict. In politically volatile New York, populated with many Democrats, George Putnam remained ardently committed to the Republican Party, though not a radical abolitionist. He knew the 1860 election was pivotal and, although he first supported Seward, he was captivated by Abraham Lincoln at Cooper Union the night of his famous speech. During the war, he worked to forward the Union cause, helping to recruit, house, and supply troops with both rations and reading material. He acted as a reporter, publishing accounts of the first battle of Bull Run. He also took on leadership roles in several organizations, including the Union League Club of New York, the United States Sanitary Commission, the Metropolitan Fair Association, and the Loyal National League. As George Putnam's biographer Ezra Greenspan has shown, the publisher blurred his professional life with public service.[95] George Putnam's children followed in his footsteps with their own war work. His son, Haven, volunteered for the Union army, and his second daughter, Edith, signed up to teach the freedmen. Mary followed them both, first to Union-occupied New Orleans in 1863 and then to Norfolk, Virginia, in 1864.

Mary Putnam first confronted the human toll of the conflict in southern Louisiana when she went in search of Haven, whose regiment of northern volunteers had been assigned the difficult task of capturing New Orleans.[96] The army hoped to gain control of the Mississippi River and connect Union forces in the South with those in the West and North. In the torrential rains and swamplands of Louisiana, Haven and his troops had difficulty keeping their camps dry and many men succumbed to malaria.[97]

Traveling alone to the front lines of the war was a bold move for an unaccompanied young woman. Shocked by her arrival, Haven remembered, "I do not know why my father should ever have given his consent to the plan. There were various difficulties in the way of the journey to New Orleans and much more serious obstacles to prevent a civilian, and a girl at that, from securing transportation and protection from New Orleans to the front."[98] Haven was a little dismayed and annoyed about her decision to come since, ultimately, "her presence might not prove of any real service." He recalled, "My condition was not such as to call for any immediate anxiety. Minnie was, therefore, free to amuse herself as opportunity might present."[99] Haven realized that a nursing mission had turned into an adventure for his older sister, who managed to "enjoy herself pretty thoroughly."[100] Personally close to her younger brother, Mary was determined to care for him, but his illness was also a ticket into unmapped territory.

Mary Putnam, "the only lady within sight," stood out as one of the few white women at Haven's headquarters in Brashear City.[101] In these circumstances, her race, class, and gender shaped the conditions of her stay. For her service and protection, officers outfitted Mary with her own tent and assigned her a black servant, who doubled as an escort. The servant later accompanied her on her return north, and became known to the family as "Sarah Contraband." At the same time, Mary Putnam attended and spoke during at least one camp meeting of freed and runaway slaves during her visit. Haven remembered hearing from his own servant that "young Missus, she did preach right powerful."[102] Although no record survives of her speech that evening, we can guess that Putnam "preached" about something more political than spiritual: a Union win and an end to slavery.

While the Putnams were antislavery, Mary and Haven acquired black servants, likely former slaves, to attend to their needs. As white, northern, educated elites, their social stature afforded them privileges that did not disappear in time of war. Dedicated to the Union, they opposed slavery as the basis for southern economic expansion and influence. They deplored slavery as an immoral institution and fought for the rights of the freedmen. But, ultimately, they upheld social hierarchies through their socioeconomic status and notions of European "civilization" and superiority. Many reformers and writers viewed slaves as victims of a cruel system who were in need of social uplift and reform, but they did not think of African Americans as their absolute equals.

Mary Putnam remained with the army for two weeks until news of a Confederate assault forced her back to New Orleans. Her quick departure brought some relief to Haven, who was uncomfortable with his sister staying at the post closest to Rebel lines. Again, citing her gender, he remembered, "This was evidently not a proper place for a civilian girl who had no duties at the post."[103] Mary spent the remainder of the summer living with the family of Quartermaster General Samuel B. Holabird, who were social acquaintances from New York. She stayed there two months, tutoring their young son in exchange for her board. She was also occupied with "medical reading" and sought remuneration for her writing while she awaited news from the lines about her brother.[104] It seemed that Mary was not "ready to go back to the comparative uneventfulness of the home in New York."[105]

During a confrontation with the Confederates at Brashear City, Haven was taken prisoner. However, when struck with gangrene, he was allowed to recover at the home of another local family.[106] Once he recovered and was released, Haven reenlisted and became a commissioned officer, a status that allowed him to make several visits to the Holabirds' home and have contact with his sister. Believing her brother was well and secure, Mary left New Orleans in the fall of 1863 for New York, with plans to then move on to Philadelphia for medical school.[107] She would return only a few years later to, again, stay with the Holabirds, where she earned extra income by tutoring their son and writing a series of columns called "Sketches of Character" for the *New Orleans Times*.[108]

Mary's efforts on behalf of her brother did not end with her departure from New Orleans. Haven was captured again the following year, and the family began their own campaign to see him released. After being home on leave, Haven joined Union troops fighting in the Shenandoah Valley, and was taken prisoner during the battle of Cedar Creek. He was eventually sent to Danville Prison in Virginia.[109] Enduring poor conditions and living off spare rations, Haven's experience was miserable. His father lobbied hard to have his son released, using every possible business and family connection in both the Union and the Confederacy. Mary, too, did her part, calling on the Sanitary Commission to send supplies to soldiers in southern prisons, knowing that her brother must have been living in the bleakest conditions.[110] Ultimately, Haven was not released until March 1865, near the war's end.

In December of 1864, as the family eagerly awaited news about Haven, another family illness called Mary to travel, which provided her with a chance to directly engage with war work as a teacher to the freedmen. She traveled to Norfolk to take care of her sister, Edith, who was ill with typhoid fever. Edith had volunteered to teach freed slaves for the Freedmen's Bureau but faced scant resources and poor conditions. Her illness required Mary to stay with her into January 1865.[111] Mary's visit to Norfolk was inspired by both familial obligations and political motivations. She had decided to aid the freedmen during her stay in Virginia and officially registered as a teacher with the National Freedmen's Relief Association in New York before her departure on 22 December 1864.[112] But the association asked her to do more than just manage lessons; it encouraged all teachers "to interest themselves in the moral, religious, and social improvement of the families of their pupils, to visit them in their homes, [and] to instruct the women and girls in sewing and domestic economy." With its broad aim to reform and uplift former slaves, the Freedmen's Association may also have brought Mary to work as a medical provider. Mary may have registered to teach the freedmen in order to gain permission and funding for a passage to visit her sister in Norfolk.[113] But, ultimately, helping the freedmen fit with the family's antislavery stance and belief in "uplifting" the less fortunate. It also provided another mission in which Mary could apply her new medical knowledge.

As Mary Putnam's experience reaffirms, the political crisis of the 1860s was also a "crisis of gender," as it required women to move beyond their assigned social roles.[114] The war served as a major catalyst for engaging middle-class women in the healing professions. Through such organizations as the Sanitary Commission, many women became active in public health and hygiene efforts. Other women directly supported the troops as nurses, becoming part of a growing, feminized profession. Nursing was acceptable war work for women because it seemed to utilize women's domestic knowledge and natural abilities as caregivers. And yet it required that they take on new roles and that the nation suspend the gendered definitions of work that governed society in peacetime. As a medical woman, traveling alone in time of war, Putnam, too, disrupted social expectations for women and gained such a strong sense of autonomy that there was no turning back.

For Putnam, the war also reaffirmed her faith in science as the best source to bring immediate relief to the nation's physical damage. Many observers shared her views. Although Union and Confederate alike believed that God was on their side, and Americans remained very religious, the tremendous bloodshed of the war would ultimately persuade them to put physical suffering in the hands of doctors rather than clergymen.

The Proof Is in the Spleen

In the midst of war, between traveling to New Orleans and Norfolk, Putnam decided to take another step to advance her medical education and enrolled at the Female Medical College of Pennsylvania in the fall of 1863. But after less than a year in Philadelphia, Putnam sought a quick exit and requested permission to graduate early and receive her diploma. To prove her knowledge and readiness as a physician, she submitted a thesis, "Theories with Regard to the Function of the Spleen," composed in Latin, the root language of medicine. She also used her thesis to pontificate about the value of science, and thus, begin to create her own scientific identity.

The main goal of science, she argued, was to revise old ideas and present new information: "New discoveries fulfill ancient ones. . . . Untiring labor seeks new worlds, and expansive darkness is borne through by incredible vivacity and effort."[115] For Putnam, "knowing" the natural world was a human endeavor, not a divine process; knowledge was not stagnant but evolved through continuous and renewed investigation. The job of medical science was to disrupt old intellectual habits and clarify physiological problems that were both

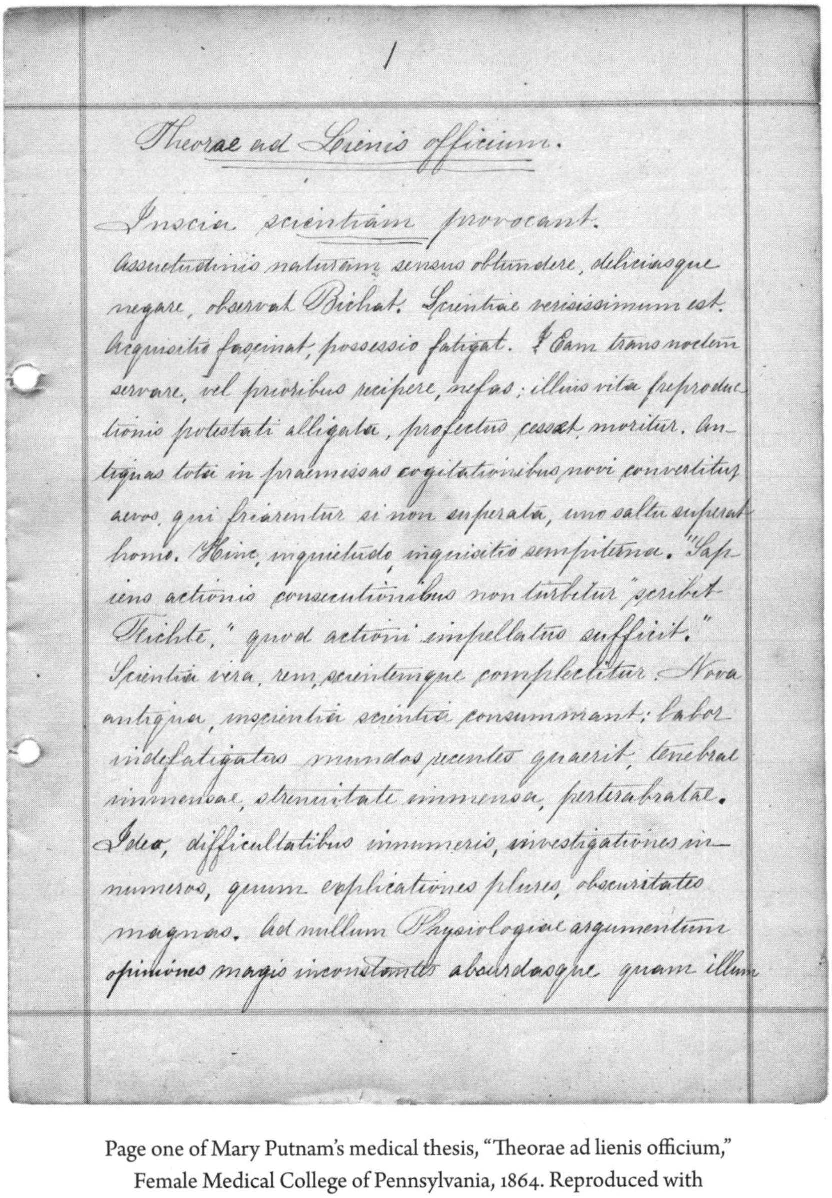

1

Theorae ad Lienis officium.

Inscia scientiam provocant.

Assuetudinis naturam sensus obtundere, deliciasque negare, observat Bichat. Scientiae verissimum est. Acquisitio fascinat, possessio fatigat. Eam trans noctem servare, vel prioribus recipere, nefas; illius vita reproductionis potestati alligata, profectus cessat, moritur. Antiquas totas in praemissas cogitationibus novi convertitur aevos, qui fricarentur si non superata, uno saltu superat homo. Hinc, inquietudo inquisitio sempiterna. "Sapiens actionis consecutionibus non turbetur" scribit Fichte, "quod actioni impellatus sufficit." Scientia vera, rem, scientemque complectitur. Nova antiqua, inscientia scientia consummant; labor indefatigatus mundos recentes quaerit; tenebrae immensae, strenuitate immensa, perterebratae. Ideo, difficultatibus innumeris, investigationes innumeros, quum explicationes plures, obscuritates magnas. Ad nullum Physiologiae argumentum opiniones magis inconstantes absurdasque quam illum

Page one of Mary Putnam's medical thesis, "Theorae ad lienis officium," Female Medical College of Pennsylvania, 1864. Reproduced with permission of the Archives and Special Collections on Women in Medicine and Homeopathy, Drexel University College of Medicine.

obscure and mysterious. With the completion of her thesis, Putnam produced a document that officially concluded her spiritual journey; it also identified her with the scientific project.

Putnam focused her thesis on the spleen because the organ had historically been tied to the emotional and spiritual world. "When dealing with physiology," she said, "there are no more unsettling and absurd ideas than those which have tried to explain the function of the spleen."[116] She referenced these older views in her text dismissively: "Loemmering voices the unsavory view that the spleen is the center of the soul, the fountainhead of laughter, the cause of sleep, and the origin of some humor that is sent to the liver. It does not suit our present purpose to go into any great detail about these."[117] By contrast, she examined the function of the spleen from an anatomical and physiological perspective, recounting theories and evidence drawn from experiments and autopsies. Like some other students at the Female Medical College, she chose to focus on a specific organ, rather than health advice or hygiene.[118]

Putnam also chose the spleen as a topic because it took her to the center of long-standing questions surrounding cell theory, histology, and cellular pathology. The function of the spleen had been the subject of medical debate and confusion since the time of Galen.[119] The ancients described the spleen as a digestive organ related to the liver that was integral to the humoral system. The Renaissance anatomist Andreas Vesalius used his anatomical studies to argue that the spleen served as a blood filter that separated blood from black bile. In the early 1600s, William Harvey also argued that the spleen modified blood, but he began to step away from humoral interpretations. "Pre-modern" ideas about the spleen also claimed that the organ was the seat of emotions, passions, violence, and laughter.[120]

In the mid-nineteenth century, new knowledge of the spleen emerged from the expansion of the rise of cellular biology and the making of histological knowledge. Between 1830 and 1860, a number of laboratory scientists in Europe focused their energies on understanding cellular structure and the production and nature of human tissues. Cellular theory, the concept associated with the work of Theodor Schwann and Matthias Schleiden, which defined cells as the main units of human life, was of great significance. Schleiden and Schwann built on cell theory by researching cellular genesis, arguing that nurturing fluids in cells generated new cells. However, it was Rudolf Virchow who became associated with cytogenesis, the idea that cells are produced from preexisting cells. Virchow also became famous for his studies of cellular pathology, which attributed certain diseases to cellular abnormalities.[121] By the time Putnam entered pharmacy and medical school, knowledge of the function of the spleen sat squarely within medical discussions surrounding the production of cells.

Historically associated with the filtering of blood, the spleen seemed to play a key role in the production and destruction of red and white blood cells. Rudolf Albert von Kölliker's (aka Albert Kölliker) histological studies of the spleen were of great importance; he argued that by normal processes, cells are both destroyed and renewed in the spleen. The abnormal destruction of cells occupied the interests of cellular pathologists who, taking the lead from Virchow, looked to the spleen as one origin of blood-related diseases. Virchow blamed a diseased spleen on the destruction of red cells that created an imbalance and an overabundance of white cells resulting in what he described as "leukemia." Virchow's research contributed to a reorientation of pathological studies to the cellular level and convinced many physicians that patients could be cured of leukemia through splenectomy.[122] These debates — over whether the spleen was a site of cell production or destruction and whether cell destruction was pathological — caught the attention of Mary Putnam.

Putnam's 1864 thesis was an overview of what she called the "whole recent controversy" about the spleen, including debates over its role in the manufacture of blood. She summarized the spleen's structure and characteristics but focused on summarizing research on its function in the body. Referencing Köllicker and Virchow, as well as J. H. Bennett, Henry Gray, and William Twining, she concluded that the spleen had a threefold function: (1) it received excess blood from the abdominal vessels, as a result of digestion; (2) it reserved stores of albumen; and (3) it was the location where red corpuscles and white corpuscles dissipated. She pointed out evidence that corpuscles are generated in the spleen as well.[123] She addressed the etiology of leukemia and, through her reading of the leading scientists, came to the conclusion that an enlarged spleen was responsible for its onset. She explained that an enlarged spleen produced a surplus of corpuscles, so that white cells highly outnumbered red cells, causing a severe imbalance. Taking her cue from research by Twining, who linked an enlarged spleen to leukemia, she argued, "This enlargement, although it does not always mark the beginning of illness, generally accelerates the onset of illness with its horrific power."[124] Putnam used the spleen to engage with debates at the center of laboratory science, and formed her opinions within the disciplinary questions emerging over cells and their relationship to disease.

Cell theory was also of critical importance to Putnam because it formed the scientific basis of her conversion narrative. In the years to come, cell theory played an even larger role in her life and career, becoming a central component of her histological studies in Paris, and a foundation for her physiological theories and experiments. It signaled the type of medicine that would consume not only her education in Europe but her research at home. By no means a practical thesis on therapeutics, Putnam's study on the spleen focused on the science of disease rather than care for a disease. She believed that the expertise expressed in her thesis surpassed any level of knowledge she could acquire in courses at the Female Medical College.

Putnam's attempt to expedite her course of study ignited a battle over the definition of medical competency within a college trying to legitimate itself and a profession determined to raise the standards of medical education across the board. The Female Medical College believed that a complete course of study within the walls of the institution was the only way to produce qualified women doctors. Putnam believed she had completed enough of the institution's sub-par instruction and, more importantly, that her study on the spleen proved that she had exemplary knowledge of medicine. She maintained that her thesis was evidence for her own competence, and thus her ticket out of the institution. Putnam and the Female Medical College faculty's disagreements reflected tensions over the professionalization of women in medicine and, more importantly, tensions over how to legitimate women doctors in the face of so much opposition.

The college faculty worried that Putnam was insufficiently prepared to be a doctor because she did not have the courses to graduate. As the country's major medical schools lodged criticism at "irregular" (considered non-orthodox) practitioners and inadequate women physicians, the Female Medical College of Pennsylvania felt intense pressure to raise standards. Allowing unqualified students to pass through, with degree in hand, threatened to undermine the institution's goals and exacerbate its already questionable reputation among regular physicians.[125] Considering there were strong efforts in the profession to improve medical education, eliminate sectarianism, and bar women, some members of the faculty stood their ground and defended their requirements. Putnam's effort to graduate prematurely during a critical moment in the history of the institution propelled the faculty to reflect on the conflicts between its mission to produce more women doctors and its commitment to join the ranks of quality medical schools.

When Putnam entered the school in 1863, the administration was striving to build up the college as an institution for women that, although separate, was equal to orthodox schools. Course curricula at the college reflected the move toward more "scientific instruction," including the use of papier-mâché models, drawings, microscopes, and "natural preparations" for lectures and demonstrations. The school strove to raise the standards of medical education so that alumnae could feel "so thoroughly fitted for their work as to claim and receive the confidence and respect of the community and the profession." According to the Female Medical College of Pennsylvania, courses equaled competency. Hoping to become one of "the best Medical Schools in the country," it required its students to study medicine for three years and attend two courses of lectures in all of the following subjects: chemistry and toxicology, anatomy and histology, materia medica and general therapeutics, physiology and hygiene, principles and practice of medicine and surgery, obstetrics and diseases of women and children, and practical anatomy. To graduate, students were also required to produce a thesis demonstrating their command of a particular medical topic.[126]

Considering the opposition to women in medicine, Putnam had very few options and little choice when she selected an institution. Certainly, many women interested in the healing arts made their home in schools of homeopathy, hydropathy, and eclectic medicine. As part of a health reform movement against "heroic" medicine, women sought training from sectarians who aimed to restore "natural" forms of healing and put an end to the extreme practices of bleeding and purging. Many of these women pursued medicine as a female calling and viewed it as an extension of their "natural" abilities and their domestic orientation. Some women in the antebellum period also tied their work to their evangelical religious commitments and social reform.[127]

Putnam, instead, desired an orthodox medical education accompanied by complete training in the sciences. Barred by men from entering most orthodox institutions, women who wanted to become full-fledged members of the "regular" profession were forced to form separate institutions. By 1863, two single-sex schools had been established: the New England Female Medical College in Boston and the Female Medical College of Pennsylvania in Philadelphia. Samuel Gregory founded the New England school in the early 1850s to train women to treat other women, to critique "man midwives," and to restore propriety to obstetrical care. Physician Marie Zakrzewska joined the staff in 1859 and soon became critical of the inferior education at the institution. Resistant to the introduction of laboratory studies and expansion of clinical training, Gregory firmly held the school to what Zakrzewska believed were antiquated practices. She resigned out of frustration in 1862 to devote herself to clinical work based on scientific principles by forming the New England Hospital for

Women and Children. Gregory's Boston school, held in poor regard by 1863, did not attract women students like Mary Putnam who prioritized a scientific curriculum.[128]

Discouraged by the reputation of the New England school, many young women turned to the Female Medical College of Pennsylvania.[129] Born out of Quaker traditions and the social reform movements of antebellum Philadelphia, the college set out to train women to become competent physicians and to produce graduates who would stand on an equal footing with men trained in orthodox schools. The school closed temporarily after the start of the Civil War in spring 1861 but reopened the following year with the intention of raising its standards and incorporating elements of an orthodox medical education, such as clinical instruction and surgical training.[130]

Putnam tried to prove her expertise on her own terms to graduate early. She submitted her thesis and tickets representing lectures she attended at the Female Medical College of Pennsylvania, as well as the New York College of Pharmacy and the New York Medical College. After reviewing her request on 3 February 1864, the faculty found her application for graduation deficient because she provided no evidence of completing requisite lectures in anatomy, chemistry, and the practice of medicine and physiology.[131] She admittedly had not completed all of her coursework in Philadelphia and tried to apply her training in New York to qualify for graduation. Total confusion arose over the nature of Putnam's prior training and her missing tickets, and her degree was in jeopardy as the faculty contemplated her questionable evidence and decided her fate at the institution.

At a meeting with college administrators, she failed to convince the committee that she fulfilled her requirements. When pushed by the faculty to explain herself, Putnam pointed to the New York institutions involved, claiming she had no documentation because tickets had not been issued to students.[132] Although she attended some lectures in chemistry at the New York Medical College, she "found them so poor that she did not care to complete the course."[133] As part of the investigation, Dean Edwin Fussell wrote letters of inquiry to Doctors Blackwell and Percy in New York as well as the dean of the New York Medical College, asking them to confirm Putnam's account of her training there.[134] The faculty never heard from Dr. Blackwell, but they did hear from others who confirmed that Mary Putnam had attained her lecture tickets legitimately and had, more importantly, "made most excellent dissections" in courses with Dr. Samuel R. Percy.[135]

Dean Fussell nevertheless led a protest against her graduation.[136] A staunch antebellum reform activist and supporter of women in medicine, Fussell had an unbending commitment to raising standards of female education at the college.[137] He accused Putnam and her former teachers of fraudulently representing her coursework. Any confusion, he argued, "was *not* a 'misunderstanding' but [a] *misstatement* on the part of the applicant."[138] Despite all of Fussell's protests, Putnam proceeded with her examinations, and, on 12 March 1864, the faculty voted in her favor, recommending graduation with a vote of sixty-one to nine.[139]

Upon Putnam's departure, the faculty recommitted themselves to the requirements and written rules of the institution. But in granting Putnam a medical degree, the college nearly lost Edwin Fussell, one of its chief instructors, who resigned after the decision to graduate Putnam. "Sadly," he wrote, "I write the word farewell. . . . Bitterly I regret that after full discussion there should be such irreconcilable differences of view in a matter which to my mind effects our integrity. I say it in sorrow, not in anger. I think this College is disgraced and I should feel myself degraded did I remain longer in connection with it."[140] His resignation spurred the faculty to create a series of resolutions intended to promote his return and to retain the honor of the college. "[W]e sympathize with the spirit that appears to have activated him," they said, and further, "we are anew impressed with the necessity of withholding our votes from incompetent applicants for the honors of this College."[141] With the faculty pleading for his return, Fussell withdrew his resignation on 20 April and returned to serve as dean, with the understanding that the college would adhere to stricter procedures. In his introductory address to the entering class of 1864, Fussell was firm in his judgment that only a select and dedicated group of women should study medicine. In what was perhaps a veiled reference to the Putnam case, he warned, "I hope there are none of you in a great hurry to 'get through!' . . . there are some things which require *time*, and among these is the study of medicine."[142]

Ironically, Putnam went on to become one of the premier doctors of her generation. Later in her career, she expressed sincere disappointment with the Philadelphia school. Reflecting on women's work in the medical profession, she criticized the poor state of women's education in her early years. She blamed poor resources and the hostility toward women medical students in Philadelphia. But she also described the Female Medical College of Pennsylvania in unflattering terms: "The instruction consisted of rambling lectures, given by gentlemen of good intentions but imperfect fitness, to women whose previous education left them utterly unprepared to enter a learned profession, and many of whom were really, and in the ordinary sense, illiterate."[143] Although she would become an active member of the college's Alumnae Association in the late 1880s and the 1890s, she looked back on her experience as a student with great frustration.[144]

Mary Putnam's dissatisfaction with the college and her troubled departure ultimately worked to her advantage, for it convinced her of the necessity of a European education. Putnam appreciated the guidance of her leading mentor at the school, Emeline Horton Cleveland. She admired Cleveland, calling her a woman of "real ability" who had received a real education in Paris.[145] Cleveland's influence on Putnam was significant, planting the seed for her to expand her education in France. But her short stay in Philadelphia clarified her intellectual expectations and exposed her to the disadvantages of female institutions. Despite all of the efforts by the faculty to reform the Female Medical College, Putnam believed that the regular institutions for men had higher standards, and that only integration — not separatism — could provide women with a true scientific way of life. The Philadelphia experience, and her thesis, provided her with an opportunity to differentiate herself from other women students, and even some of her male instructors. It also introduced her to a new method for measuring the quality of American medical education, as European medicine became her yardstick.

Marie Zakrzewska and her colleagues at the New England Hospital for Women and Children in Boston provided added encouragement for a European education. From April to August of 1864, Putnam served as an intern at the hospital and had a positive experience, despite the fact that it was another all-female environment. Zakrzewska's hospital produced some of America's most noteworthy women physicians and provided them with a network of professional support. In her history of women in medicine, Putnam recalled the "magnetism" and "personal influence" of Zakrzewska, who gathered a number of talented women who "banded together for life."[146] A German-born physician and leading medical activist, Zakrzewska left a lasting impression on Putnam. She not only insisted on the importance of the natural sciences in medical education, but she also showed Putnam that women should engage in the same type of medicine as men, and that medicine played a critical role in the struggle for female equality.[147] Moreover, almost all of the early staff of the New England Hospital studied abroad in some capacity.[148] Among the most influential for Putnam was Lucy Sewall, who studied in Paris, and Susan Dimock, who studied in Zurich. In the 1860s, several American women, including Putnam, looked to Europe for a more extensive education that remained inaccessible to them in the United States.[149]

✷. MARY PUTNAM did not venture to Paris for nearly two years after her graduation from the Female Medical College of Pennsylvania. She remained in the United States until 1866, attempting to form a small private practice and continuing her scientific studies. Back in New York, she took private chemistry lessons from Ferdinand F. Mayer, her former professor of chemistry and materia medica at the New York College of Pharmacy.[150] Mary was at first intellectually attracted to Mayer, who shared her scientific worldview. Their hours of study soon turned into a courtship, and the two became engaged. Generally disinterested in marriage, Putnam shocked her parents with this decision. George and Victorine Putnam never envisioned their daughter marrying a "foreigner," an immigrant teacher of German Jewish descent who was "poor, as a scientific man most often is."[151]

Months later, the engagement ended when Putnam realized that she had become "quite indifferent" to Mayer, who did not guide, challenge, or inspire her. She sometimes found him "narrow," "childish," even boring, and preferred to have a partner that "magnetized" her rather than one who made her feel "vexed, annoyed, tied down" by his excessive attention. Moreover, although Mayer was a scientist, their marriage would stand in the way of her professional pursuits. "Do I not above all things need freedom of action, and power to carry out the intellectual schemes that are so dear to me?" she wrote her father.[152] Looking forward to Paris, Putnam realized that in the future, she would need to find a partner who not only shared her intellectual passion but also would support her in both marriage and medicine. As for Mayer, he disappeared and was last seen in December of 1869, after suffering deeply from "neuralgia"; his colleagues assumed that he was dead, possibly by suicide.[153]

As Mary Putnam moved ahead with her medical education, her identity as a woman in medicine, committed to science, came into conflict with the expectations of her family and her culture. George Putnam had always supported his daughter's intellectual development, but he hesitated to support her "repulsive pursuit."[154] He found medicine inappropriate for his daughter because it was an affront to conventional Victorian codes of femininity and was assumed to be a path to single life. When Mary Putnam departed for Philadelphia, her father begged her to "preserve your feminine character" and "be a lady."[155] He knew she had an independent spirit, one that often inspired her to ignore the division between masculine and feminine, write in the voice of a man, or take on what were considered masculine roles. He warned: "*Don't* let yourself be absorbed and gobbled up in that branch of the animal kingdom ordinarily called strong minded women! *Don't* let them intensify your self-will and independence for they are strong enough already. *Don't* be congealed or fossilized into a hard, tenacious, unbending personification of intellectual conceit, however strongly fortified you feel sure that you are."[156] Concerned she would be hardened further, George Putnam worried that medical studies would undermine his daughter's remaining feminine qualities.

Mary Putnam was well aware of the accusations that certain types of education and work would "unsex" women. She refuted them by remaining feminine while doing "unfeminine" work. Her answer was not to deny womanhood but to reassert it and reinvent it, normalizing women as physicians and urging a new type of femininity, one based on logic, reason, and independence rather than religion, domesticity, fashion, or frivolity. Women would remain women; they would just share much more in common with men, and vice versa. Putnam learned to carefully negotiate her gender identity, realizing its flexibility and adaptability in different environments. Her performance of gender would be critical to her acceptance in circles of medical men.

Certainly, she had her work cut out for her; there was still intense opposition to women becoming physicians in the United States. Despite the strong medical and cultural barriers, women, like Putnam, found ways to obtain medical training and carve a place for themselves in the healing professions, even if it meant crossing the Atlantic. In Europe, Putnam used her outsider status to get inside the well-fortified bastions of medicine and science.

ON THE BORDERLAND

A Medical and Political Education in Paris

In 1868, in a letter to her father, Mary Putnam described her experiences living in Paris and defended her interest in socialism, stating, "It is precisely on the borderland that we find what is profound and new and stirring." She tried to reassure her worried family that she had not been indoctrinated by fanatics but had become engrossed in a set of political ideas that promised to shake the very foundation of French society. She reminded her father that it was not in her character to accept the status quo and that, quoting poet Robert Browning, "our interests lie on the dangerous edge of things."[1] While Putnam had come to study in one of the medical centers of the world, she found her political inspiration on its intellectual periphery, inspired by radical politics on the city's ideological "borderlands." Pursuing the complete medical education she was denied in the United States, she simultaneously experienced a personal and political awakening that launched her lifetime commitment to science and activism.

Putnam stood on the gendered "borderlands" of Paris as she gained access to a medical world that had historically been preserved for men. Knowing her pursuit of medicine in Paris was a challenge to French sex norms and laws of the empire, Putnam carefully devised her identity as a foreign woman entering masculine territory and gained acceptance. Her admission to the École de Médecine was historic and part of a broader political process, as leaders sought to reform the Second Empire in the late 1860s. Arriving at a critical moment of political change, she witnessed and was a centerpiece in French disputes over gender, power, and knowledge.

Putnam's French education incorporated both political lessons and scientific training, blurring the boundaries between science and politics, both in theory and in practice. In addition to her intense focus on clinical training, Putnam's interest in science was renewed and reinforced at dissecting tables and in microbiology laboratories. Her technical training went hand in hand with her belief in the social value of science, which she formulated into a positivist worldview. In Paris, she embraced several facets of Auguste Comte's positivist doctrine, believing all knowledge should be based on observable phenomenon, that faith in "humanity" should replace metaphysics and become a new "religion," and that science offered the solutions for reforming the social order.[2] While the Second Empire of Napoléon III, from 1852 to 1870, is known for its political conservatism, it has also been called "the age of positivism," when intellectuals used the burgeoning of scientific knowledge to question religion and metaphysics. Although there was great resistance to positivist philosophy, it appealed to artists, philosophers, and scientists, who adapted it to their own ideological positions.[3]

Influenced by Élisée Reclus, a renowned geographer and later a leading anarchist, Putnam learned how to meld science and politics in the production of knowledge about the natural world. Beginning in October 1869, she lived with the Reclus family, a group of socialists interested in political reform and women's rights, and witnessed the Franco-Prussian War and the Paris Commune. She became enamored of socialist principles and voiced her support for the goals of republicanism in France. With Reclus as her intellectual mentor, Putnam decided that if positivist science promised to deliver the "truth" about nature and society, then it could be used to legitimate a new model for gender relations as well.

Putnam occupied complex national identities in Paris, as both an American and an admirer of French socialism and republicanism. In many ways, her own metaphor of "borderlands" describes not only the political fringes of Paris but also the ideological space she occupied between nations. Putnam became an important agent of intellectual exchange in which she constructed transnational connections through her public and private letters, her fiction, and her published political commentaries. Through articles in American magazines, newspapers, and medical journals, she conveyed a picture of Paris constructed from her identity as an American woman. Putnam's transnational experience provides a poignant example of the type of political and scientific exchange of knowledge that occurred across the Atlantic in the late nineteenth century.[4]

Putnam's Paris experience served as a critical turning point in her intellec-

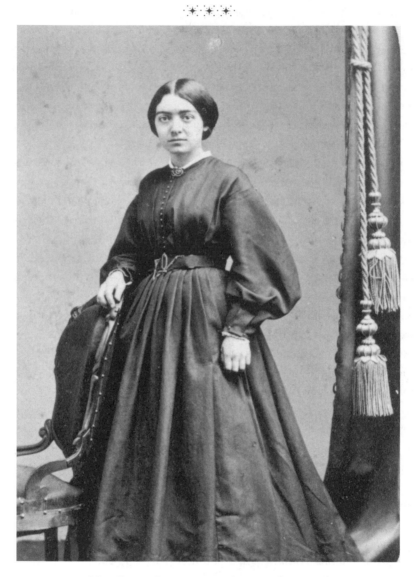

Mary Corinna Putnam, c. 1866. Courtesy of Prints and
Photographs Division, Library of Congress.

tual and political development, inspiring her career later as an activist in New York. Working at both the centers of orthodox medicine and the locales of women's rights activism in America, Putnam merged medicine and politics, a process she began as a young student in the French capital, living on its ideological borderlands.[5]

Accessing the Medical Capital

In September of 1866, at the age of twenty-four, Mary Putnam left New York City for Paris in search of greater educational opportunities. Paris offered Putnam no certain promises, since men dominated the academies of Paris and worked consciously to exclude French women. But as one of the world's medical capitals, the city carried tremendous symbolic power. Many American physicians believed that to study in Paris was to be at the center of the scientific world.[6] American men of medicine had traveled to Paris since the antebellum period to gain a competitive edge, believing that they were acquiring the latest medical knowledge. Most importantly, they wanted greater access to bodies, either in the clinic or on the dissecting tables.[7] A fashionable destination for American physicians and New York's elite, Paris, with all its medical and cultural offerings, had great appeal. At the end of the Second Empire, political change was imminent in France, and new possibilities for intellectual advancement emerged for Mary Putnam as an American woman.

While many students came to Paris in search of patients and cadavers, by midcentury, they took part in the expansion of laboratory studies in clinical medicine. American medical students in the early to mid-nineteenth century prioritized hands-on experience and clinical practice in making empirical judgments about patients' conditions.[8] But by the mid-1860s, the French empirical model was now on the decline in favor of a model that linked experimental laboratory sciences with the clinic. The unification of knowledge from the laboratory and the bedside, a model associated with German science, was also prominent in Paris.[9] In 1865, the French physiologist Claude Bernard published *An Introduction to the Study of Experimental Medicine*, which soon became the platform for medical reform in Europe and across the Atlantic.[10] Bernard called for the direct application of experimental methods, that is, microscopy, chemistry, and, above all, physiology, to clinical medicine. Through his studies, he described the concept of *milieu intérieur*, or how the body maintained its internal environment and processes, what we now call homeostasis. Putnam arrived just in time to feel the impact of Bernard's ideas, absorbing his message on experimentalism and the "independence" of organisms by way of internal regulation.

While Paris medicine offered great opportunities for men, it was less welcoming to women. Until the 1860s, women were barred from the orthodox training schools of Paris — most importantly, the École de Médecine. In fact, women generally had very few educational opportunities in France until the liberalization of education at the end of the Second Empire. French culture in the nineteenth century idealized women and their moral superiority but also regarded them as childlike, dependent, and subordinate to men. Gender norms defined the female role as domestic and limited women's educational sphere to the teaching of children in the home. The Napoleonic Code legally ensured the social subordination of women, granting men control over family affairs, including property, work, domestic finances, and the lives of children. The Catholic Church reinforced patriarchy and maintained that "nature" determined women's roles as obedient wives and mothers.[11] French women's secondary status, enforced by laws, religion, and cultural norms, also hindered the expansion of their educational opportunities.

In the 1860s, French opposition to female physicians emerged from concerns about the disruption of the family and social order in French life, as critics argued that women physicians posed a threat to the nation's moral health. According to critics, female doctors threatened the equilibrium of French life, as their practice of medicine challenged all of the "natural" roles of women. Dr. Henri Montanier, for example, argued that nature intended women to be mothers, wives, and the caretakers of the home, and that medical work upset female delicacy and modesty.[12] Some of the strongest opposition to women physicians came from the ranks of medical men, who for the most part refused to admit women into their medical circles. Like their American counterparts, physicians in France produced scientific knowledge that demonstrated women's physical and mental weakness, and they attempted to prove their cognitive and emotional inability to practice medicine. Physicians borrowed from new theories of evolutionary biology to argue for female inferiority and used medical knowledge on mental illness to characterize women as hysterical and unfit for higher learning or medical practice.[13] While medical arguments against women physicians were far more popular in America, French critics also linked the education of women to the moral and physical decline of French civilization.

At the heart of the "woman question," the debate over women physicians sat at the crossroads of larger debates over gender norms and national identity. There was great cultural resistance in France to women practicing medicine because female physicians challenged family ideals, and definitions of women's nature. As in Great Britain and the United States, opponents in France expressed their disapproval through arguments that reflected larger anxieties about the prospects of altering gender roles and the impact of social change on the state of the nation.

Beginning in the 1830s, French women with socialist leanings called for the expansion of their rights and worked for economic independence, the freedom to marry and divorce, and participation in public life. Feminists were active during the 1848 revolutions, thereafter calling upon leaders to grant women the vote. But, despite these efforts, women did not achieve suffrage rights, and they made little progress by midcentury in regard to education and professional training. In the conservative political climate after the 1848 revolutions, women's voices were repressed by state censorship while patriarchal discourse dominated the reign of Napoléon III.[14] It was not until near the end of the Second Empire in the late 1860s that signs of change began to appear.

Mary Putnam arrived in France at an opportune time. Toward the end of Napoléon III's rule, the French state began to institute reform laws, allowing more freedom of the press and expanding rights of assembly. The voices of feminists and socialists were being heard, and many assumptions about gender were thrown into question. Strong conservative opinions, like those of writer Jules Michelet, who insisted that French women were "naturally" wives and mothers, certainly supported traditional gender roles for women.[15] But the Ministry of Education, now governed by a few liberal-minded men, contemplated the possibility of admitting women to schools of higher learning and medical training. This reconsideration of women's education, and the debates that ensued, provided Putnam with great opportunity.

Putnam, attuned to the fact that fears about women physicians differed when one crossed national borders, also took advantage of her national identity as an American woman. She remarked, "An Englishman would say that it was indelicate to admit women to study medicine, a Frenchman, that it was dangerous."[16] In France, critics were most concerned with how the medical woman posed an internal threat, challenging French notions of women's roles in society and the family. Putnam seemed aware of this cultural concern in her decision to go to Paris, and she decided to use her outsider status as an asset rather than a liability.

Putnam also realized that a female physician "was never heard of" because the French believed it was unnatural, indelicate, and, as Putnam insinuated, dangerously provocative to have women in the close company of men. Knowing that it was difficult to be "delicate" at the dissecting table, she recognized that foreign women had a better chance of dispelling the myth that women doctors posed a threat to French society. She explained, "I knew well enough that I was not 'dangerous,' and that Frenchmen would instantly perceive that I was not, and when once that first difficulty was overcome, that I could be much more at ease here." The French "disbelief" in women was so deeply "rooted," observed Putnam, that "their whole social system is constructed so entirely on the principle of keeping young men and women as far apart as flame and gunpowder." But as an American woman, with "greater coldness of temperament and reliability of character," she did not threaten to spark inappropriate relations.[17] Maintaining a strong deportment, and "not flirting with the [other] students," worked in her favor.[18] To the French, American women like Putnam seemed less feminine and lacking passion, and, therefore, less of a temptation to men. Ironically, American women in medicine became acceptable in France for the same reason female professionals became unacceptable in the United States: they appeared less womanly.

Putnam balanced a strong professional air with the demeanor of a respectable lady, negotiating a place for her own style of femininity within a masculine medical culture. She rejected feminine norms in her adopted nation and constructed a different identity as an American. Emphasizing character over appearance, modesty over fashion, French observers saw Putnam as more "*gentille*" than beautiful, which was to her advantage, since "much prettiness would be in the way of attending, or, in fact, receiving permission to attend the hospitals."[19] Describing herself as a "boy-girl" to her family, she knew that she was combining qualities of both genders, and upsetting traditional roles both at home and abroad. She tried to calm her parents, who worried about their daughter acting "more like a son." She told them not to worry about her with such "feminine perversity," that she would find a way to remain respectable yet resilient in her attempts to access the education she so desired.[20] French physicians may have had doubts about Putnam, but ultimately, she gained admission to Parisian clinics and laboratories, and eventually, the École de Médecine. Putnam was accepted because she did not pose a serious risk to the French social order, or so it seemed.

An American "Boy-Girl" in Paris

When Putnam first arrived in Paris in September 1866, she was in awe of her new home, preoccupied with the beauty of the city. Her temporary lodgings on the Rue de Rivoli gave her easy access to the architecture, art, and fashion that would first absorb her curious mind. Strolling in the Tuileries gardens, down the boulevards, and over the bridges of the Seine, Putnam was completely enchanted with the statues, the monuments, and the fountains that decorated Paris. At the same time, the young traveler was already aware, and a little skeptical, of the emperor's grand plans for organizing and beautifying the city, pondering what lay behind its extravagant facades. Overjoyed by her new city, Putnam wrote to her sister Edith, "You have no idea of the overwhelming effect of Paris upon a person coming for the first time. For the first few days I was as one intoxicated. . . ."[21]

While the city excited her senses and fed her intellect, Putnam was conscious of her professional mission to expand her scientific education. For guidance, she soon turned to a fellow woman physician, Elizabeth Blackwell, who was in Paris at the time and helped her acclimate to her new surroundings.[22] Blackwell secured more permanent lodging for Putnam, who rented a "tiny bedroom" from a family who resided on Rue Monsieur le Prince in the Latin Quarter. Living near the Luxembourg Garden, Putnam found herself pleasantly situated and her knowledge of French improving every day. The Latin Quarter also had its professional advantages; Putnam's lodgings on the Left Bank placed her in the heart of the Parisian academic and medical community, situated in the same neighborhood as the École de Médecine, the École Pratique, and some of the city's major hospitals. She followed in the footsteps of many male medical students, French and American, who formed the community of scientific scholars on the Left Bank.

Shortly after her arrival, Putnam followed the lead of other medical women in Paris and made inquiries about working at the Hôpital de la Maternité, the large lying-in hospital and training school for midwives. When Elizabeth Blackwell first came to Paris in 1849, the Maternité had provided female practitioners with the best opportunity for acquiring "practical" medical training. Blackwell, like her male counterparts, traveled to Paris to acquire greater clinical experience.[23] Although the living and working conditions were poor, Blackwell recalled, "My residence there was an invaluable one at that stage of the medical campaign, when no hospitals, dispensaries, or practical *cliniques* were open to women."[24] Arriving more than fifteen years later, Putnam decided not to resign herself to working at the Maternité, for it was a "gloomy establishment." "I was in no hurry to seal my fate by entering that detestable place," Putnam stated.[25] She realized that training at the Maternité limited her options because she would then be labeled a midwife, relegated to obstetric work, and denied a full scientific and clinical education.

Upon departing from New York, Putnam claimed to be "undecided" about how to focus her career. Would she choose to be a physician, or would she become a research scientist? By November 1866, just two months after arriving in Paris, she came to a decision. In a letter to her mother, she confirmed that she would study "chemistry as subordinate to medicine."[26] Committed to pleasing her parents, who supported her financially and preferred that she become a "practical physician," Putnam recognized the greater remunerative possibilities available to a physician than those available to a woman scientist. Although she had already cultivated a love for science and would continue her chemical and physiological pursuits, she agreed to prioritize clinical training.

She soon received helpful introductions from Elizabeth Blackwell and the letters of Lucy Sewall from the New England Hospital for Women and Children. She met a key ally, Dr. Benjamin Ball, an English physician in Paris.[27] Ball first tried to help Putnam get permission to attend lectures at the École de Médecine, but he did not succeed. He did receive permission for Putnam to "follow" hospital clinics at two of the city's most important institutions. She was one of twenty "internes" at the Lariboisière, a general hospital, where she worked in service of Dr. Hippolyte-Victor Hérard. An "agreeable" man, Putnam said, Hérard "keeps me by his side so that I can see everything most distinctly and takes pains to explain matters to me as he goes along."[28] Putnam received numerous opportunities to observe Hérard in the clinics, according to her published reports in the New York *Medical Record*. For example, she recounted Hérard's opinions on the relationship between pneumonia and pulmonary consumption and observed his treatment of syphilis with mercury during pregnancy and his use of hydrochloric acid to treat dyspepsia (indigestion).[29] Putnam's service to Hérard provided her a critical entrée into the centers of Paris medicine.

Thanks also to Benjamin Ball, Putnam gained access to clinics at the Salpêtrière, the hospital for the insane made famous by the hysteria studies of Jean-Martin Charcot.[30] Like the Lariboisière, the Salpêtrière was located away from the city's medical schools, and was therefore less popular with medical students. Although it was a long walk for Putnam, the Salpêtrière offered her unrivaled access to patients, many with hysteria, and clinical instruction. Working for the physician Jacques-Joseph Moreau de Tours was "quite like taking private lessons," she said.[31] Furthermore, working with Moreau exposed Putnam to theories and treatments of nervous diseases.[32] Although remembered for his studies on hashish and hysteria, Moreau was also interested in hereditary insanity and other etiological questions about common neuroses.[33] Putnam's experience at the Salpêtrière was a prelude to a career-long interest in issues of insanity and nervous disease.

By the spring of 1867, Putnam had a full schedule of hospital visits. She spent three to five hours a day in clinics on topics that ranged from the specific (for example, diseases of the larynx or surgical) to the general (for example, practical diagnosis). In the typical format for the teaching clinic, instructors and students together observed and examined patients. Instructors then called upon the students for their evaluations and opinions. At other times, students examined patients before the group rounds, and made reports on the cases.[34] Putnam was pleased with her work in the clinics and believed she performed as well as those who had already completed their medical education. She claimed, "I made a careful comparison of my own mistakes with theirs, (*internes* and *externs* together,) and the strictest impartiality would decide, I think, that there is no difference either in their quality or quantity." Putnam bragged about receiving feedback from the faculty of physicians, who, she said, "place me on a level with their good students."[35] The confident young doctor once boasted to her parents, "Friday I was particularly exultant at the fact that in our auscultation class at Lariboissière [*sic*], I was in the right three times, when every one else was wrong."[36] After braving an environment dominated by men, Putnam expressed haughty satisfaction about her intellectual triumphs.

Along with her clinical rounds, Putnam also attended clinical lectures in surgery, a development that gave her new hope for gaining admission to medical school in Paris. In April 1867, she attended her first surgical lecture in an amphitheater and met a professor from the faculty of medicine for the first time.[37] In May, she began to "assist" at the surgical lectures of Jean-François Jarjavay at the Beaujon.[38] She wrote to her sister expectantly, "Since I am moreover in *two* different courses of young men, one for anatomy, the other for the microscope ... perhaps, next fall I could use these and other facts for stepping-stones and make a fresh attempt to attend lectures at the École de Médecine."[39] Putnam's strategy was a good one; her presence in lectures and performance in the clinics did, indeed, help her admission to the school of medicine.

Putnam soon found ways to build a scientific curriculum within her clinical schedule, and to combine the study of science with clinical medicine. Upon first arriving in Paris, she believed "it is true that a purely scientific life would suit me better than any other." But she found "less facility for it" and complained to her mother, "I have been much exasperated lately by the difficulties I have encountered in finding a laboratory where I can pursue certain chemico-medical analyses."[40] This changed in the spring of 1867 when Putnam started working a couple of hours every day at the microbiology lab of Louis-Antoine Ranvier, an assistant to Claude Bernard, and André-Victor Cornil, who impressed her as "really distinguished and scientific men."[41] Working with Bernard's assistant meant Putnam gained access to the scientific culture of the city and was exposed to the most important developments in histology and microscopy.[42] In 1869, Ranvier and Cornil published the *Manual of Pathological Histology*, which described and classified morbid tissue conditions as seen under the microscope. "Paying little attention to naked-eye descriptions," this manual represented the laboratory investigations of the two scientists and their students, who may have included Mary Putnam.[43]

Putnam's work in Ranvier and Cornil's laboratory informed her thesis research, which she used to complete her degree later at the École de Médecine. Based on several of her own chemical investigations and experiments using human livers (from autopsy subjects) and animal livers (rabbits, pigs, and cats), she examined how the fatty degeneration of tissue cells resulted from failed "nutrition" of the body. Through her experiments, Putnam showed how the "lessening in assimilation and disassimilation," that is, the absorption and breakdown of food materials, caused fatty degeneration of tissue cells. Ultimately she verified the work of Ranvier, arguing that the formation of fat in cells, visible under the microscope, depended on chemical reactions or the influence of other fats already present in cells. Recalling her knowledge of Virchow and principles of cellular pathology, her French thesis addressed the physiological impact of cellular degeneration and how cellular nutrition effected a body's general health and "vital powers."[44] Such investigations, Putnam believed, were essential for determining sources of illness and designating therapeutic regimens. Working alongside some of the leading figures behind the promotion of laboratory science in medicine, Putnam's experience with Ranvier influenced her own medical philosophy, shaping her commitment to the integration of microscopy and chemistry into medical practice.

At about the same time, Putnam used her access to clinics and laboratories to report medical news from Paris to American physicians, becoming the "special correspondent" for the *Medical Record*.[45] In her column "Medical

Matters in Paris," she described the latest clinical reports, medical theories, and debates being published in French medical journals and gazettes. Using the pseudonym P. C. M. (a reversal of her initials), Putnam disguised herself, and her gender, to her reading audience. George Frederick Shrady, founder and editor of the *Medical Record*, accepted her first report in June of 1867 and published her columns regularly for the next two years. A respected surgeon and leading medical journalist in Manhattan, Shrady served as medical editor for the *New York Herald* for many years and probably had professional ties to Mary's father.[46]

Eager to secure funds for her education, Putnam wrote for American publications in order to finance her continuing stay in France. For most of 1867, she sent correspondence to the *New York Evening Post*, summarizing French news, including scientific developments. But the paper wanted Putnam to lighten the content and focus more on "gossip" and "scandalous stories," which she found a "dreadful bore."[47] Frustrated with the *Post*, she decided to contribute fiction and social commentary to her father's own *Putnam's Monthly*.[48] One tale, called "A Martyr to Science," tells of a man who takes medical experimentation too far. This physician, who also has a crisis of religious faith, rejects Catholicism in favor of science. In the name of "supreme heroism," the physician wanted "undying fame," to sacrifice himself to science and be remembered with a "reverent homage." He plans a vivisection on himself, but before he can become a martyr to science, his students place him in an asylum.[49] In this dark yet amusing mad-scientist story, Putnam scoffed at her character's egotism but showed some understanding for the all-consuming desire for discovery. She used science as a subject for her fiction, but she found her medical communications more productive for her studies and most personally satisfying. She knew that as a medical correspondent, she was an important agent of scientific exchange across the Atlantic.

Speaking to American men of medicine, many of whom had studied in Paris and pursued the empirical model of medicine, Putnam's articles in the *Medical Record* described the technical and theoretical developments emerging from the Paris clinics.[50] She conveyed her firsthand observations of working on clinical rounds with Hérard and relayed the methods, procedures, and approaches of her other instructors.[51] Putnam praised the teaching clinics and said the system was "admirable . . . for its democratic equity in throwing open the best clinical advantages to all who choose to try for them."[52] This appreciation for "equity" certainly reflected her appreciation for opportunities granted to her as a woman. At the same time, it emerged from her critique of the American system, which offered limited opportunities for hospital study, especially for women. She remarked, "No one can observe the working of the method without wishing for its introduction at home."[53]

Putnam's letters to the *Medical Record* focused on clinical reports, but they also addressed matters of pathology and developments in the laboratory. In her reporting on the debate over Bright's disease (a disease of the kidney characterized by a renal lesion, albuminuria, and dropsy), for example, Putnam described microscopical investigations, including those by Cornil, to illustrate debates over whether certain physical conditions represented distinct diseases or steps in the evolution of a chronic disease. Her coverage of this debate over disease specificity spoke to her growing interest in the laboratory as a locale for diagnosis.[54]

In the spring of 1867, Putnam had new hope for entering the school of medicine. Ranvier arranged for her to have "private entrée" into the "grand library" of the École de Médecine. At the very same time, she received word that she would be allowed to attend a fall class in operative surgery at the École Pratique. This was significant, Putnam recognized, because the "École [Pratique] is literally and figuratively, at the very doors of the École de Médecine and is one of the institutions that Dr. Blackwell prophesised that I could not enter."[55] Surpassing Blackwell and the efforts made by previous women, Putnam seemed on the road to admission.

Months later, Putnam had new indications that she could be admitted to the École de Médecine. She discussed the prospects of her admission with the secretary of the faculty of medicine, who offered Putnam great hope for admission and urged her to apply. To her astonishment, he stated, "'If you wish yourself to take out inscriptions and graduate with our degree, nothing is easier!'"[56] The secretary then admitted that he had been responsible for rejecting her requests to attend lectures the previous year but had a change of heart. Putnam would later learn that the decision did not rest solely with the secretary but was part of a larger reconsideration of women in medicine within the Ministry of Education.[57]

Strongly encouraged by this personal exchange, Putnam believed her admission was almost a "settled fact." She officially submitted an application, applying under the title of "foreign physician."[58] Like many of her American male counterparts, Putnam requested that her American degrees fulfill the prerequisite training required by the faculty of medicine, including a total of sixteen "inscriptions," or course registrations, and three preliminary first-year examinations. The secretary of the faculty again assisted her, this time in preparing a statement for the minister, which was accompanied by her diplomas from the United States and a certificate of citizenship prepared by the American ambassador. With great expectations, already assuming her acceptance, she explained, "This official recognition of an American degree is a great thing for the medical education of all women, and I feel singularly honored that the recognition should have been conferred upon them in me." Convinced that she was already "in for it," she began to make her preparations for examinations to attain the degree.[59]

Putnam's words of celebration were premature. The faculty of medicine at the École de Médecine rejected her application during its meeting on 23 November 1867, linking her fate to the fate of French women. Minutes from that meeting reveal that participants addressed key issues at the heart of the woman question in France. The Commission Scolaire, having met separately, rejected Putnam's application requesting permission to take exams at the École de Médecine, and denied her exemption from sixteen inscriptions. Some members of the faculty supported this decision and spoke against her admission. Dr. Charles-Pierre Denonvilliers stated that "the Council on Public Instruction has always been of the opinion to rule out women from the practice of medicine in France." According to Denonvilliers, the law granting the right for women to practice midwifery remained silent (*muette*) on the issue of women practicing medicine because it "seems so contrary to our customs and our social conditions." Dr. Behier expanded on the legal impediments; he explained that women, if married, are minors (*mineure*) under French law and "escape all personal responsibilities." Consequently, he concluded, "the adoption of the request of Mademoiselle Putnam could lead to grave complications."[60]

One member then rose in her defense. The dean of the faculty, Adolphe Wurtz, pointed out that the law had great ambiguity, and was silent on the issue of women practicing medicine, stating, "There is no more reason to interpret it in the negative than the positive." Wurtz pushed even further, stating that the minister of education had already authorized Madeleine Bres, a French woman with medical ambitions, to take her inscriptions and seemed "to have decided the question" in the positive. Nevertheless, the faculty refused to accept the request of Mary Putnam.[61] Clearly, a divide had emerged in her case that represented contrasting French political perspectives on the debate over the "woman question."

Following the "blunt" rejection of her application, Putnam reverted to her own original plan: first to apply for admission to attend classes at the École de Médecine and then request examinations later. With this strategy, Putnam

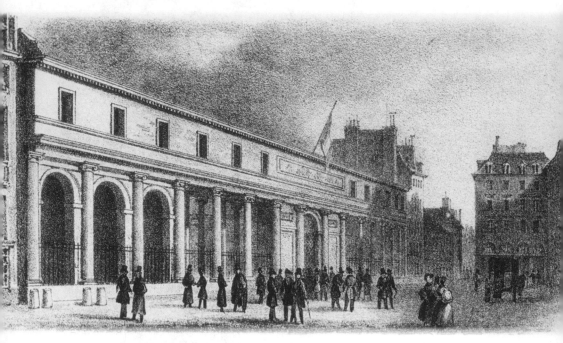

École de Médecine, Paris. Courtesy of the National Library of Medicine.

⋅✦⋅✦⋅✦⋅

hoped that the faculty and students would grow accustomed to her presence in courses, see that she was not a danger but rather a serious student, and ultimately permit her to take examinations. A slower, more pragmatic approach was hailed by the secretary of public instruction. Dining with him at the home of a friend, Putnam asked for his support to attend the famous histology course given by Charles Robin at the École de Médecine.[62] After a month of work, the secretary successfully acquired authorization for Putnam to attend Robin's course and officially become a student at the École de Médecine.

"A Petticoat in the Amphitheatre"

In a letter to her parents on 25 January 1868, Putnam announced her groundbreaking news: "For the first time since its foundation several centuries ago, a petticoat might be seen in the august amphitheatre of the *École de Médecine*. That petticoat enrobed the form of your most obedient servant and dutiful daughter!"[63] Putnam recognized and celebrated the fact that her admission was historic. Careful not to alarm her parents, she reminded them that she was a respectful and loyal daughter and, ultimately, still a lady; she even wore proper feminine undergarments. The "petticoat" became an important symbol for women physicians who wanted to prove that they maintained their femininity while surrounded by men.[64]

Despite the shocking presence of a "petticoat" in the medical amphitheater, Putnam tried to "feel as much at home as if [she] had been there all of [her] life." When she began to attend Robin's course, she entered the amphitheater through a side door, a separate entrance from the other students, and seated herself in a special chair near the professor. Putnam reported that she felt at ease in the course, but her presence was indeed, as she put it, "a considerable triumph." Although nurses sometimes assisted physicians, the medical amphitheater had been designated a masculine domain. The amphitheater itself was a symbol of medical knowledge, and students watched the drama of a surgery or examination unfold on the medical stage as the professor conducted the procedure. Putnam was happy to disprove all the "humbug" and predictions that a "*tapage*" (furor) would break out among the students upon her admission. Her successful attendance and peaceful reception, she thought, were the result of a "practical stratagem executed upon the Faculty, whose lines have been turned by an adroit maneuver."[65] Putnam recognized that, with the help of several supportive physicians and officials, she had carried out a serious coup.

As Putnam continued her courses, she hoped she would soon take her examinations and earn the degree. She realized that her opportunities depended on administrators who were sympathetic to her cause. In letters home to her family, Putnam recounted her campaign to take her exams. When she felt "half prepared," she took some brave steps on her own behalf. She wrote to Joseph-Arsène Danton, the secretary of the minister of education, requesting to take her exams and warning that she would appeal to the faculty or directly to the minister himself, if need be.[66] Knowing full well that Putnam would have support from the minister and less from the faculty, dean Adolphe Wurtz suggested that she appeal directly to Minister Victor Duruy. Putnam admitted that going to the highest levels of government "scared [her] a little," but she did not retreat, submitted a request, and began to study intensely.[67] Ultimately, she received approval by the minister of education himself.

Putnam described the drama of learning the good news by underscoring her bold moves and relaying a public moment of triumph. Growing impatient after only four days, she marched down to the Sorbonne to demand an answer to her request. On her way, she encountered the secretary of the faculty, Monsieur Forget, who had her authorization in hand. The official note conveyed the decision of the minister, Victor Duruy, and stated that it was he who granted Putnam permission to take her exams and exemption from the sixteen inscriptions and three exams required of other applicants.[68] The faculty officially accepted Putnam's degrees from the Female Medical College of Pennsylvania and the New York College of Pharmacy in place of other courses and training, as noted on her matriculation record.[69] Upon greeting Putnam with the letter of authorization, Forget invited her to stroll with him around the Luxembourg Garden. Later Putnam wrote of "the evident astonishment of the numerous bands of students" that watched the victory lap. It was a welcome gesture, which Putnam called a "public demonstration that he was on my side."[70]

Mary Putnam's admission to the École de Médecine resulted from a long process that rested on personal connections.[71] Her social network of medical women helped pave her way in to the world of Paris medicine. Elizabeth Blackwell, Lucy Sewall, and the English doctor Elizabeth Garrett all offered important connections to physicians and professors who were sympathetic to female practitioners. After working directly with Putnam, these men of medicine supported her endeavors, including her clinical observations and laboratory studies. Even Putnam's official application and ultimate acceptance to the École de Médecine were facilitated by personal connections. But it was also the political positions and ideologies of the people in the network that facilitated her admission and the changes that ensued.

Putnam's admission to the École de Médecine only materialized with the support of an important set of liberal-minded men who occupied powerful positions within the École de Médecine and the Ministry of Education as well as within a broader context of social change. While the Second Empire of Napoléon III is not remembered for its liberalism, nor for its support of feminist concerns, significant changes did occur in the 1860s to relax the authoritarian style of the regime and challenge the dominance of conservative forces. The election of 1863 marked an important turning point, for it was then that the liberals and republicans won twelve seats in the 282-seat Corps Législatif. Although far from achieving a majority, French voters communicated their decreasing tolerance for imperial policies and their desires for reform. In response to the election, and the need to appear more lenient, Napoléon III appointed liberals to various key posts in the cabinet. These new officials had a profound effect on helping to open up the press, extend the right to assembly, and expand the educational system; some of them were even sympathetic to the interests of women.[72]

One of the most important of these reformers was Victor Duruy, who became minister of public instruction soon after the election of 1863. Called "the major liberal of the empire" by his biographer, Duruy put forth great efforts to reform and expand French education in the 1860s. After inheriting an elitist system, he set out to increase literacy and extend public education to the French masses. Duruy is also widely recognized for his efforts on behalf of women and girls. In 1867, he successfully enacted the "Duruy law," which gave girls' primary schools legal equality with boys' schools, and improved the working and living conditions for teachers. He then attempted to construct a system of public secondary schools for girls. Justifying his plans to the Empress Eugenie, he argued that the education of women and girls would greatly benefit society and the state, and enhance family life, as mothers could teach their sons.[73] Critics and clerics saw his proposal for secondary girls' education as antireligious policy that defied gender norms, even if he did maintain that he was not interested in making girls into "bluestockings." Although dissenters eventually stopped Duruy from carrying out his plans, feminists welcomed his efforts.

Duruy was also a strong supporter of women's medical education, evidenced by his decision to admit Putnam to the École de Médecine. He reversed a long tradition of denying women higher education and medical training and opened the school to the admission of other women in the future. The English woman Elizabeth Garrett was admitted soon after Putnam and became the first woman to graduate from the École de Médecine. A Russian woman, Ekaterina Goncharova, followed next. Finally, Madeleine Bres was the first French woman to matriculate in 1868, after years of studying as a midwife and lobbying for admission. But in the next twenty years, foreign women dominated the list of those admitted to the École de Médecine.[74] Certainly, the prior education of Putnam, Garrett, and Goncharova, facilitated their admission; French women had little access to education and therefore could not provide the same qualifications.[75] In addition, the École de Médecine admitted more foreign women because an atypical, talented female visitor from a foreign land was far easier to accept as a physician than a French woman who seemed to be challenging the essence of French civilization. Foreign women did not directly disrupt the integrity of French femininity; nor did they threaten to undermine family norms.

The tolerance, and ultimate acceptance, of women into the École de

Médecine was also part of a broader set of reforms in the French government directed at Algeria. Duruy used concerns about women's health in the colonies as an opportunity to train women in medicine at home. With the encouragement of Empress Eugenie, he proposed a school for women, arguing that Arab women would benefit from treatment by a practitioner of the same sex, who could more easily access their homes, going where a male doctor "could never enter." As in the United States, the propriety of same-sex medical care worked in favor of women doctors. The empress believed that female practitioners were an important colonial initiative, vital for "attaching us to the Arabs, and to spread our influence in the Orient."[76] Although she and Duruy claimed their plan was benevolent, their program functioned to extend French oversight of colonial subjects into their most private lives and domestic spaces.

The empress also recognized that developing a medical training school for women would also benefit the nation at home. A medical training school for women would "give to our midwives superior instruction," she believed, and would give the Sisters of Charity "better knowledge of the medicines they often distribute to poor families."[77] Training medical women became a matter of national pride and identity and, according to Duruy, was "patriotique." In 1870, Le Figaro announced that Russia had authorized women to practice medicine, although they were not allowed to earn degrees. Not wanting to be upstaged by the Russians, Eugenie wrote to Duruy and urged him to work quickly, saying that the French needed "to allow ourselves to advance after having the first idea."[78] Eugenie, of course, was not a feminist or a liberal reformer herself. Colonial interests and nationalism inspired her to support educational reforms. However, the empress's support for medical women, in conjunction with the reforms of Duruy, contributed to the expansion of medical opportunities for women in France.

From the highest ranks of the empire — the empress and the Ministry of Education — came the approval and promotion of women physicians and the general broadening of women's education. At the same time, after an era of imposed silence, feminist activists were speaking out on the needs and rights of women. The period from 1867 to 1870 marked an important resurgence of feminism that coincided with a critical reconsideration of women's education. Putnam's historic admission to the École de Médecine emerged from this context of change and simultaneously fueled it. A woman who began her career in Paris as an anomaly and an outsider ultimately became a catalyst for the acceptance of medical women in the Paris clinics.

Science and Socialism

Putnam's triumphant admission to the *cours* at the École de Médecine coincided with her political awakening and introduction to radical politics. In the
first months of 1868, Putnam began to attend Robin's course on histology,
continued her work in the laboratories of Cornil and the anatomist Marie
Philibert Constant Sappey, prepared for her examinations, and worked on
her thesis. At the same time, she became deeply occupied with the turbulent
political changes and social hardships that accompanied the Franco-Prussian
War, and the rise and fall of the Paris Commune. As she progressed with her
scientific agenda, she simultaneously grew as a political thinker, and began to
see herself also as a political actor.

With the Reclus family, Putnam associated with some of the key figures
in leftist politics in Paris, and absorbed their energy and ideas about social
change.[79] They shaped her opinions about state politics, religion, the bour-
geoisie, and the value of socialism. Most importantly, as a geographer and
scientist himself, Élisée Reclus drew parallels between the natural world and
the political, influencing Putnam, who later overlapped her views about the
physiological body and an egalitarian body politic. He also expressed support
for women's rights, as he backed the efforts of La Société de la Revendication
de Droits de la Femme (Society for the Vindication of the Rights of Woman),
an organization attended by his brother Élie and sister-in-law Noémi.[80]

Putnam met the Reclus family's two eldest brothers, Élie and Élisée, in
the spring of 1868, on the heels of her admission to the École de Médecine.
She immediately wrote to her sister to sing their praises. Despite their modest means, Putnam was deeply impressed by the family's "vigor and finesse
of the intellect" because they had a "kind of perfect cultivation united with
a certain buoyant heroism." She was captivated by the family's relationship,
which was "so warm and demonstrative, as to be an astonishing revelation
in the midst of cool, polite Paris." In addition to the family's personal appeal,
Putnam found them intellectually rich and unattached to the material possessions that were so important to "vain and dependent people."[81] The Reclus
family introduced her to a society of reformers and radical republicans that
met regularly to discuss politics and social reform. The family also brought her
along to Vascoeuil, the country estate of Alfred Dumesnil, brother-in-law of
Élie and Élisée Reclus, where family and friends retreated for relaxation and
more political conversation. Putnam greatly enjoyed visits to this rural salon

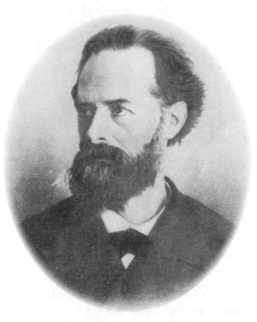

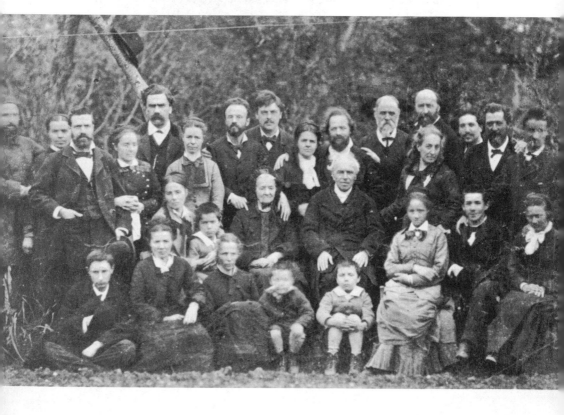

in eastern Normandy, where she read in the countryside, wrote in the tower of the château, and engaged in "gay and animated" conversations.[82] She admired the intellectual vivaciousness and philosophical commitments of the Reclus circle, though some of their beliefs seemed, at first, to be extreme and idealistic. Intrigued, she said their ideas "are strange and fresh and vivid, and the people whom they inspire, live in them and by them and would die for them if need be."[83] The family also nurtured her unconventional views about women's roles in society, especially Élie and his wife and cousin, Noémi Reclus. Inspired by her new social life with radicals, Putnam relished her friendship with a family that seemed so different from her own.

During her stay at the Reclus home, Putnam also developed a relationship with a young physician, referred to only in family correspondence as "Monsieur M." Little is known about this personal dimension of Putnam's life in wartime Paris. The couple courted and became engaged at the beginning of the war, before he was sent to the front. Upon his return, they decided to break their engagement so that they both could pursue medicine in their home countries. As Noémi Reclus explained to Putnam's parents, "I said to your daughter . . . 'If you should consent to stay in France, you would simply be the wife of Monsieur M., which would not suit either your ambitions or your scheme of life.'"[84] Although Putnam put her professional goals and familial duties first, she felt this man "suited" her perfectly, professing, "I believe in him. *Voila tout.*" It is clear that Putnam's fiancé offered her more than just romance. A young physician and intellectual, "Monsieur M." played an important part in her political awakening. As she said, their relationship was "something that has completely revolutionized me."[85]

In this company, Putnam had entered a circle of the most important radical French thinkers of the time. Élie and Élisée Reclus were significant activists, journalists, and political theorists who offered the ideological underpinnings for social revolution in France. For this activism, the Reclus brothers became symbols of the Commune. Although there is no evidence that they fought at the barricades, they were important icons of socialism, and later anarchism, and remain so today.

Élie and Élisée Reclus both began their careers as journalists and expanded their professional work in concert with their political activism. Élie wrote on a variety of social and political topics and became famous for his account of the Commune, *La Commune de Paris au jour le jour: 19 mars–28 mai, 1871.*[86] Although he did not fight in the Commune, he became the director of the Bibliothèque Nationale during the insurrection in April and May of 1871. Élie was a committed socialist who took part in various associations of workers and radical republicans. But it was his brother and comrade, Élisée, who was the more significant political player in French radical politics.

Élisée Reclus was one of the chief architects of radical thought in France during the resurgence of socialist activity in late-nineteenth-century Europe. In the late 1860s, he participated in a number of related movements and associations, including the cooperative movement, Freemasonry, the Free Thinkers, and the International Working Men's Association. A friend and political ally of socialist leader Michael Bakunin, he was involved with the League of Peace and Freedom, an organization aimed to unite Europe under a single republican government.[87] Reclus worked within the existing political and social structures to promote an evolution in social thinking that would lead to revolution, the overthrow of the emperor, and the establishment of a government led by the people's associations. Although Élisée Reclus became an anarchist after 1871, he was a revolutionary socialist in the years leading up to the Franco-Prussian War; he hoped for the establishment of a "social republic" in France and abroad that would end the tyranny of centralized government and allow people to directly govern themselves through communal associations.[88]

The study of geography was an integral component of Élisée Reclus's political activism. Reclus, once called "the father of modern geography in France," made his field central to the study of the relationship between humans and the physical world. Reclus first developed an interest in geography during his travels in the 1850s, especially on his trip to the American South, where he saw the cruelties of slavery and the plantation system.[89] In the 1860s, his political activism increased and he began to compose his most significant earth studies. In 1868, he published *La Terre*, his first major geographical work, and in 1876, he began work on *La Nouvelle Géographie Universelle*, a nineteen-volume chronicle that he completed in 1894. At the time of completion, his political orientation had shifted to anarchism. As one of his biographers argues, Reclus was one of the first scholars to study "human geography" and merge ideologies of science with anarchism.[90]

A scientific understanding and positivist approach guided Reclus's studies of the earth and its relationship to humans and their political structures.[91] Reclus studied nature with positivist, scientific methods, employing direct observation to produce knowledge about the earth and its peoples. A critic of nationalism, Reclus believed that people should be organized according to "natural" boundaries rather that state boundaries. For example, during the Franco-Prussian War, Reclus did not support French efforts to keep the Alsace and Lorraine regions, for he believed that each geographical territory had a right to determine its own fate. "Natural" processes also governed progress and the social and political structures of the future, he said. Darwinian thinking informed his belief that human biology and human society would evolve toward progress. And the evolution of humans would lead to the obligatory reformation of their environment toward revolutionary ends. Submitting to the laws of nature, Reclus argued, would undermine state structures and lead to social liberation. According to one biographer, Reclus and other anarchists were confident "that anarchy was a theoretically possible human condition, because it represented the fulfillment of laws which were immanent in human nature."[92]

Putnam's time with Reclus had a profound effect on her own integration of politics and science because he cultivated and reinforced her interest in rationalism and, more importantly, positivism. During her stay in Paris, Putnam energetically read French philosophy, especially the works of Enlightenment thinkers, such as Rousseau and Voltaire. She also studied Comte, whose writings on science and society would long inspire her. She had started reading Comte before arriving in France and discussed his work at length with her brother, Haven.[93] But, it was in Paris that positivism became the philosophical underpinning of her daily studies of medical science. Putnam, like many physicians and scientists of her generation, selectively adopted Comtean principles, embracing his ideals of observation and investigation and neglecting his criticisms of experimentation and statistics. Moved by Comte's unification of science and faith, she interpreted his thought to create an epistemological foundation for her work in Paris, and later in New York.[94]

As Reclus mapped the earth to reflect socialist principles, Putnam learned to construct the human body as an ideal representation of human relations. Inspired by Comte, she began to see that the sociopolitical body, or social organism, grew, functioned, and sustained itself much like living organisms, through the contributions of all its interdependent parts. Nature, in other words, required the inclusion and work of all people, including those who had been on the margins, especially women. It also meant that all parts of the social organism had a stake and a role in shaping society. Putnam grew to understand nature as a model for collectivism and republicanism, a metaphor for Reclus's social republic.

Feminism and socialism came together for Putnam during her time with the Reclus family. Their support for women's rights and education affirmed her both personally and intellectually, as they strongly encouraged her academic and scientific pursuits. In their company, she also studied the work of utopian socialist Charles Fourier, a vocal critic of industrialism, Catholicism, patriarchy, marriage, and the traditional family structure, and an advocate of female emancipation. He believed humanity was evolving toward "Harmony," a state of being characterized by equality between the sexes in which men and women would be similarly educated, productive, and free to express their "passions." Harmony could be achieved through "associationist communities," in which all members contributed equal labor, and through the liberation of women, who would lead the task of social reform.[95] Putnam was very intrigued with Fourier's ideas and planned to write an article about him in September 1868 during a stay at Vascoeuil.[96] His idea that men and women were born equal but made unequal by society resonated with her and had the greatest long-term impact. When she returned to New York, she made several references to him in both her private correspondence and her published writings, particularly her book on positivism.[97] His influence can also be seen in her studies of female physiology and her arguments for male/female similarities.

Putnam's interest in socialism and feminism can also be seen in her rejection of the materialistic orientation of French bourgeois culture. Her Calvinist background had taught her to value simplicity and spirituality over goods and wealth. She had a deep respect for the Reclus's domestic values and modest, intellectual lifestyle. She was annoyed by men she considered "thoroughly *bourgeois*," meaning one "particularly bent on making himself comfortable, and absorbed in no wider ideal, political, social, religious, literary, or scientific."[98] Putnam's critique of bourgeois culture and her passion for the world of ideas were critical components of her political awakening.

Putnam also developed a critical stance against the Catholic Church and its ties to the French state, voiced after a visit to Vascoeuil in the fall of 1868. Putnam articulated her distaste for religious ceremony in her reportage of two rituals: a funeral and a wedding. When Dumesnil's father died, he chose to have an *enterrement civil*, a civil burial, which offended a number of Catholics who attended the service. By contrast, Putnam was impressed: "I cannot convey to you the full impression made upon me by the solemnity, simplicity, and sincerity of this ceremony."[99] She then proceeded to criticize a Catholic wedding she attended with the Dumesnil family, devoting several pages to the lavish decorations and the extravagant party that followed. Putnam paid critical attention to the bride, describing her derisively as a nineteen-year-old "damsel" who made "pretty" speeches and changed clothes six times. Putnam had visited the marriage chamber, and she commented condescendingly on the couple's embroidered sleeping gowns and the crucifix that lay on the bed. The ceremony, she said, "in a miserable little country church, with staring artificial flowers, and extremely ugly wooden images," was full of "insignificance — all at once tawdry and naïve — you cannot imagine how ridiculous it all is."[100]

By contrast, she admired Élisée Reclus's wedding to his second wife, Fanny L'Herminez, in 1870. In a radical departure for the period, Élisée and Fanny did not have a clergyman at their wedding, nor is it clear that they even had a magistrate. The couple affirmed their union with a written statement, signed by all of those in attendance, including Mary Putnam. The couple stated that they entered into the marriage as an "act of free will," without ceremony or superstition, and without religious or legal affiliation.[101]

Élisée's union with Fanny L'Herminez gave Putnam new faith in the institution of marriage. In her midtwenties, Putnam was wary of marriage because it would interfere with her work as a physician. In a letter home in January 1868, she firmly stated, "As to my marrying, even at forty, it is absurd, it would be horridly inconvenient." She also rejected common assumptions about the social and economic purposes of marriage. She complained that young American women who entered marriage to elevate their social status represented "the last vice of civilization." Such decisions led to "mercenary marriages," she said, which were "the ruin of France." Putnam equated adulthood not with marriage but with the nourishment of the mind, which came from "studying, observing, not rushing prematurely into society."[102] Putnam gained new respect for marriage from Élisée Reclus, whose second marriage offered her a new model. A union made of "free will" and independent of religious affiliation was very appealing to her. In a letter of congratulations to Élisée after the wedding, Putnam said she was happy to be a witness at their service, and she praised him for his "*courage moral*" and a celebration that did not fit the "standard rules of society."[103] Putnam's perceptions of marriage, colored by a rejection of religion and materialistic inclinations, were central to her politicization, as she incorporated socialist beliefs into her perceptions of social customs and gender relations.

Putnam combined her criticism of the Catholic Church with her new enthusiasm for socialism in a short story, "A Sermon at Notre Dame," published in her father's own *Putnam's Monthly* in December of 1868 and February of 1869.[104] This fable, set in Paris during the onslaught of a cholera epidemic, describes the failures of organized religion and the triumph of public health measures. The story opens at the Notre Dame Cathedral, where one of the city's most famous preachers delivers a sermon on the immortality of the soul.

The preacher calls upon the people to ignore "materialists and men of science," who believe that human life centers in the observable, material world of the body, not the spiritual realm of the soul. "For all morality, justice, virtue, is rooted in the hope of immortality," says the preacher. The service ends, and as the congregation leaves the cathedral, they witness a scuffle between a police- man and a young man posting placards that read: "Cholera!!! Citizens, the plague has broken out in our midst. . . ." Signed by a Volunteer Board of Health, these posters call on citizens to stop the epidemic. As the crowd erupts in a panic and the preacher tries to suppress their fears, the government ministers and the citizens "recognized at that moment none of them believed in the Im- mortality of the Soul." Then a leader emerges from the crowd and calls upon the people to defend themselves against the plague just as they would defend themselves against a foreign invader. He is not there to comfort them, as the priest had, but to mobilize the people, including the poor and the weak, to carry out a "gigantic plan for arresting the cholera." For seven days and seven nights, the people work to depopulate the city, remove its "pestilence," and transport people to the countryside. Committees were enthusiastically born and organized, "with as much effective precision as organs shape themselves out of the fluid mass of an embryonic body," wrote Putnam. In the story, the people save themselves and the city, for, as the narrator remarks, "life alone, intense, mobile, overflowing, could resist the threatened stagnation and pa- ralysis of death."[105] The people then gather before the cathedral to sing a "new hymn" and rejoice in the power of humanity. "It was a new Elevation of the Host."

Putnam's "Sermon at Notre Dame" promoted faith in socialism and sci- ence over faith in religion. It is "the people" and not a preacher, public health measures, not passive prayer, that ultimately resolve an impending health crisis. Despite the preacher's attack on "materialists," it is material knowledge and science that triumph in the story. Putnam's positivist tale of a Parisian health crisis directly criticized the strong links between the French church and the state and endorsed a new alliance between science and the government, run by the people. It also served to illustrate that only socialism had the power to secure the future of France. In a letter to her father, Putnam explained that "the single saving element of France at this moment lies in the direction of Socialism," and when it has had "full play," "a new religion will spring up, that shall spontaneously recreate belief in another life."[106]

Putnam clearly wanted Americans to know that "it [was] the hour of Socialism" in France. Her short story was such a strong critique of French society and religious faith that George Palmer Putnam at first hesitated to publish his daughter's piece, but he ultimately printed it. In an attempt to pacify her father, she explained, "*Of course*, I did not mean to say that no one in the world believed in the immortality of the soul, for such a statement would be a palpable absurdity." Instead, she said, her intention was to show that "all the pomp and circumstance of the established Church only serve to conceal inward rottenness, that it is maintained by the state simply as a question of expediency, and that even its most vital doctrines have ceased to constitute an effective force, and have no hold upon any of importance in the country."[107] Putnam's story portrayed France as a country burdened by its religious institutions; it also served as a warning to those Americans who privileged religious interpretations over scientific and positivist readings of nature.

Putnam's interest in socialism paralleled her growing dislike for the French government and its monarchy. In fact, her cynicism toward the emperor Napoléon III turned into outright disdain. She reported to her family: "I am accumulating as deliberate and unqualified hatred against . . . Louis Napoléon as I am capable of entertaining against a human being." Putnam's anger arose from covert attempts by the emperor to censor the press. Behind a facade of reform, the emperor silenced newspapers through government indictments to quell opposition to his regime. "The country is literally and insolently gagged," she reported, "and its entire intellect chained, trodden underfoot by this upstart traitor and usurper."[108] As the daughter of a publisher and, potentially, a new consumer of radical journals in Paris, Putnam took offense to the emperor's interventions and his efforts to disrupt the circulation of ideas. As Putnam carried on her medical studies, she became more attuned to political problems, and more hopeful about revolution in France.

By November 1869, Putnam was preparing for her third examination, living in the Reclus home, and working at the Hôtel Dieu, the famous Parisian hospital adjacent to the Notre Dame Cathedral. In a letter to her mother, she mentioned the numerous strikes occurring in Paris and her hopes for a collective uprising by the people. "The Revolution is advancing rapidly in France as in England. . . . I should be much disappointed not to be here to see it," she stated with great optimism.[109] Believing that the emperor's "funeral" was less than six months away, Putnam rejoiced over the prospect of social revolution in France, as her anger toward the imperial government swelled with the coming of the Franco-Prussian War.

"Vive la République"

Not long after war was declared against Prussia in July 1870, the French army began to struggle at the front and suffer severe losses. In Paris, people grew impatient with the emperor, becoming unsettled by French defeats and believing the nation ill-prepared for possible invasion. Putnam reported: "The day that the first news of defeat arrived, Paris was in a regular panic. I went upon the boulevards in the evening with Élie Reclus, and it was curious to see the soldiers stationed with arms, ready to fire upon the people. There was much more fear of insurrection at Paris than of the enemy."[110] Apparently, Napoléon III was so fearful of his own people that he kept thousands of troops in Paris instead of sending them to the front. He then proceeded to hide the fact that French soldiers, bourgeois and poor alike, were suffering tremendous losses to the Prussians. With defeat imminent, Putnam hoped that the people of France would revolt and put an end to the war themselves.

In September 1870, the French army surrendered, the emperor was captured, and a republic was declared in Paris. In a joyous letter to her father, Putnam announced: "I write the date to my letter with precision, for it is a great day. I have heard the Republic proclaimed in Paris!" Her father published that letter in the November issue of his magazine, enabling his daughter to be an important narrator of events to American audiences, reporting the celebrations and political confusion that followed the fall of the emperor. Putnam's piece outlined the military losses and the emperor's political mishandlings that led to his downfall; she also described the actions of the assembly, the Corps Législatif, as deputies decided how to proceed with government. But, most of all, she described the revelry at the fall of the empire, and the numerous exclamations of "Vive la République!" during celebrations at the Place de la Concorde. Putnam was impressed with the degree to which the country embraced the idea of a republic: "It is the feeling of tenderness, of affection, with which the Republic is welcomed, that is most touching. A lost ideal refound."[111] She did her utmost to convince American readers that France was ready to reclaim the ideals of 1789 that had been lost under the empire. Reminding Americans of their shared ideological history with France, Putnam persuaded her readers to accept, sympathize, and support the "revolution" that she experienced in Paris.

Thereafter, Putnam became more than a witness to political events. She inserted herself into the conflict and fashioned herself as an active participant. In her accounts, she described herself as part of the effort to establish a republic in France, situating herself within broad political conflicts. At times, she was an American witness and ambassador to a foreign land, determined to uphold true republican principles. At other times, she appeared more French than American in her firsthand knowledge of the conflict and her deep personal investment. During the war and uprisings in Paris, Putnam stood on the borderlands between French and American national identities.

When the Prussian army threatened to seize Paris, the government ordered all noncombatants to leave the city. Putnam, however, remained in Paris with the Reclus family, determined to finish her studies and support the republic. "I feel really quite ready to die in its defense," she stated with dramatic commitment, "especially if in so doing I could help the Réclus."[112] She remained in Paris during the siege and suffered all the hardships that ensued. It was a cold winter, and the Reclus family was short of fuel and had a limited supply of food. In a letter to her father, Mary described the harrowing nights of the Prussian attack on Paris: "When the bombardment arrived, we were obliged to decamp, for the bombs rained around our house and a number of persons were killed in the neighborhood. . . . I stayed with some friends in the north of Paris, — the Reclus were dispersed in different directions. One night I slept in the vaults of the Panthéon to 'see the elephant,' — it being a place of refuge of four or five hundred people in the neighborhood. It was singularly dramatic, — the tombs of Voltaire and Rousseau sheltering the victims of the Prussian barbarians."[113] In her retelling of these events, Putnam romanticized her night in the Panthéon, braving the bombardment and sleeping among the graves of the Enlightenment thinkers and icons of positivism. Immersing herself in the politics of her adopted nation, Putnam was willing to withstand the siege and brave the consequences of her affiliation with revolutionaries. She proudly took responsibility for her role, saying, "*We* become more belligerent every day."[114] Putnam's parents worried about their independent daughter, but she adamantly defended her decision. "I did not stay in Paris for the empty bravado of playing at heroics," she explained, but to help save the Republic, appealing to her father's own republican ideals and his political commitments to the Union during the Civil War. Putnam described the experience as momentous: "I would not have missed the occasion for anything in the world."[115]

Beyond her allegiance to the republic, she also remained in Paris because of medical commitments. Despite the bombardments, Putnam refused to postpone her studies and abandon her thesis. She continued to work in the hospitals during the siege but soon resigned from her surgical post because the surgeon had "monarchical opinions."[116]

Putnam's strong support for the French republic reflected her experience in France as well as her knowledge of American politics. She said the "cause of the French republic" resembled the way "the North fought in the war of Secession."[117] Putnam's experiences during the American Civil War buttressed her commitment to the republican cause in France. Moreover, like other American observers, she read the founding of the French republic as a struggle for popular sovereignty and republican government that mirrored events in American history: the revolution against the British monarchy and, more importantly, efforts to preserve the Union.[118]

The declaration of the republic inspired hope among the people of Paris, as radicals and moderate republicans joined together to support the provisional government.[119] As the Prussians surrounded the city and began their bombardments, a political divide ruptured the unity of the government, as moderate and revolutionary republicans disagreed about how to proceed and blamed each other for military failures. Parisians began to suffer due to dwindling provisions of fuel and food. The government pursued an end to the war and signed the armistice in January 1871, but an unpopular armistice led to widespread reaction against the republicans in government. To the dismay of working-class and some bourgeois Parisians, the monarchists won a majority in the National Assembly with the support of rural voters. The chief executive of the national government, Adolphe Thiers, bowed to conservative forces, moved the government to Versailles, and tried to disarm the National Guard and stop the growing revolutionary movement.

Radical republicans resisted the Thiers government and seized power in Paris, proclaiming the Paris Commune on 18 March 1871. The Commune government, installed in the Hotel de Ville, was represented by members with various political positions on the left, from reformist republicans to revolutionary socialists. During its short-lived reign of Paris, the Commune tried to institute reforms and aimed to expand workers' rights, officially separate church and state, grant education to women, and grant direct government representation to the people of Paris. Notably, several women, with a range of socialist and feminist principles, took part in supporting and defending the Commune.[120] But the Commune lacked strong leadership and accomplished few of its aims. After seventy-two days, the government of Versailles defeated the Communards and destroyed the revolutionary government, executing and jailing tens of thousands of participants and sympathizers.[121]

Putnam expressed great frustration with the failure of the republic and the fall of the Commune. During the winter of 1870–1871, as the new republican government faltered, she wrote "Some of the French Leaders," which was published in *Scribner's Monthly* in 1871, after the fall of the Commune.[122] She condemned the new government for its weak leadership and subservience to imperial interests, and explained the turn of events this way: "These men, who had represented the Republic under the Empire, well-nigh represented the Empire under the Republic."[123] After providing detailed biographical information on each leader, she then attacked them, criticizing their lack of passion, their weak commitment, and their lack of vision for the republic. Ultimately, she concluded: "The crowning defeat of the Provisional Government lay in the inadequacy of its conceptions; — an inadequate conception of the abomination of the Empire, the greatness of the Republic, of the resources of Paris, of the urgency of the crisis, of the solemnity of its relations to the past, of the tremendous questions for the future involved in the solution. . . . What wonder, then, if that epoch were sterile?"[124] In this piece, written for American consumption, Putnam explained the fall of the republic as the failure of particular individuals, not the French people. Ultimately, her article critiqued the weaknesses of the republican government and legitimized the Communards, who stood firm and defended republican principles. America was a nation both fascinated and perplexed by the flamboyant political conflicts in Paris.[125] As a firsthand observer, Putnam described the conflicts with the hope of persuading readers to sympathize with all forms of the republican cause. Putnam's commentary on the fiery situation in France had the critical and authoritative tone of a Parisian and seemed so "French" that *The Nation* later accused her of publishing a translation of an article by another author.[126] While advice from French friends may have influenced the article, Putnam clearly understood the political conflict and had formulated a strong position on the problems. Her editor at *Scribner's Monthly* defended her work's authenticity, calling *The Nation* "ignorant" and "prejudiced" and praising Putnam's article as "one of the ablest ever printed in an American magazine, and intelligent people recognize that fact."[127]

While many Americans in Paris condemned the French civil war, Putnam supported the Commune as a continuation of efforts to defend the republic. She described the Commune as an attempt to defend Parisian municipal rights and avoid reducing Paris to "a state of nullity as under the Empire." Putnam had hope in the Commune and told her father, "It is extremely interesting to compare the vivacity, oddity, picturesque and original character of the situation during the second siege, with the pallor and mediocrity which the Provisional Government imposed on the first." But she clearly predicted that it would come to a disappointing end: "a mild edition of '93, minus, decidedly minus, the guillotine."[128]

On 7 May 1871, in the last volatile days of the Commune, Mary Putnam managed to send a letter home. "I am thoroughly imprisoned ... [in] Paris," she said, again inserting herself as an actor in the conflict.[129] Putnam was trapped in the city, and her studies were interrupted due to the political chaos and the closing of the École de Médecine. Élisée Reclus was literally imprisoned. He had registered to serve in the National Guard and defend the Commune but was jailed by Thiers before he could actually fight. Élisée Reclus was imprisoned for his intent to defend the Commune and remained in jail for refusing to renounce his revolutionary goals.[130] Soon after, the Commune came to a horrific end and Parisians suffered greatly.

Putnam, undoubtedly, saw the fall of the Commune as a disappointing conclusion to the French struggle for republican government. In many ways she made the struggle her own and equated the Parisian fight for sovereignty with the pursuit of her own rights and autonomy as a woman in medicine. Élisée Reclus recognized this himself. Writing his wife from prison in June 1871, he hailed Putnam's medical studies as a "scientific triumph" and praised her for "fighting a good battle."[131] While the larger battle for socialism had been temporarily lost, Reclus saw progress in the movement for women's rights through the success of his friend and fellow political activist.

"Eminently Scientific"

At the end of the Commune, Mary Putnam left France and traveled to London, where she spent the next couple of months waiting for the École de Médecine to reopen so she could take her final examinations. With the dispersal of the Reclus family from their home and Paris in poor shape after the war, Putnam sought respite in London. She spent her days walking in Hyde Park and visiting the British Museum, awaiting the restoration of order at the Paris academy. She also contemplated her second failed marriage engagement. Noémi Reclus acknowledged to Putnam's parents that the couple's separation "was infinitely painful to her," but she expressed hope that Mary's time in London and the distraction of her exams would help pass her grief.[132]

In July, a month before her twenty-ninth birthday, Putnam returned to Paris and passed her final examination, proudly proclaiming to be "now *docteur en médecine de la Faculté de Paris*."[133] After passing five required exams and receiving marks higher than did many of her male colleagues, she submitted and defended her thesis on the nature of fatty acids, "De la graisse neutre et des acides gras."[134] Applauded by her colleagues at commencement and awarded a bronze medal for her thesis, Putnam — only the second woman to graduate from the École de Médecine — had good reason to celebrate.

Indeed, Putnam left Paris committed to promulgating the idea that "good medicine" was "scientific." Her thesis argued for the importance of chemical and physiological investigations for medical practice. Pathological studies were not enough; according to Putnam, one must study chemical phenomena to comprehend the true nature of disease. Arguing for the inextricable connection between empirical observation and molecular investigation, Putnam explained her medical ideology: "It seems to me that medical thought can be represented by a pyramid. The base of it is constituted by some fact, visible to the naked eye, like the problems with blood circulation in the veins. The top of the pyramid, sharpened to a point, would be represented by some molecular phenomenon — the nutritive culmination — of great circular alterations. Whatever would be the studies done on the mechanical, physical, or morphological aspects of the organs' lesions, it is necessary that we make them all come between two lines which converge below the top."[135] Putnam's thesis also addressed ongoing debates about the relationship between chemistry and physiology in the science of nutrition. Since the 1840s, scientists had debated whether chemical or physiological investigations should be privileged in the study of respiration, digestion, and nutrition. Followers of Antoine Lavoisier argued that chemical knowledge provided the key to understanding vital phenomena. Members of the physiological school, led by Claude Bernard and focused on anatomy and vivisection, believed that chemical analyses were informative but secondary to physiological knowledge; chemistry provided useful information but was abstract unless understood through physiological analysis of living beings.[136]

With access to histological laboratories in Paris, Putnam carried out mainly chemical analyses in her French thesis. But in the years to come, she based much of her nutritional research on an interactive model of physiology and chemistry, integrating Bernard's concepts of experimentalism into her own research and teaching. Furthermore, she also transported the medical environment of Paris to New York, by making Bernard's concept of the *milieu intérieur* fundamental to her ongoing research on women's health. Studying the body's internal environment, regulated by way of nutrition, or the building and depletion of tissues, was critical to understanding female health and the essential characteristics of the sexes. It also had symbolic significance: "The constancy of the internal environment is the condition for free and independent life," said Bernard.[137] From Putnam's perspective, this freedom existed both physiologically and politically, for both men and women.

As she finished her studies in Paris, it was important to Putnam that she identify herself, and be identified with, science in medicine. She took special note that her thesis received praise from her examiners for its "'eminently scientific tone.'"[138] A writer from the medical journal *Archives de Médecine* also commented that her thesis demonstrated "the scientific faith which [had] inspired her."[139] Combining clinical and laboratory studies in her own education, Putnam pursued a type of medicine that would soon become a model for American physicians. But Putnam worried that she would suffer in the less rigorous medical world of New York City. Reluctant to work at a woman's hospital or medical college, she was concerned about her prospects for continuing a scientific brand of medicine in New York. From Paris, she wrote to her mother: "I have already sufficient terror of the demoralization imminent from the atmosphere of New York, with its very slack interest in medical science or progress, its deficient libraries, badly organized schools and hospitals, etc."[140] With high expectations and such foreboding, Putnam upheld the notion that Paris was the center of the medical universe.

Despite the opposition to women and medicine in the United States, several American newspapers recognized Mary Putnam's graduation as a significant occasion. New York, especially, celebrated the achievements of the publishing king's daughter. Both the *New York Evening Post* and the *New York Tribune* announced her achievement with reprints of articles from *Le Figaro*, which reported the commencement and described Putnam's unique place among the crowd of male graduates.[141] In Paris, the *Archives de Médecine* also published a lengthy commentary about Putnam's degree in July 1871, citing it as proof that "women are not only fitted for learning but also for the application and practice of medicine." The author, possibly a fellow student, stated that the matter of admitting women to the profession had been "solved" in Paris, and the door would remain open for others who wanted to follow in Putnam's footsteps.[142]

Putnam recognized her own significance for the "woman question." She was self-conscious about her anomalous position at the École de Médecine, as well as her role in the larger social and political struggle for women's medical education. Not surprisingly, when she completed her thesis, she inscribed it with political meaning. She used its dedication to acknowledge the medical men who mentored her, and one who decided her fate: "To the professor, whose name I do not know, who was the only one to vote in favor of my admission to the school, thus protesting against the prejudice which wanted to exclude women from advanced studies."[143] Published in France, her thesis both represented her new knowledge and documented her vital role in disrupting the rules of gender in French medicine and beyond.

In the fall of 1871, Putnam left Paris, a city in both physical and political disarray. Following the Commune, she assessed the damage to her adopted city and foresaw a dark political future in France: "The material ruins of Paris are not as formidable as you may suppose. The real misery of the situation does not lie on the surface, but it is profound. The situation is horrible, and no one knows what will come of it."[144] With Élisée Reclus in prison and the rise of conservative forces in state politics, she saw little hope for the republic and the fulfillment of a socialist vision. With the defeat of the Commune and repression of socialism, Putnam also worried about the future of women's rights in France. Although the disappointments left a lasting impression, she also had new hope that social change was possible, and she returned to the United States with a new sense of mission.

As she sailed across the Atlantic, Putnam carried more than a diploma from the École de Médecine. She returned with a set of philosophical commitments that would inspire three decades of activism in the United States. The fusion of science and politics in France set the stage for her activism in the 1870s and 1880s in the United States, where she made the advancement of science and the advancement of women interrelated projects, and often treated them as one and the same.

SCIENCE AND SOCIAL EMANCIPATION

In the fall of 1871, after spending a good portion of her young adult years in France, Mary Putnam returned to Manhattan. Now almost thirty years old, she came home with a list of ambitious goals. She wanted to gain admission to the New York Academy of Medicine, study experimental therapeutics, and acquire a teaching position where she could offer young women "rigid" medical training that mirrored her own in Paris. But she was also on a mission to create "a scientific spirit . . . among women," in medicine and beyond, for science was the key to women's advancement in American society, she believed.[1]

Putnam quickly became part of New York's growing medical community. She set up a small private office in the basement of her parent's home on East Fifteenth Street near Stuyvesant Square. Her father, now in the last year of his life, had conceded to his daughter's unusual ambitions and reportedly nailed up a plaque, reading: "Dr. Mary Putnam."[2] Despite her earlier claim that "I should stifle in clover at a girls' college," she accepted a teaching position at a single-sex institution, the Woman's Medical College of the New York Infirmary, where she served first as a lecturer and later became professor of materia medica and therapeutics.[3] As she taught, she treated patients at the New York Infirmary and published on medical subjects, reporting her cases and findings to the *Medical Record*.[4] She also sought membership in the city's most influential medical societies, gaining admission to the Medical Society of the County of New York, an organization newly open to women thanks to Abraham Jacobi, its progressive president.[5] It was through the Society that the couple met, and they eventually married in July of 1873.[6] Henceforth, she used the name Mary Putnam Jacobi. While other politically conscious women (the prominent suffragist Lucy Stone, for example) chose not to change their names, she recognized the advantages of being identified with both her family's business and her new husband's medical reputation in New York.

In the 1870s and 1880s, Mary Putnam Jacobi applied the political and medical lessons of Paris to the American context. She translated the revolutionary socialism of the Commune era into a democratic socialism based on republican government and a unified social order. She transported French positivism to American soil, replacing Élisée Reclus's geological approach with a physiological model for social relations. Jacobi also converted the gender politics of radical Parisians into an American feminist agenda and came to believe that positivist understandings of the physiological body would justify women's greater place in the body politic.

In these years, Jacobi used positivism, medical school reforms, and experimentalism as political tools in the struggle for gender equality. She made scientific medicine a feminist venture, daring to use the study, practice, and ideologies of science as forms of women's rights activism. She believed that medicine, more than suffrage and legal rights, had the power to remake social relations in American society, for it could create "a full equality and independence for women as nothing else ever had or perhaps could: an intellectual, practical, and social emancipation."[7] In her efforts toward "the creation of a scientific spirit," she sought to uplift the status of her sex by downplaying the very relevance of sex in scientific practice.

Positivism: New York Style

Although Paris had a strong hold on Mary Putnam Jacobi, New York had much to offer, for Manhattan was becoming the nucleus of American intellectual life. It was the center of American literary culture as well as the publishing capital, due in part to George Putnam's contributions in the previous decades. New York was the locale of a growing academic community, led by the expansion of the city's universities. And it was a medical mecca due to its growing hospitals, medical societies, and public health movements after the Civil War.[8] New York City was also becoming a prominent urban center of American women's rights activism, a movement that started in Seneca Falls in 1848. After belonging to such vibrant intellectual circles in Paris, Jacobi sought out like-minded intellectuals and professionals in New York, and did not need to look far.[9]

Shortly after her arrival, Jacobi became involved in the New York Positivist Society, a loose-knit group of the city's intelligentsia dedicated to the ideas of August Comte. At bi-weekly meetings, middle- and upper-class writers, artists, and professionals met in parlors or lecture rooms to philosophize about the problems that plagued modern industrial society and to construct programs of social reform.[10] These American disciples of Comte focused on two key positivist principles. First, they believed that all knowledge should be based on observable phenomena derived from empirical, scientific investigation. As David G. Croly, head of the New York Positivist Society, put it, "Our faith is . . . based upon demonstrated truths, not upon authority or tradition, or mere subjective conceptions, but upon objective realities which can be seen and known of all men."[11] Rejecting the atheist label, positivists insisted, "Our Supreme Being is Humanity, which we affirm is the only God man ever could or ever can know."[12] Second, they viewed society as an organism that mirrored both the family structure and the human body with its interrelated and interdependent parts. In the positivist view, all members and sectors of society, like all parts of an organism, should work in concert for the broader good. The philosophy translated neatly into middle-class visions of social reform in the post–Civil War era, for positivists believed professionals could eradicate social problems, and a new moral order would emerge where citizens worshipped humanity and directed their spirituality toward social improvement.[13]

New York intellectuals turned to the philosophical systems of Comte to resolve the "spiritual crisis of the Gilded Age."[14] The post–Civil War period was a time of both religious enthusiasm and skepticism. While some Americans questioned the tenets of traditional theologies, others embraced spirituality and religion with new energy. Modernization and new forces of secularization, including systems of mass education and developments in science — especially Darwin's theories of evolution — disrupted long-held assumptions about the origins of human life and engendered a "crisis" of faith. For men and women who felt spiritually disillusioned, positivist philosophy provided a spiritual middle ground, particularly when it integrated religious ceremony and scientific principles, as it did in New York.

At meetings of the New York Positivist Society, members celebrated positivism as a "religion." These gatherings involved a series of toasts, speeches, and rituals that resembled Christian ceremonies. Participants were given sacraments, and new members were "baptized" into the community. They mimicked communion by ingesting crusts, instead of traditional hosts, and drinking water instead of wine, in honor of the poor. Members also worshipped positivist "saints," honoring men like Plato, Hippocrates, and Voltaire in addition to Darwin and Spencer. Positivist worship of humanity offered a new form of faith and a direct critique of traditional religious worship, especially Catholic ceremonies, rites, and mystical beliefs. Catholicism, practiced by thousands of new immigrants in New York, offended positivists who had traditional Protestant temperaments or secular leanings. By co-opting Catholic rituals for the worship of humanity and science, positivists attempted to symbolically redirect American faith toward human action rather than church doctrines. As one outside observer noted, "Their faith seems on the surface to consist of the lack of faith, and . . . they seem to make of science a demi-god. . . . Yet, on the other hand, they . . . practically exhibit so high a faith in human nature, and such a conception of man's responsibility and duty, that their practice redeems their principles."[15]

The New York Positivist Society drew in "a number of ladies" to its meetings, chief among them, Mary Putnam Jacobi. She addressed the group and, at one meeting, called on her friends to "live in the open air" and express in vocal and material ways knowledge about the world. She joined other American women who translated the French philosophy into an ideological foundation for women's rights.[16] As historian William Leach has shown, a number of activists, including Elizabeth Cady Stanton, incorporated positivism into their political visions, arguing against individualism and on behalf of social reform rooted in the application of natural science methods.[17] Going far beyond most feminists, Jacobi actually did the physical and mental work of science while formulating a feminist positivism that linked science and gender equality.

Jacobi also employed positivism to criticize "the limitations of Christianity" for women. In contrast to the evangelical position that Christianity elevated women, she believed that it degraded them. Christianity accepted the "biological inferiority of women," she complained, despite the fact that the faith was founded on so-called feminine virtues of compassion, purity, patience, and fortitude. Jacobi blamed Christianity for using the female body to perpetuate women's subjugation; she also objected to the ways women were assigned blame for the world's sin and temptation. While some women used Christian doctrine to affirm their moral superiority, she believed that, over the centuries, this same doctrine produced negative female archetypes, defining woman as either the temptress or the "Virgin, the wife, the Madonna." Historically, religion had a strong hand in binding women to the home and made it "almost impossible for the modern woman to escape" the "restrictions and disabilities" heaved upon her. Jacobi refused to accept that woman's "original" fall from innocence guaranteed her, and humanity, a sinful future.[18]

Jacobi also criticized Christianity's inability to seek out and reveal "truth." Positivism gave her a new sense of history because, for the first time, a "new view of Truth came into the world only with the rise of positive science, which substituted laborious research and tests for the easier method of dogmatic assertion professing to be inspired," she explained. Christianity, alienated from the "real" world, impaired the progress of social reform. Science in conjunction with socialism, she said, would mobilize individuals to serve institutions and seek knowledge for the broader good, which would ultimately provide a way for people to escape being "slaves of abstract ideas," to "see truthfully what is," and to seek viable solutions to society's ills.[19]

In the late 1870s, positivism came under fire from several critics, including William Hurrell Mallock, a Catholic writer from England. In his 1878 essays and 1879 book, *Is Life Worth Living?*, he attacked positivists for their lack of faith, charging that a disbelief in the supernatural and the unknown amounted to disbelief in God.[20] Mallock predicted that the rise of positivism would lead to the degeneration of human life since it questioned and diminished morality and spirituality, privileging materiality. Although positivism resolved the spiritual "crisis" for some believers, it produced serious anxiety among faithful Protestants and Catholics, like Mallock, who held tightly to their religious ideologies.

While positivist ideas permeated Jacobi's writings, her treatise *The Value of Life: A Reply to Mallock's Essay* (1879) was her strongest effort to disseminate positivist principles and launch a counterattack against critics.[21] Jacobi defended positivism by outlining the flaws in Mallock's argument and critiquing his disregard for Comte and other "true positivists," who, she insisted, never abandoned spirituality completely. She maintained that positivism "propos[ed] a systematic substitution of science for faith," whereby people could emerge more faithful in humankind.[22] Rather than living by the "imagination," as Catholics allegedly did, Jacobi privileged the "realities of existence" as revealed by the positivist method.[23] She claimed to represent true positivism, but it is clear that her version of the philosophy was shaped by her community in New York. While Comte himself did not completely condemn the Catholic Church, but rather condemned its belief in the supernatural, New York positivists tended to be both anti-Catholic and disillusioned with the style of evangelicalism so popular in nineteenth-century America.[24]

In her positivist writings, Jacobi argued for the primacy of observable facts over metaphysics and unseen phenomena. "The great Positivist doctrine about truth," she argued, "is that it is always an expression of relations existing between the human mind and the object that is contemplated by it. Things are not known in themselves, but only as they affect us and as we can perceive them. What is true for us is what we see to be true, and any other truth is inconceivable by our minds."[25] With such discourse, positivists forged a link between their method of "truth seeking" and a mandate for social reform. The Comtean creed, rather than religious teachings, they believed, should direct the course of society, since only observable facts could produce material change.

Laboratory studies, in Jacobi's view, represented the ultimate positivist exercise, as she insisted on the centrality of laboratory knowledge for the positivist project. "It is in the life of the laboratory," she argued, "where the secrets of nature are not only divined but reproduced, that the true joy of knowledge can best be learned."[26] While Comte emphasized empirical observation, Jacobi idealized experimentalism. She believed the laboratory was the best venue for discovering the most accurate and vivid knowledge of the human body and made it a central component of her medical practice.

The laboratory provided the means for observing and monitoring the interior functions of the human body, particularly the process of nutrition. A central concept in late-nineteenth-century physiology and histology, "nutrition" referred to the organic changes of substances in the body, and the building and depletion of body tissues. Physiologically, nutrition did not refer simply to the consumption of food or to dietary regimens, as it most commonly does today. Rather, it described the process by which cells and tissues were continuously destroyed and then regenerated to sustain life. Cells were nourished through the circulation of blood by bodily "force," and blood delivered the chemical substances needed for growth, a process of internal regulation fundamental to Bernard's concept of the *milieu intérieur*.[27] Jacobi believed that bodily health rested on normal nutrition and that illness was often a manifestation of failed nutrition. She used this conceptual thread to explain a variety of conditions associated with women. Beyond its physiological and chemical processes, nutrition had symbolic meanings as well.

Jacobi advanced an organic image of American society based on a human biological model. Conflating the social body and the human body, she compared people to cells, families to tissues, and larger groups and classes to human organs. Likening the individual person to the human cell, she explained that an individual "cannot be thought of without the correlative of other persons, and of a larger social life whose central events dominate the local events around each individual."[28] Just as the human body failed without nutrition, the social organism broke down when all of its members did not participate, particularly women. She viewed citizens as integral parts of an interdependent, cooperative unit. She argued that human beings, like human cells, required physical and mental nutrition, in the form of education and meaningful work, to reproduce and function.[29] She explained, "The nutrition of a human being must be divided into two kinds: the nutrition of the body and that of the soul, or in other words, satisfaction of physical, and satisfaction of mental or spiritual wants." It was in this system that the "life of society is immediately carried on."[30] But just as cells are not all the same, neither are people. The coal heaver and the secretary of state, for example, are both "indispensable to the welfare of society," but these two men "differ as widely in each case as the nutrition and function of connective tissue cells differ from those of ganglionic bodies."[31] Here, Jacobi used cellular variations in the body to explain away the uneven positions of people in different occupations, social classes, and educational rank.

The concept of the social organism was popular among many positivists and socialists at the end of the nineteenth century because it privileged the needs of a unified social order over the needs of the individual. Many socialists found inspiration in Herbert Spencer's evolutionary model and his notion of the social body. In his 1860 work, "The Social Organism," Spencer described how society functioned like an animal or plant, not a machine; as a living body received nourishment and grew, so did society evolve and progress, he said. Spencer's ideas inspired evolutionary socialism and the belief that the social body would evolve toward collectivism.[32] Influenced by this mode of thought, as well as Reclus's notion of social evolution/revolution, Jacobi, too, used several organic and evolutionary metaphors as she merged socialist thought with biological principles.

The cooperative interrelationship of cells and organisms, individuals and society, also reflected Jacobi's admiration for French utopian socialists such as Claude-Henri de Saint-Simon (father of Saint-Simonian feminism) and Charles Fourier, who envisioned alternative communities based on social and gender equality. In the early nineteenth century, Saint-Simon described human society as an organic body, one with natural laws to be studied via positive science. He predicted that a "social physiology," a biological/social discipline of study, would emerge to reform the "social organization," create harmony among workers and industry, and move humanity toward progress. His ideas inspired feminists, who drew from his principles as well as a new church of humanity as an alternative to Christianity. In the same period, Fourier gained a following for his notions of human "passions" and for tying individual happiness to the greater needs of society. He condemned the government, law, and church for supporting female inferiority. Equality between the sexes was necessary, he argued, because "the extension of the privileges of women is the fundamental cause of social progress."[33] Jacobi admired Fourier, calling him the "most sagacious of modern Socialists."[34] She applauded his critiques of the subordination of women in the capitalist labor system and hailed his proposition that women could acquire the same qualities and skills as men. Although she did not join American utopian communities inspired by Fourier, she agreed with his ideas about creating social cooperation through scientific methods and diminishing the ill effects of competitive industrial capitalism for the good of the social organism.

Certainly, positivism itself, as defined by Comte, had a conservative undertone and did not support true social equality, particularly gender equality. Comte believed women contributed to the social order but that they did so within the confines of the domestic sphere. In the United States, some positivists tried to translate Comte's ideas into a more democratic vision for social change. American feminists, in particular, saw great potential in positivism and reconfigured it into a justification for women's political participation.

Although many women activists like Jacobi tailored Comte to their own advantage, they did not account for the different needs of other disempowered groups and were unable to construct immigrants, African Americans, or the laboring classes as equal members of the social organism. Many socialists influenced by the utopian ideas and intellectual movements of Europe also worked for reform on behalf of the working class, not alongside them. They believed that reform led by experts, from the top town, would have the greatest impact on creating a just society. In a preview of Progressivism, bourgeois professionals appointed themselves as the vanguard of reform and created social programs that reflected their own values, which were at once conservative and forward-thinking.[35]

The organism concept justified reform projects for the greater good, but positivism could also reinforce social hierarchies of race, class, and culture. Comte's notion of the social organism referred only to civilizations of Europe and the Mediterranean, Jacobi explained. To illustrate, she used an example from nature, comparing the earth to a gigantic bird ovum. The embryo of the egg, the germinal area, represented Europe; the yolk represented colonial Asia and Africa, which were "the subordinate civilizations and barbarisms which in various ways nourish the life of Europe, and are probably destined to be absorbed by it." Buried in the appendix of her positivist manifesto, Jacobi's egg analogy suggested that the social organism consisted of "civilizations" hatched out of Europe.[36]

Despite these limitations, positivist science did have adherents among minority groups and marginalized peoples. African American and Jewish writers countered scientific racism by using discourses of science, especially evolution, to challenge racial hierarchies.[37] Some African American leaders incorporated evolution into their ideas about social progress.[38] Members of different Jewish communities held a range of interpretations on evolution, from all-out refutation, to acceptance, to adaptation.[39] Native-born and immigrant, white and nonwhite, found evolutionary theory useful for either reinforcing or rejecting long-held beliefs about race, class, and religion. As we will see, critics and supporters of women's rights also used science to argue in favor of or against new roles for women.

Positivism united science, socialism, and feminism as the basis of Jacobi's activism. Mixing together the social and scientific allowed thinkers like Jacobi to join science and politics into common cause, and equate gender equality with biological fact. Positivism promised to free women from the false barriers established by churches, laws, and American culture, for it provided the tools and methods for delivering supposedly accurate representations of nature. Natural law did not confine women from public life, Jacobi believed; rather, it required them to be full participants in the social organism. This biological requirement was especially true in the realm of work, and in the professions of science.

Women's "Special Destinies"

In 1873, in the company of women's rights activists, Mary Putnam Jacobi contemplated the subordinate status of American women. Women held secondary positions because of a false, but popular, "public sentiment": reproduction superseded all other activities of the female sex. "It is so far from true," she continued, "that the bearing and rearing of children suffices to absorb the energies of the whole female sex, that a large surplus of feminine activity has always remained to be absorbed in other than these primitive directions."[40] According to Jacobi, women had a surplus of unused energy that could be diverted from the "primitive" to the productive, and divided between the private world of home and family and the public world of higher education and professional work. Women needed to be contributing members of society, intellectually engaged, and devoted to the greater good. This was not a choice; the health of women depended on it.

For Jacobi, women's work was a matter of health, but it was also a tool of liberation, an equalizing force that could grant women financial independence and social autonomy. Work could prove women's economic and intellectual worth while granting personal freedom. Women had always worked, she said, "but they demand now, and simply, some opportunity for a free choice in the kind of work, which, apart from the care of children, they may perform."[41] She respected all forms of work, but professional careers held a special advantage because they provided a lifetime of economic autonomy, not temporary compensation. The professions allowed women to have "separate resources" from men, meaning fathers and spouses. In marriage, they could create what she called an "equitable monetary division between husband and wife."[42] Professional work was not indulgent; rather, it was "only the natural result of the double pressure of an economic and of a psychological necessity."[43]

Jacobi argued that the professions provided women with financial security, particularly during the childbearing years. Pregnancy was temporary in a woman's life, she explained; afterward, women should return to an occupation that was both "useful" and "pecuniary."[44] Normally, the type of work available to women between pregnancies was limited and transitory and was neither intellectually stimulating nor reliable long-term. Most temporary work was physically wearing and personally unrewarding. Most importantly, it locked women into subordinate positions; women work as "hirelings and drudges, but rarely as masters and controllers," Jacobi said.[45] But work in the professions could raise the status of laboring women to the "higher ranks," on the same level as men, she maintained. It also could allow working-class women to raise their incomes and their social status.

The medical profession, in particular, could potentially liberate women from what Jacobi described as a "narrow and trivial existence."[46] She realized that not all women were cut out to practice medicine. She often said so, referring to the lack of quality education for women, particularly in the sciences. But for qualified women with access to proper training, medical practice was economically and intellectually ideal. Medicine could provide women with a source of steady income; it could also stimulate their minds. By improving their knowledge and cognitive abilities with medical study, women could then prove the intellectual potential of their sex, which would work toward "dissipating the stupid prejudices" of a public resistant to female higher education. Through their own example, women physicians would lead the movement for changes in education, she said.[47]

Jacobi also believed that professional success in medicine translated into political power. She insisted that injustices against women would only be diminished as women demonstrated their competence. This could be achieved through work and entrance into the professions: "If women are ever to obtain a voice and place in the government of society, it will only be when they have demonstrated their ability to act independently *in* society, under the government that now exists."[48] Women could gain political influence, she argued, not through revolutionary means but through professional work in medicine.

Jacobi's faith in the political power of science extended beyond medicine to social reform and women's public service. "The creation of a class of women especially devoted to biological studies," she claimed, "is the surest way of opening sociological studies to the larger class of women destined to occupy themselves with social reform." Addressing social work directly at a congress of the Association for the Advancement of Women in 1874, Jacobi asked women to redirect their efforts and formulate their reform activities according to scientific principles. She urged women to create a sisterhood in the professions rather than to become members of a church or a denomination. Social reform work had been "ineffective," she claimed, because it had been "uninformed by scientific study of the social conditions with which it had to cope."[49] Here, Jacobi sold the value of science to women already committed to social activism. Her rhetoric reflected the coming unification of reform and social science that would later characterize women's work in the Progressive Era.

Jacobi also believed that women physicians should teach other women how to apply science to domesticity and the care of children: "The enlightenment of mothers and of mistresses of households depends upon securing more definite instruction in the science of life and of living bodies, that can be best imparted by duly educated women physicians."[50] She argued that teaching women scientific principles would ultimately lead to their "enlightenment," or their emancipation. This call for applied science in the domestic sphere predicated by several years and facilitated the coming of "scientific motherhood."[51] Although she believed the real medical care of children should be left to pediatric experts, knowledge of science was necessary for motherhood in the modern world.

In Jacobi's view, women physicians should become leaders in the struggle for gender equality. Calling them "heroic," she compared women medical students to the founders of the American colonies, those men who created the commonwealth and built the foundation for the Revolution.[52] Women's work in science and medicine, she suggested, was a doorway to emancipation, for it would propel "a radical change in the views now held about the relations of women to work."[53]

The expansion of scientific education to both sexes would also transform the lives of all middle-class women, she argued. As mothers and caregivers, women dealt with health and human bodies every day; they were consumed with "anxieties" about illness in their families. And yet the average woman was, in general, "profoundly ignorant" of science. With scientific knowledge, women would maintain the health of their own families, and then use that information for the good of humanity. This knowledge would "overfl[ow] the limits of the personal household, and [lead] the intelligent mother to interest herself in the injured households of the poor and unintelligent; to busy herself in their education, physical as well as moral; to participate in sanitary investigation and enterprises; to take her place on health boards; to assume her lawful responsibility in shielding tender and defenceless human lives from the pressure of greed and ambition and industrial rapacity!"[54] In other words, science could make all women into social reformers. And although scientific thought seemed foreign in female circles, Jacobi predicted it would one day be part of women's "special destinies," and she envisioned a future where the majority of middle-class women would acquire scientific knowledge: "I [am] convinced that one day, instruction in biological science will be diffused among women in at least the ratio in which musical education is at the present day. For men, this branch of knowledge may remain a specialty or an exceptional accomplishment; but for women, it will be seen proper to place it at the very core of their education." Jacobi hoped that by replacing music with biology in women's education, women would surpass men with their expertise, diminishing men's interest in the biological sciences to a hobby, like music. And by defining science as women's true calling and downplaying the role of men, she offered a radical revision of womanhood itself. With biological education, "for the first time . . . the influence of women on the amelioration of human life [will] be . . . made justly apparent."[55]

Despite the revolutionary potential of science, according to Jacobi, most women did not have the education, skills, drive, or initiative to be physicians. They had not adequately cultivated their intelligence in the direction of science, nor prepared themselves for the physical work of medicine, since many had been pampered and accustomed to "soft living." A certain degree of "refinement" was necessary in a woman physician, but so was the "tenacity of purpose," bravery, endurance, and strength, characteristics of any good physician.[56] To be successful, women needed to leave their emotionality and religious views behind.

Jacobi believed women's "natural" healing and sympathetic qualities would not benefit them as physicians. Rather, it was the ability to apply science in therapeutics that characterized "good medicine." She said emotions had no place in the examination of bodies and the treatment of diseases. Instead, physicians should read a patient's maladies through an "objective" lens and analyze them with medical knowledge gained through the combination of laboratory and clinical training. Anecdotal and empirical information was not enough; the doctor must respond based on knowledge of the sciences: anatomy, physiology, physics, chemistry, pathology, and histology. The most important qualities of a physician, she argued, involved the ability to synthesize medical knowledge and to act on it immediately.[57]

In direct opposition to the sympathetic model of treatment, Jacobi recommended that physicians be impassive and directive with patients.[58] She advocated treatment programs based on medical expertise rather than on what patients disclosed about their conditions: "At the very outset of clinical study it is well to be impressed with this fact: namely, that what the patient has to tell you constitutes precisely the least important part of what you must learn about him in order to be able to understand his case, and to do him any good."[59] Uninterested in the voices of patients and their families, Jacobi advised physicians to abandon interactive clinical models. A physician, she maintained, must "enforce his directions, in spite of the reluctance, or indifference, or carelessness, or stupidity, or forgetfulness of his patients." A physician could have sympathy, but the sympathy must be disguised and controlled, be "fine, and not blubbering . . . it must manifest itself in deeds, not in words; in defatigable efforts to accomplish the essential, not in rambling talk about irrelevant trifles, even when, to the sick person, these seem to be the most important." For this reason, while the patient might be considered a "personal friend," he should also be considered a "possible enemy" in his own treatment, for he may try to persuade and negotiate with the doctor, who should be in control and be considered the "superior person." Physicians must convince a patient that "notwithstanding this personal sympathy, the physician is studying his case as coolly, impartially, abstractly, as if it were a problem in algebra."[60]

Women physicians needed to fit the learned and detached image of the modern doctor, Jacobi believed, or they would not be successful in the new scientific paradigm. She reinforced a medical hierarchy, drawing solid boundaries between women doctors and women nurses. She associated nursing with caring duties as opposed to curing: "It is impossible to be a physician on the basis of personal sympathies alone. . . . [The patient] may gain a nurse, but he loses a physician."[61] Nursing, a feminized profession growing rapidly in the post–Civil War period, offered many women a path into medicine that combined "sympathy and science." Although Jacobi recognized the important roles played by nurses, and believed women doctors should care about the welfare of patients, she stressed that physicians should occupy a commanding position and not show emotion.

Jacobi believed that women physicians should also avoid intense religiosity and instead put their faith in science and positivism. Elizabeth Blackwell's own religious inclinations were extremely irritating to Jacobi, who once wrote to the elder doctor, condemning her "transcendental method of arriving at conclusions" and her refusal to "submit these to tests of verification."[62] Jacobi was most bothered by Blackwell's lack of "proof" to support her assertions. "Now I have always thought . . . you had a large mind," she commented, "but one relatively untrained in technicalities."[63] Jacobi's antagonism toward Blackwell's spirituality was also a broader criticism against women who espoused religion as part of healing. She urged women to internalize a positivist, scientific model of medicine and embody a new type of womanhood to avoid some of the most common criticisms of women physicians.

The belief that medical women, through laborious study, would become ill, sterile, and "unsexed" was alive and well in popular literature and inside the profession. She was fully aware of this "bugbear" that plagued all working women, debunking the charge that they would become "an extraordinary transmutation of species that out-Darwins Darwin, cease to be women, and become a nondescript, unpleasant race, hateful to men, and not over-agreeable to one another. Monstrous impossibility!"[64] In Paris, she strategically accessed the École de Médecine as an American woman with a strong countenance and "passionless" manner. In the United States, facing fears of invalidism and "race suicide," women could take a different approach, by remaining healthy and robust, and by marrying and having children. As a mother and wife in good health, and a believer in the physical benefits of childbearing, Jacobi remained safely feminine in America, avoiding the label "unsexed."

But above all, to become a strong force in the profession, women also needed to acquire a more rigorous education, Jacobi believed. Historically denied the same educational options as men, women as a group did not have the same knowledge base as their male counterparts. They were severely hindered by the strong opposition to women in medicine and the generally poor state of American medical education, especially in some women's schools. She set out to ensure that American women received the highest quality training, and she began her mission at her home institution, the Woman's Medical College of the New York Infirmary.

The Woman's Medical College

At the Woman's Medical College of the New York Infirmary, Jacobi applied her Paris training to constructing her courses in therapeutics. Although she taught at a single-sex institution, her curriculum was not geared toward women. Rather, she endorsed the same type of medicine for men and women, based on her positivist philosophy and integrating the laboratory and experimentalism into the clinic. While the content of her courses elided gender distinctions, her work at the Woman's Medical College was steeped in the gender politics of the time, as she sought to produce graduates who equaled or surpassed men in their knowledge and abilities. This involved simultaneous efforts to shape the curriculum and to mold the gender identities of women physicians to reflect a scientific model of medicine.

Jacobi played a significant role at the Woman's Medical College as well as the New York Infirmary. Between 1871 and 1897, she held the positions of visiting, attending, and consulting physician at the New York Infirmary, spending almost three decades treating patients in the hospital and the dispensary, and producing medical research from her cases. As a member of its medical board, she was also involved in the institution's management. In 1886, she formed a children's ward at the New York Infirmary, taking part in the movement to treat children separately and differently from adults, an effort she started years earlier at Mt. Sinai Hospital, in cooperation with Abraham Jacobi and Dr. Anne Angel.[65]

At the Woman's Medical College, beyond teaching, she was a public advocate, serving as president of the Association for the Advancement of the Medical Education of Women, a fund-raising organization for the school. So personally invested in the college, she donated her own money to acquire and sustain needed faculty. She was aggressive in shaping the curriculum and raising standards.[66] But sometimes her tenacity brought her into conflict with fellow faculty. One disagreement, in fact, led to her resignation in 1889. When her course in therapeutics was "relegate[d]" to the second year, to make room for a new professor of physiology and to avoid content overlap, Jacobi protested and announced her departure. She devoted many years of service and left a significant imprint on the college, but not without some controversy.[67]

Soon after her arrival in 1871, Jacobi's (then Putnam's) first months of teaching were riddled with "trouble." She expressed "'malignant criticism'" of her students and felt "'thorough contempt for [her] class,'" believing they were unprepared to study medicine and ill-equipped to be doctors.[68] Records show that thirteen students from her materia medica class submitted a petition to the faculty, possibly a complaint, but the contents are unknown. At the end of her first term, it was unclear whether she would return to teach. Elizabeth Blackwell, who founded the college, was alarmed at the news of these frustrations. From London, Blackwell wrote to the younger doctor, "You have lived so long away from America and have become so much of a French woman, that you really must go to school and relearn your own country, before you will be able to teach acceptably."[69] However, it was difficult for Jacobi to shed the parts of her that had become "French." Instead, she tried to replicate her European education at the Woman's Medical College by reforming it into a "scientific" institution inspired by positivist values.

Despite Jacobi's negative reaction to her students, the Woman's Medical College was, actually, a strong institution that equaled and even surpassed some male-only medical schools. As Regina Morantz-Sanchez has shown, it maintained the highest standards and earned the respect of physicians profession-wide, instituting curricular improvements and extending requirements years before such changes had been made at Harvard.[70] And still, Jacobi complained and worried about the quality and content of the education offered by her institution. Her critical voice reflects less about the actual quality of the Woman's Medical College and more about the strategies she employed in the battle over the exclusion of women in medicine. She set the bar extremely high for both men and women physicians and, in her criticisms of both, tried to wipe away gender distinctions. Her approach, at times, clashed with Elizabeth Blackwell's vision for the institution.

Blackwell practiced and taught medicine based on scientific principles, but she and Jacobi, like many physicians of the time, male and female, disagreed on what they meant by "science."[71] Moralistic and maternalistic, Blackwell believed women should be taught the natural sciences so that they would better understand patient suffering, not simply the physical science itself. She lamented the ascendance of experimental knowledge, not sharing Jacobi's respect for Claude Bernard, whose work, she said, lacked clinical application and concrete therapeutic benefit. "Experimenters were simply accumulating facts," not producing solutions to ease human suffering. Trained in the older French empirical method, Blackwell believed in the importance of observation and individual evaluation, approaching illness in what we might call a "holistic" manner. In her view, science was not "unbiased" but shaped by a clear desire to improve human welfare. In her "sympathetic" approach, she tried to associate the combined art of caring and curing with feminine virtue.[72]

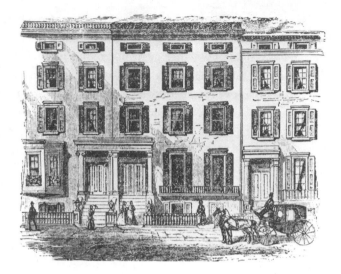

The New York Infirmary for Women and Children, 126 Second Avenue,
New York, N.Y. Reprinted by permission of the New York Downtown
Hospital. Reproduced from Wilson, *Lone Woman*.

·✦··✦··✦·

Blackwell's Woman's Medical College opened in 1868, emerging out of the
New York Infirmary for Women and Children. The infirmary was established
in 1853 in a one-room office near Tompkins Square Park, south of Fourteenth
Street and near the East River; the following year Elizabeth Blackwell officially
opened it as the New York Dispensary for Poor Women and Children. The
dispensary served a dense population, mainly of immigrants, who crowded
into tenements in the Eleventh Ward. Although the city's poor were often
unfairly associated and equated with disease, their living conditions were, in
fact, conducive to disease. The neighborhood was squalid, exacerbated by
the large number of slaughterhouses and horse stables in the area. The close
quarters and poor ventilation of the tenements, with contaminated drinking
water and negligible sanitation, was a recipe for the spread of diseases such as
cholera and tuberculosis. As a result, Blackwell's dispensary grew quickly as
it provided much-needed medical care to poor women and children in lower
Manhattan.[73]

In 1857, Blackwell, with the help of her sister, Emily Blackwell, and Marie
Zakrzewska, established a hospital, the New York Infirmary for Indigent
Women and Children on 64 Bleecker Street at Crosby, near the Five Points.
There, needy women and children received care free of charge, supported by

donations and fees from patients who could afford to pay. With only about sixteen beds, the infirmary cared for a limited number of patients in-house, treating most people in the dispensary. With its growing clientele, the infirmary moved in 1861 just blocks away, to 126 Second Avenue.

By the early 1870s, when Jacobi arrived, the infirmary had become a critical source of medical care for women in New York, providing services to between 6,000 and 7,000 patients per year.[74] Families sought care for a number of ailments, from respiratory disease to gastrointestinal disorders, from eye and ear problems to bone fractures and breaks. Matters of female reproductive health drew many women to the infirmary because they could receive treatment by members of their own sex. They sought relief from gynecological pain and discomfort, as well as assistance with childbirth. Each year the Blackwell hospital handled an increasing number of patients and later provided medical assistance through home visits, which were run by what was known as the "Out-door Department." Patients seen at the infirmary provided students at the college with a constant stream of cases to observe and analyze in the teaching clinics. Designed and staffed by women, the infirmary provided a much-needed place for women to learn and practice medicine.[75]

When Jacobi started teaching, the Woman's Medical College already had a strong reputation, enrolling twenty-five to forty students and graduating five to ten students per year. For admission, students had to be twenty-one years of age, "be of good moral character, and have received a good general education."[76] To receive a degree, they had to complete three years of instruction and compose a thesis. Subjects were introduced in a graduated system. In the first year, students studied the "elementary branches" of the sciences, including anatomy, physiology, materia medica, chemistry, and pharmacy, along with doing "practical work" (dissection) in the anatomical rooms. Students continued this line of study in the second year, with added instruction in surgery and obstetrics. In the third year, they took part in clinical instruction and learned to evaluate cases and write clinical reports. During their entire course of instruction, women learned general hygiene, focusing on personal and domestic cleanliness, water and food purity, and the prevention of contagious diseases. In addition to the daily clinics held at the infirmary, students also could attend clinical lectures at other New York institutions. Although women doctors did not receive hospital appointments, they could attend lectures for instructional purposes at some of the city's most respected and populated hospitals.[77]

There was greater fluidity between the men's and women's medical communities than one might expect, particularly in New York. For example, students at the Woman's Medical College of the New York Infirmary could attend clinical lectures at Bellevue Hospital, which claimed to have the largest collection of medical and surgical cases in the country. They could also attend clinics at the nearby New York Eye and Ear Infirmary, the Nursery and Child's Hospital, the Presbyterian Hospital, Mt. Sinai Hospital, and city dispensaries. As a college announcement stated, "The liberal sentiment of New York has opened to women the great City Hospitals and Dispensaries, with their admirable clinical lectures."[78] Several leading male physicians, who served on the staff at these hospitals, supported the aims of the Woman's Medical College and welcomed women students into their clinics.[79] Greatly admired in the city, Elizabeth Blackwell drew the support of several medical men. New York, populated with many politically minded male physicians, including Abraham Jacobi, offered women professional opportunities not available in other cities.[80]

Although the curriculum set out by the Blackwells matched that of many other medical schools in the country, it faced extra scrutiny as a woman's institution, particularly in light of the economic and curricular problems at other American medical schools at midcentury.[81] In the antebellum period, several new "regular" schools with orthodox curricula emerged and competition for students increased, but standards weakened. Reduced requirements for admission and graduation resulted in practitioners with very little training. The American Medical Association recognized this problem as early as 1847 and again in 1867, when it issued guidelines for improving the nation's medical institutions. Recommendations included expanding the terms and length of study, adding dissection and clinical requirements, instituting faculty quotas, and requiring higher standards for admission.[82] Many of these standards had been put in place by the Woman's Medical College, and yet Jacobi remained critical.

Soon after her arrival, Jacobi tried to make concrete alterations to the college curriculum. Specifically, she wanted to separate the study of materia medica, the chemical properties of drugs, from the study of therapeutic physiology, so that students acquired chemical knowledge first, before applying it to patients. Not long after she arrived, she complained about how these subjects, taught in tandem, did not prepare students to understand the action of drugs and how to navigate "the labyrinth of therapeutical problems."[83] Elizabeth Blackwell, writing to her novice teacher from London, begged Jacobi to stick with the established curriculum and to "give the short condensed and routine course of materia medica, which all are accustomed to."[84] In other words, she asked her to fashion her courses to match students' needs, not her own expectations.

More importantly, Blackwell did not want to isolate laboratory instruction, so that students learned medicine at a distance from patients. Knowing Jacobi played a critical role in the future of the college, Blackwell also pleaded: "Do, my dear Mary, be very prudent and patient! You are young enough to wait for brilliant success, *but you must not fail now*."[85] Jacobi was not patient, and she moved forward to revise the curriculum. By her second year of teaching, Jacobi ended the "illogical" system of teaching materia medica to students who had no knowledge of pathology or physiology.[86] By creating two distinct courses, materia medica and therapeutics, she created a graduated, sequenced system of study that organized students into elementary and advanced courses. Students first learned the properties of drugs and how to formulate them. Then, advanced students practiced administering these drugs to animals in the laboratory and patients in the clinic.

Jacobi, no doubt, rejoiced in the growth of laboratory work at the college and announced these changes to the *Medical Record*, telling a largely male readership that a school for women outpaced male orthodox schools in restructuring its curriculum and expanding its emphasis in laboratory studies.[87] "Progress in Medical Education — The Women Taking the Lead," announced Jacobi, boasting that the Woman's Medical College offered separate courses in chemistry and materia medica. Describing the program of laboratory work, she said, "I think it worth while to call attention to this feature of our course, for it is an entirely original one, and entirely peculiar to our school, yet it is certainly eminently rational."[88] With this type of publication she simultaneously promoted women doctors and her preferred brand of medicine, and strategically associated women and science in the pages of a widely read New York medical journal.

Jacobi insisted on the centrality of laboratory work for medical education: medicine must be learned not only at the bedside but simultaneously in the laboratory. In a fund-raising speech on behalf of the Woman's Medical College, she explained, "The processes that go on in the animal body all involve multiple changes in the composition of its tissues, which can only be studied by means of the science of chemistry. And this again can only be understood by practical work in a laboratory. Some knowledge of the sciences of botany, physics, histology, is equally indispensable, and again can only be obtained by laboratory work."[89] Jacobi persistently argued that students needed to be working with real bodies in order to have real knowledge of medicine.

Not surprisingly, the laboratory played a crucial role in Jacobi's teaching, and reflected not only her Paris education but also her early medical training in pharmacy. In materia medica courses, students worked in the pharmaceutical laboratory, learning the physical and chemical components of drugs and how to prepare them for medicinal use. From describing the structure of roots, leaves, and minerals, to preparing forms of glycerine, iron, camphor, mercury, alcohol, and ether, students learned how to formulate drugs. In her course on therapeutics, women studied the "physiological action" of different therapies on living bodies, studying how and when to use various remedies. They also studied how to use electricity to relieve pain and treat a variety of conditions.[90] Students watched Jacobi perform physiological experiments, modeling how to study both animal and human subjects, administer medicines, and interpret physical responses.

Besides Jacobi, several instructors at the Woman's Medical College included laboratory work in their courses. For the study of chemistry, students were required to spend six hours a week in the laboratory doing "qualitative chemical analysis," and extra hours on "quantitative" analysis, measuring, for example, the elements in urine. To learn pathological anatomy, students conducted microscopical tissue studies to witness cellular and chemical changes.[91] Dissection was an important illustrative tool for the professor during lectures and a tactile experience for the student, who was required to spend two to six hours dissecting and to do two dissections of "every part of the human body."[92] As Susan Wells has argued, many women physicians believed dissection was critical to their study of physiology, for it satisfied their desire to see and "know" the interior structure of the body.[93] Since it was a central component of anatomical instruction, the college advised first-year students to start dissection work in the summer with "the lower animals," cats and dogs, to prepare for their upcoming year of course work. They recommended either attending anatomy lectures at Cornell University by Professor Burt Wilder or using his book on the anatomy of a cat, which provided "excellent guidance to those who pursue such dissection at their own homes."[94] Certainly, Victorian mothers could not have relished the idea of their daughters dissecting cats in the sanctity of their households.[95]

Anatomical dissections were also a critical act of belonging for women physicians trying to access the profession. By the post–Civil War era, dissection had become standard and mandatory in medical schools, after years of public controversy. The manipulation of dead bodies, an affront to gentile sensibilities and the spiritual body, became a critical tool in the acquisition and dissemination of biological knowledge. The physical deconstruction of a cadaver was also part of the masculine claim to medical authority. Most medical men believed it "endangered the 'delicate' sensibilities and health that were the defining characteristic of refined womanhood."[96] Therefore, as women dissected to learn anatomy, they physically rejected the gendering of medicine and exercised their own medical authority.

Live subject experiments were even more controversial. With the expansion of laboratories at the Woman's Medical College, professors now taught physiology with animal vivisections, "when needed."[97] Jacobi supported this development and claimed physiological experiments were essential for all medical students: "To really study [physiology], people should engage for months and years in the most delicate and difficult experiments upon animals and human beings. They must unravel the modes in which the heart beats, and the lungs breathe, and the nerve feels, and the brain thinks."[98]

But in the late nineteenth century, human and animal experimentation was a source of great controversy in American medicine and culture. While most physicians supported laboratory instruction in medical school, some practitioners rejected animal vivisection as a pedagogical method. They also disliked turning patients into research subjects. Movements to regulate animal experimentation took many forms, and were engineered inside and outside of the profession, by both men and women. But women most vocally opposed vivisection, connecting protective, maternal gender attributes to saving innocent animals.

Elizabeth Blackwell stridently opposed vivisection, arguing that experiments on humans and animals corrupted the medical profession and devalued patients by turning them into objects of inquiry. With regard to human subjects, she had serious concern for the abuse of the poor, claiming that the laboratory turned indigent patients into "clinical material."[99] For nonhuman subjects, she believed the "destructive experimentation on helpless animals, not for their own benefit, is a demoralizing practice." She could not fathom how physicians could engage in acts so "morally dangerous" and exhibit such "atrocious cruelty" toward animals.[100]

Elizabeth Blackwell especially feared the use of vivisection at her own medical college in New York. In a letter to her sister Emily in 1869 from Britain, she argued against the instructional use of vivisection at the institution. Calling vivisection pure "mischief," Blackwell insisted that it was "morally degrading to students and as intellectually degrading to prof[essors]."[101] Blackwell continued, unsuccessfully, to oppose the practice in New York from across the Atlantic. She responded sharply to news that the Woman's Medical College had plans to expand its physiological laboratories and had hired a famous

"New York Vivisector" to oversee the facilities.[102] Vivisection was illegitimate as an educational tool, she argued, because of the vast physical differences between humans and animals. In other words, one could not acquire substantial knowledge about humans from dogs. Experiments on living animals posed a great "moral danger" to medical students, especially women students, she believed.[103] "Animal torture" privileged materialism over spiritual life and threatened to destroy womanhood: "The excuse or toleration of cruelty by a woman upon any living creature is a deadly sin against the grandest force in creation — maternal love."[104] Finally, Blackwell lamented that experimentalism had become "a widespread reproach to many of the *young* members of our most honourable and merciful profession."[105] Blackwell's reference to young physicians was likely a reference to Jacobi, her junior colleague, who disagreed with her, time and again, on this issue.

Despite the concerns of Elizabeth Blackwell, by the mid-1880s, the Woman's Medical College required students to have extensive laboratory instruction, some of which involved vivisection.[106] In fact, laboratory exercises became an integral part of the college's teaching philosophy. "The *laboratory work* not only supplies the practical method indispensable to the prosecution of all physical science," read the college's annual catalogue and announcement, "but drills students and prepares them for the more complex work of clinical observation."[107] While Blackwell remained opposed to vivisection, Jacobi claimed it was invaluable for medical education and individual experiments.[108] Defending the practice, she wrote to Blackwell in 1888: "Of course, as you know, in regard to the vivisection question I should oppose you." Clearly impatient with her senior colleague, she continued, "I am tolerably confident that I am the only woman in the United States who experiments on animals!"[109] Certainly, Jacobi was not alone in using animals for medical purposes. Out of frustration, she self-consciously presented herself as an experimental maverick, a woman set apart from sentimentalists like Blackwell who were unwilling to sacrifice animals for human good.

Emily Blackwell, dean of faculty of the Woman's Medical College, supported vivisection as an instructional exercise. Writing in *The Woman's Journal*, Emily Blackwell defended the practice, stating that it did not amount to cruelty but showed great humanity. She explained that colleagues purchased stray dogs and cats from the pound that were already condemned to death. At the college, "without violence or terror, [they are] quietly etherized, just as a patient would be for an operation, and before the anesthesia is carried to the fatal degree, the professor, by surgical operation, illustrates some point of physiological function or structure; then the animal is allowed to die by profound etherization. There is no suffering. . . . For the animal itself, it substitutes a quiet and merciful death for the terror and suffering of the public pound and drowning."[110] In a strategic defense, the younger Blackwell claimed that experimentation at the college was merciful rather than horrific. Although Emily Blackwell believed that vivisection advanced medical knowledge, she tried to garner support by couching her defense of the practice in the language of compassion rather than cruelty.

While critics attacked human and animal experimentation as immoral, inhumane, and unwomanly, Jacobi equated her scientific practice with an act of faith and used religious terminology to describe anatomical investigations: "The study of the mechanism of the human body is not mere dirty work, but one of the most *sublime* occupations."[111] These were not sacrilegious acts but acts of worship in honor of humanity. "Mysteries are not *sacred*," she continued, "but embarrassing masses of ignorance destined to be dispelled; that the sensuous disgust attendant on anatomical and physiological research can be, and is, completely consumed in the *divine* flame of an idea; that human life is more precious and more deserving of *reverence* than any of the accidents, physical or social, by which it is environed."[112] Drawing on her positivist principles, Jacobi connected vivisection and humanitarianism, arguing that physicians were dedicated to saving people through scientific study of animals. Women, especially, did not destroy their morality with such work, nor did they "unsex" themselves, as critics charged. They remained women, dedicated to improving human life through medical means, in the same manner as their male counterparts. She impressed this belief upon her students and carried it out in her own research, making experimentalism central to her personal identity as a physician.

The Female Experimenter

Rejecting the notion that medicine and science were somehow "male" in nature, Jacobi proceeded to experiment as if the laboratory doors were wide open to women. However, the investigative enterprise had historically been constructed as an arena where women had no place.[113] The laboratory was considered a place of order, logic, and process; it was also a place of body fluids and severed bodies. The graphic and grisly nature of anatomy and the physiological study of live subjects were antithetical to late-nineteenth-century Victorian notions of femininity. By doing vivisection, Jacobi and other women

rejected growing masculine associations with experimentalism and symbolically laid claim to gender equality.

Just as the profession debated the role of science in medicine, Jacobi blurred
the gender boundaries of the laboratory. Men added to the gender confusion
as well. While some members of the profession tried to link experimentation
and masculinity, some men associated their manhood with an older model of
medicine based on skillful work at the bedside and protecting the dignity of
patients and medical subjects, human and animal.[114] In this transitional moment, Jacobi resisted efforts to associate experimental practices with masculinity and certain healing techniques with femininity. She most forcefully resisted
the gendering of experimentalism vis-à-vis the controversial act of live-subject
experimentation.

Jacobi engaged with a broad spectrum of experimental practices, reflecting her teaching and research in materia medica, neurology, physiology, and
pathology. On several occasions, she studied animals in order to test therapies
and drug dosages to gauge the impact on humans. For example, she examined
the effects of atropine on pulse rates, and recounted giving large amounts of
the drug to a rabbit, which she "sacrificed" and then dissected to find that "the
pia-meter of the brain and cord were . . . engorged with blood."[115] She also
studied the effect of nitrate of silver for treating infections and "morbid tissue"
that she related to diseases of the nervous system. She tested the drug on dogs
and rabbits, applying it to recently killed animals and also living animals, which
then died after the experiment. To measure her results, she conducted full
autopsies on the animals and examined their tissues under a microscope.[116]

Certainly, Jacobi was not the only woman doing experimental work. Several
women practiced animal experimentation and dissection as part of their medical education and ongoing accumulation of knowledge. It was controversial,
particularly when women attended clinical lectures and studied the body in
public. Nevertheless, Jacobi announced her practices in medical journals to
illustrate her willingness to use animals for drug-related experiments and study
them postmortem.

Early in her career, Jacobi made vivisection part of her experimental repertoire. She conducted several neurological studies on animals in her laboratory,
performing surgical procedures on the brains of live dogs and rabbits. She
and her colleagues cut into the animals' cerebella to study how inhibiting one
part of the brain impacted muscle coordination and equilibrium. The results
were unpleasant. The dogs could not stand and were afflicted with spasms
and a "convulsive tremor" in the days that followed the procedure. One rabbit

was "rolling over and over on the floor," and another "leaped sideways," the left side of his body unable to function.[117] Although the animals were very disturbed, Jacobi was not, and she stoically presented her cases to a medical society meeting in 1873. She compared her studies with the findings of the leading French neurologists, Jean-Martin Charcot and Charles Édouard Brown-Séquard. Abraham Jacobi, then her future husband, sat in the audience and offered feedback on her animal studies. He was simultaneously courting the young doctor, beginning their professional and romantic partnership in the context of a graphic medical discussion.[118]

For Mary Putnam Jacobi, dissecting live animals was the most "practical" way to acquire accurate physiological knowledge. While vivisection repelled some witnesses, it was inspiring for her as a practitioner. She recalled one of her experiments on a frog. After opening the animal, she focused her lens to capture the "streaming movement" inside him. In her eyes, the view was remarkable: "The microscopic shred of tissue from the insignificant animal seemed for the moment to give a glimpse of a mighty vision of endless life, streaming infinite energy into the minutest particles of an infinitive universe. The impression was indescribably powerful."[119] Witnessing the internal movements of live animals was both educational and inspirational for medical students, she maintained. Without that experience, they would be left ignorant to the real workings of physiology in animals and, consequently, humans.

Jacobi researched the physiological impact of drugs on patients through laboratory tests on animals.[120] In a lecture printed in the *Medical Record*, she described investigations with rabbits that examined the degree to which atropine accelerated or decelerated the pulse, and the relationship between pulse rate and arterial tension, a topic of debate.[121] Despite some instances where atropine had a paralyzing effect, Jacobi corroborated that pulse rates accelerated with it. Testing the drug on rabbits demonstrated a dilation of the cerebral blood vessels, a result which led Jacobi to administer the drug as a therapy for "cerebral anemia" to a human: a woman who fell and suffered from a concussion three weeks after giving birth. The drug had some bothersome side effects, initial dizziness and "mental apprehensiveness," but Jacobi believed the drug restored the woman to health.[122] These investigations in therapeutic physiology laid the groundwork for her later studies on pulse and nutrition.

Experiments on animals did not rule out investigations with human subjects in an era when human experimentation was still unregulated.[123] For Jacobi, laboratory studies on human patients were commonplace, as she often reported taking blood and urine samples in her published studies, samples that she used both for diagnostics and for experimental data. In her famous menstruation studies in particular she collected and evaluated her female patients' bodily fluids.[124] Always in dialogue with colleagues, she reported unusual clinical cases to the medical journals and presented specimens from human autopsies at medical society meetings. Sometimes patients accompanied her to meetings so that she could use living examples to illustrate problems or findings to fellow physicians. In these cases, she publicly integrated therapeutics and the process of medical investigation.

In her pediatric practice, Jacobi carried out pathological studies, using the laboratory to explain the deaths of her young patients. In an 1878 article, she described diagnosing an infant's illness based on an autopsy rather than her clinical observation, and contrasted an emotional scene from the sickroom with a more sober analysis from the laboratory.[125] A patient, Mrs. H., had experienced five pregnancies, four of which involved serious complications and the infants died. During the sixth pregnancy, she consulted Jacobi. Upon examination, the doctor found the child's heart to be in poor shape, so she induced labor with the hope of saving him. The baby was born alive but immediately began to hemorrhage from the umbilical chord. The strength of the infant's initial cries convinced Mrs. H. that her child would recover, but when the child stopped crying, Jacobi found him in a dire condition: "The quiet was ominous, and on approaching the child I found that the face had again become perfectly white, and that it had ceased to cry because it had ceased to breathe. The heart still beat feebly, but in a few minutes its pulsations also ceased, and life was completely extinct."[126] Although the infant's bleeding navel drew Jacobi's attention in the clinic, "the real cause of death," Jacobi explained, "was revealed at the autopsy made twenty-four hours later." Examinations of heart tissues under a microscope revealed an "excessive abundance" of fat-granules in the heart muscle due to a "direct arrest of nutrition, by arrest of vascular blood supply," from a lesion in the placenta.[127] The origin of the infant's illness was resolved not through direct contact with the dying infant but through the eye of the microscope.

Jacobi blurred the line between therapeutics and scientific study by transforming some of her patients into experimental subjects at the New York Infirmary and the Mt. Sinai Pediatric Infirmary. She used patients in her care to test out hypotheses or drugs, or to simply witness particular physiological phenomena. For example, she used a sphygmograph, an early pulse writer, to study and track patients' arterial tension and pulse rates after administering alcohol, caffeine, and a variety of drugs.[128] Notably, she studied the pulse rate of an injured Irish boy, Josie Nolan.[129] The boy had fractured his skull in an accident, and the wound had healed, but an opening in the cranial bone remained, covered by a thin membrane that, Jacobi reported, "rises and falls in regular pulsations synchronous with those of the radial artery." Jacobi placed the sphygmograph, which was customarily attached to a patient's arm, on the boy's head in order to measure his intracranial pressure under normal conditions and, then, under the influence of stimulants. Next, she tried to draw relationships between the cranial pressure and the amount of blood circulating in the boy's brain. Reporting this and other cases to the medical journals, Jacobi publicized her findings, offering it as a model of therapeutics based on science.

Although Jacobi constructed medical science as a weapon against female inequality, her concept of equality was limited and did not evenly translate to the clinic or to her vulnerable immigrant patients. Her priorities often rested on the diagnosis, treatment, or investigation itself, not the individual wishes of her subjects. Although she fought to empower women with science, she did not defend powerless animals. She justified animal vivisection for the greater good and believed that experimentation produced knowledge of benefit to humans, who were "far more valuable than the frogs and rabbits of the laboratory."[130]

Living the experimental life herself, Jacobi pushed medical men to meet the new scientific ideal. She vocally demanded that her mostly male colleagues embrace experimentalism, and she condemned those who did not. For example, Jacobi was known to critique the work of S. Weir Mitchell for lacking a scientific basis and, in the process, dismissed his theories on the etiology of female pathological conditions.[131] But she also addressed broad audiences of medical men. In 1889 she spoke to the Massachusetts Medical Society at its annual dinner in Boston, calling on all physicians and medical students to engage with physiological experimentation. Following in the footsteps of the French experimentalist icon Claude Bernard, she insisted they needed to have "fertile contact with nature." "Such contact cannot be obtained second-hand," she maintained, "but [can be acquired] only by those who, as Claude Bernard says, have in the hospital, the amphitheatre, and laboratory, with their own hands stirred the soil foetid and palpitating with life."[132] Only by seeing and touching live organisms "in the process of life" could physicians really know the human body and know how a patient would respond to drugs and health regimens. Without this firsthand knowledge of physiology, physicians risked the health of their patients. "The physician who has not learned to adjust himself to the intricate delicacies and fragilities of living organisms by laboratory study," she argued, "is condemned to take his first lessons in dealing with life upon human beings."[133]

Jacobi's Boston speech was a calculated response to physicians and laypersons alike who were demanding restraint in medical experimentation. She was fully aware of the strong animal welfare movement in Britain and the new restrictions imposed on researchers by the English parliament.[134] Correctly anticipating the resistance growing in her own country, Jacobi used her speaking engagement in Massachusetts to insist that the need for physiological experimentation was not "occasional, but permanent," not an exception to the rule, but a constant form of teaching and learning about the "Science of Life."[135] Published soon after in the *Boston Medical and Surgical Journal*, the speech gave her a very public platform to endorse a scientific model of medicine. It also gave her the opportunity to identify herself, and her womanhood, with science and, by implication, cast a shadow over those men who resisted experimentalism. This was a strategic move to benefit her career and, she hoped, the future of women in medicine.

✛ IN THE 1870S AND 1880S, Mary Putnam Jacobi achieved many of the goals she set for herself when she returned from Paris. She was the first woman to enter the New York Academy of Medicine, admitted in 1885, and she made her way into other medical societies usually reserved for men. She taught a rigorous, scientific curriculum to women at the Woman's Medical College, and found other teaching opportunities as well. She was a clinical lecturer in children's diseases at the New York Post-Graduate Medical School, "the first time a lectureship in a masculine school was ever, in this country, filled by a woman."[136] As she hoped, Jacobi also carried out research, engaging in experimental therapeutics and a range of laboratory work, presenting papers, and publishing prolifically in the most prestigious medical journals. As a female experimenter, she "embodied" a scientific identity and defied the masculine monopoly of her profession. She simultaneously promoted the laboratory and gender equality by claiming men and women should engage in the same type of medicine.

In this period, Jacobi also gave positivism, medical reforms, and experimentalism political meaning. Scientific practices, performed by women, were acts of disobedience in a culture that saw such activities as unwomanly. But preaching, teaching, and doing science were not enough to topple popular perceptions of women's mental and physical inferiority. American laws and social customs hindered women, Jacobi admitted, but "inaccurate" notions of female biological weakness crippled them most. Links between women and invalidism permeated Victorian culture. Jacobi knew that to change conventional wisdom about women's health she could not just claim women's physiological equality; she would need to prove it, and fight science with science.

✦ 4 ✦

FIGHTING SCIENCE WITH SCIENCE

"The limitations attributed to female capacity . . . are largely artificial — social, not physiological — affairs of custom based upon a highly cultivated social taste."[1] So Mary Putnam Jacobi said, arguing that the notion of female inferiority was a work of fiction, designed to attach women to a separate sphere and to bind them to an isolated physical and mental domestic existence. In reality, men and women had equal capacities; this was physically evident, she maintained, if people were willing to see it.

To bring the truth to light, Jacobi produced studies to demonstrate that women were capable of education, paid work, and political activity. In the course of her career, she tried to overthrow very powerful perceptions of the female body that relegated women to a lower caste and a separate sphere. To do so, she aimed to depathologize women's bodies and normalize women's health by rejecting the association between women and illness. Jacobi also tried to disprove the oppositional model of sex differences and present a complementary model of commonalities and differences between men and women. She set out to expand women's social roles and elevate their social status via biological knowledge.

Jacobi believed that many of the recent claims about female biological weakness had been produced by medical men whose research did not live up to scientific standards and who allowed their prejudices to taint their investigations. Critiquing their scientific failings, Jacobi often contrasted her work with the research of her theoretical rivals, asserting her own expertise and accusing them of doing "bad science." These medical men were biased against women, did not have statistical support for their theories, and did not back their ideas with experimental methods, she charged. Delineating legitimate and illegitimate knowledge, she tried to demarcate scientific from unscientific approaches as she presented more favorable interpretations of female physiology.[2] She brought the debate over science in medicine to bear on the "woman question" by associating her studies with legitimate laboratory investigations.

Jacobi drew clear boundaries around scientific medicine by demonstrating her own expertise. As some critics claimed women were incapable of scientific work, she turned the tables in the debate, displaying her own abilities and publicly holding men to higher standards. She tried to show that a woman could be a medical expert based not on her maternalism or her physical experience as a woman but on her mastery of physiology and chemistry. In the midst of gender conflicts, she overtly and intentionally exhibited her knowledge and skills while vocally denouncing what she saw as mediocre medical work.[3]

In the course of her career, Jacobi concentrated on different elements of health and illness, reflecting shifts in medical knowledge and cultural concerns of the time. In the 1870s and 1880s, she studied diseases of menstruation and the physiology of the female reproductive system, and used her findings to justify women's growing presence in higher education and the professions. By the mid-1880s, she had become deeply involved in neurological research, using the treatment of hysteria as a way to prove the necessity of mental and physical activity for female health. In the 1890s, she placed greater emphasis on sex differences and, through her treatment of a hermaphrodite, attempted to prove that men and women were physically very similar, and that their common characteristics validated their equal roles in society.

Joining forces with the women's rights movement, Jacobi used science to revise American notions of female biological destiny. To convince her audience, she also performed neutrality and objectivity in her studies by providing numeric evidence, recording and representing visual realities, and claiming to suppress emotional interference.[4] But while she claimed to do "neutral" research on women's health, her knowledge was socially and politically contingent, shaped by her understandings of nutrition and positivism, sex differences and similarities, and experimental medicine and objective science.[5] Situated in particular notions of gender and scientific practice, Jacobi introduced her own version of biological determinism, arguing that women's bodies mandated an active existence and that the social organism required equal nourishment from both sexes.

"In the Interest of Truth"

In the late nineteenth century, the image of the female invalid permeated Victorian culture. Concerned members of the middle class looked for explanations, desperate to heal their daughters and save "the race" from severe decline. Evolutionary theory fueled the concern that white American women were weak and unable to reproduce and therefore impeding biological progress. Physicians were divided over the source of female illness, many claiming that women were inherently unhealthy, or that they became so through mental and physical exertion. A cultural obsession with female frailty caused some women to focus more on their ailing bodies than their active minds. As Jacobi observed, "Too much attention is paid to women as objects, while yet they remain in too many cases insufficiently prepared to act as independent subjects."[6]

Frustrated by the preponderance of female illness, Jacobi spent her career rejecting ideas of innate frailty and studying what she considered to be the "real" social factors limiting women. Like her theoretical opponents, she worried about the evolutionary implications of female illness, or the "impairment of race vitality." She agreed with many physicians that the harsh conditions faced by New England settlers negatively affected their descendents, degenerating the (white) race and causing young women to be less vigorous than their ancestors. In education, poor "hygiene," such as inadequate food, a lack of exercise, cramming, and excessive work hours, could harm girls. However, mental work itself did not lead to degeneration. "To suppose that cerebral activity could dwarf sexual activity (which is often alleged) is absurd," Jacobi asserted. Rather, the "two poles of existence develop *pari passu* [at an equal pace]" in "highly civilized peoples." It was social constraints and "excessive luxury" that caused the most damage, Jacobi believed, and held women back from their full potential. She blamed "the refined and delicate ease of life and sensibility in which so many thousands now contrive to live" that could easily escalate into a "dangerous effeminacy." Constant worry and reflection about health also caused many young women to become "nothing but bundles of nerves."[7] As a solution, she proposed an active model of femininity, a proposal buttressed by physiological theories and evidence produced in her studies.

Jacobi tried to redirect the attention of medical men who were obsessed with ovarian and uterine disease and its connection to mental illness. She looked to nutrition instead, claiming that illness was more often a manifestation of failed nutrition, and less so about the pathology of sex organs. Concepts of nutrition, for example, were central to her interpretation of menstruation.

While some physicians viewed menstruation as a symbol of female weakness and an illness itself, Jacobi described menstruation as a "nutritive" process that sustained women's health. Rather than see menstruation as a drain of body force that taxed the system, she argued that menstruation was a sign of vitality and a time of "increased vital energy and especially of increased mental force."[8] She tried to normalize menstruation by defining it as a nutritional process, inseparable from other biological functions.[9]

Jacobi also pointed to nutrition, instead of sex organs, as the main difference between women and men. Men and women were different, she argued, not because women menstruated and men did not but because nutrition in women differed from nutrition in men. The first and most obvious difference between the two sexes, she asserted, was their muscular mass. In puberty, men developed more motor force than girls because girls' muscles "refuse to assimilate a certain proportion out of each group of nutritive molecules which is brought to them by . . . circulation." Nutrients were diverted from muscles, and an "afflux of blood to the uterus" occurred to increase the functional capacity of the uterus and prepare the body for menstruation or pregnancy. This process of nutrition in women was neither temporary nor periodic but continuous and recurring in the course of each month. Jacobi argued that women experienced "rhythmic wave[s] of nutrition," or rising levels of vital force, that gradually rose from a minimum point just after menstruation to a maximum point just before the flow; she used the concept of waves to illustrate that nutrition and vitality increased in her subjects before and during menstruation.[10] With this strategy, she challenged the notion that menstruation was tantamount to female weakness.

Jacobi, of course, was not alone in her attention to nutrition. Other nineteenth-century physicians and gynecologists believed illness resulted from a general failure of the body to build and deplete its tissues properly. She shared basic understandings of nutrition with many American physicians, particularly neurologists. For example, the writings of the famous neurologist S. Weir Mitchell related the pale and feeble characteristics of hysterics to nutritive complications.[11] The practitioner Graily Hewitt also cited the predisposing characteristics of hysteria as "defective nutrition of the nerve centres."[12] But while Jacobi and these neurologists could agree on the fundamentals of nutrition, they disagreed on how to apply them to the treatment of women.

Jacobi's focus on nutrition to define menstruation as healthy was significant: she used it to oppose ovarian determinism, a theory that said female sex organs controlled women's bodies. For this reason, she did not oppose ovarian surgery when it was necessary. She believed removing the ovaries did not unsex a woman, nor did it threaten her overall health, since nutrition was far more significant. On this matter, she disagreed with Elizabeth Blackwell, who was wary of ovariotomy. Frustrated, again, with the elder doctor, Jacobi wrote, "When you shudder at 'mutilations,' it seems to me you can never have handled a degenerate ovary or a suppurating fallopian tube." The loss of one's ovaries was not more severe than "the loss of a limb or an eye." She now famously declared, "There is no such special sanctity about the ovary!"[13]

Jacobi was certainly not the first, or the last, woman physician to offer an alternative interpretation of sex differences. Some women in the nineteenth century used medical knowledge to construct the female body in ways that corresponded to their own views of womanhood. Some shared her physiological approach, demoting the importance of reproductive organs. For example, Elizabeth Blackwell was a self-described "Christian physiologist" who focused on the moral and religious meanings of "sex" and saw men and women as complementary. But, unlike Jacobi, Blackwell focused on "corresponding" physiologies as well as the uniqueness and central importance of motherhood: "The life of sex [becomes] . . . inseparable from the woman's personal existence. Thus, all the relations of sex form a more important part of the woman's than of the man's life."[14] Physician Frances Emily White, another believer in morality and maternalism, did not deny sex differences but offered more favorable views of divergent sex roles by claiming women were the caretakers of morality and therefore deserved a prominent place in society. Civilization, she said, transformed women from inferior beings to superior beings, which would eventually lead to the "subordination of man to woman."[15]

Other women physicians tried to dismiss sex differences. Marie Zakrzewska denied the uniqueness of female biology by arguing that digestive and reproductive organs were not only related but physically linked.[16] As Arleen Tuchman shows, Zakrzewska reconceptualized the uterus, describing it as an outgrowth of the intestines. Zakrzewska compared human females to lower animal species to show that the oviduct was once connected to an intestinal canal. From different angles, Jacobi and Zakrzewska strategically took the gendered meanings out of female reproductive organs, dismantled the idea that the womb represented the totality of womanhood, and denied that sex mattered in scientific practice.[17] Surgeon Mary Dixon Jones also rejected theories that stated female reproductive organs defined women.[18] Although ovaries could be diseased, they did not determine a woman's biological destiny. For these women physicians, the challenge was to deny the relevance of sex differences without reinforcing accusations that women would pathologically "unsex" themselves by doing "men's work." This is why Jacobi turned to nutrition, a concept that allowed her to strategically delineate gender symmetry and asymmetry.

Focusing on nutrition also allowed Jacobi to associate reproduction with physiology. In her writings on women's health, she spoke of sex organs and pregnancy as part of the physiological system, rather than isolated elements that controlled the female body. She believed childbearing was necessary for good female health, not because women were biologically destined to act maternally, but because reproduction was a nutritional process that needed to be exercised by women's bodies. An equal "distribution of reproduction," or sufficient time between pregnancies, helped women avoid menstrual pain and ensured uterine and physiological strength. Excessive childbearing could be harmful, but so could childlessness and "prolonged celibacy," which caused the "contractility of uterine fibre [to] become deficient or exhausted."[19] In nineteenth-century parlance, "celibate" most commonly meant "unmarried," but it also implied sexual abstinence.

Jacobi prescribed marriage for women with chronic illness, even suggesting it to her sister Amy, seeing benefits in both reproduction and intercourse. With this recommendation, she came into conflict with women who believed celibacy was a virtue and an ingredient for good health. Educator and activist M. Carey Thomas, for example, took issue with Jacobi's marriage prescription to her friend and future partner, Mary Garrett. Thomas rejected marriage and viewed sex as "carnal" and male, preferring intimate friendships with women.[20] She believed the "constant indulgence" of married life was dangerous and that pregnancies could deplete a woman's health. She cited numerous friends who had become invalids since marriage, including Amy Putnam, and cited women in celibate marriages who faired much better, such as her own aunt. According to Thomas, Jacobi's ideas on marriage resembled not those of medical women but those of medical men, such as S. Weir Mitchell, who reportedly told a male patient that he should "marry or have a mistress to cure him of his headaches. . . ." Thomas said Jacobi's recommendations to patients were also "marked," "tinged," and could not be trusted because she had "revolting relations to Dr. [Abraham] Jacobi (so people say)."[21] While the actual "relations" of the Jacobi marriage are unknown, her prescriptions for marriage conveyed a healthful attitude toward sex and reproduction.

For these reasons and more, Mary Putnam Jacobi supported limiting the size of families, saying we "must control the great reproductive force instead of being controlled by it." Children were "beautiful," she acknowledged, but a woman's health and family income were also important considerations. She asked, "Has man, i.e. man or woman, a right to control the production of children, yes or no?" She answered, "The antique world and the modern world say emphatically, *yes*. The next question is, *how* can this be done?" The matter must be approached "scientifically" and without "sentiment," she said; women should be free to decide with their husbands when to have children while still maintaining good marriage relations. Finally, child limitation should be considered in regard to the "pressure of population," a growing concern among the white middle class, who worried about the multiplying masses. For Jacobi, controlling reproduction was both a public concern and a personal "right."[22]

Just as the nutritional process was essential to reproduction, according to Jacobi, women were an important part of the larger social organism. Women represented vital cells in clusters of tissues, not segregated, independent organs. They needed to be intellectually and physically nourished, but they also provided sustenance to the larger community. For Jacobi, nutrition was a powerful metaphor because it analogized the human body and the social body. In her vision, the social organism required the participation of both genders, but the organism itself was a gender-neutral body. In other words, society was a living, evolving being that had no sex itself.

Nutrition could also be measured and traced, according to nineteenth-century physiologists and chemists. Laboratory techniques were utilized to track pulse rates, to analyze urea, and later, to measure hemoglobin, providing visual indicators of the rate and extent to which aliments were absorbed, processed in the body, and excreted.[23] Such techniques were central both to the way Jacobi evaluated her patients and to her definition of scientific medicine. They also enabled her to produce visible evidence of female nutrition.

Jacobi was, indeed, determined to carry out her studies in the most accurate way, by conducting surveys and collecting data and designing experiments to test and prove her theories. Her menstruation studies best illustrate her performance of scientific expertise, as she consciously asserted her technical achievements and condemned the failures and inadequacies of her rivals. She directly confronted work she deemed unscientific, especially the work of the infamous Edward Clarke.

Clarke's now classic text, *Sex in Education; or, A Fair Chance for the Girls* (1873), pronounced that menstrual functions and coeducation were incompatible for young American women. Too much education and mental exertion threatened the physical development of girls, especially when undertaken during the period of menstruation. He stated, "Girls lose health, strength, blood, and nerve, by a regimen that ignores the periodical tides and [the] reproductive apparatus of their organization."[24] Young women should rest during menstruation, Clarke argued, and concentrate their energies on their reproductive health. If women pursued higher education at the same level as men, they risked sterility and hindering their reproductive functions. Although he claimed that "the relation of the sexes is one of equality," men and women were "different, widely different from each other" and should be educated accordingly.[25] Defiance of "nature" threatened to masculinize a whole generation of young women. His motto was: "Educate a man for manhood, a woman for womanhood, both for humanity. In this lies the hope of the race."[26] Couched in the language of evolutionary theory and ovarian determinism, Clarke's polemical book, published soon after his retirement from Harvard, articulated common ideas about the female body and fears about the expanding roles of women in American society.

Only one year after the publication of *Sex in Education*, Jacobi produced her first paper in defense of her theories about female physiology and women's educational rights. She joined Anna C. Brackett and other women's rights activists to challenge Clarke in a collection of essays published by her family's company, G. P. Putnam's Sons, titled *The Education of American Girls*. Jacobi's piece, "Mental Action and Physical Health," was an all-out refutation of Clarke's major claims.[27] She designed this essay to corroborate the moralistic essays of the Brackett volume with physiological evidence and to communicate medical information to a nonmedical audience. For these reasons, the piece reads more like a lecture than a medical article. And yet it was technical enough to gain the attention of physicians and to win her a prominent position in medical debates about women's health.

In the Brackett volume, Jacobi accused Clarke of overstating the incapacities of girls during menstruation and falsely attributing menstrual diseases, amenorrhea (absence of menstruation), and menorrhagia (excess of menstruation) to mental exertion. Jacobi's own study of twenty women, several of whom attended medical school and coeducational colleges, showed that only six subjects out of the twenty ever experienced menstrual pain. She argued that Clarke overprescribed rest during menstruation; her own study deemed rest unnecessary, positing that an entire week of rest was exorbitant, for her subjects never suffered enough to require such a regimen. Women did experience menstrual discomfort, Jacobi admitted, but pathologies did not result from intellectual endeavor. Rather, they arose from sedentary habits, a lack of exercise, or the interference of emotions with the intellect. While the inferiority of women seemed to be "incontrovertible" to Clarke, he had not proven his arguments sufficiently or empirically, Jacobi charged. Attuned to how conventional theories about the nature of women had been used in arguments against coeducation and women's rights, Jacobi insisted that a positivist reading of the body would demonstrate women's ability to engage in intellectual pursuits.[28]

Calling Clarke out by name, she systematically tried to undermine his authority by linking his ideas to his prejudices toward women, charging that his work "appeals to many interests besides those of scientific truth."[29] She repeatedly pointed to his lack of "experimental proof" and described his work as a pure "exaggeration of fact." She also attacked his vast audience of readers who so easily swallowed his "food for the imagination." Jacobi compared him to the French writer Jules Michelet, who claimed, "*La femme est une malade,*" associating Clarke with the most extreme claims of female inferiority and attempting to disassociate him from science. In "the interests of truth," Jacobi offered what she believed was a different science of female physiology.[30]

Despite their many differences, Jacobi and Clarke actually worked from a similar premise, reflex theory. They believed in a direct, physiological interconnection between the body and the mind, between physical development, reproduction, and mental activity. Rejecting the Cartesian model of mind/body dualism, they drew relationships between cerebral activity and the body's many functions, including those of the nervous and reproductive systems.[31] The nervous system, as it was understood, consisted of two interrelated sections: the ganglionic, made up of nerve matter, and the cerebro-spinal, which included the brain, spinal cord, and medulla oblongata. Clarke argued that mental labor (a cerebral action) and menstruation (related to ganglionic nerve force) could not occur simultaneously without causing a physical drain in women. Women's mental activity was dangerous because it diverted a limited storage of nerve force from reproductive growth and functions. In other words, intellectual work absorbed precious energy and deprived the reproductive system of vital force. Clarke believed ganglionic nerves dominated a woman's bodily functions; this view subordinated her brain and, as Jacobi quipped, "reduced her to the anatomical level of a crustacea."[32]

Jacobi argued that menstruation and mental work were compatible, as were other pairs of physiological functions. She maintained, "There is no absolute incompatibility between the evolution of nerve force at the ganglionic centres and at the cerebro-spinal." Digestion showed this to be true. Digestion and ovulation were both unconscious processes of the ganglionic system. If digestion did not necessitate rest and cause "torpor of the brain," she asked, why should menstruation? Rest was not necessary after every meal, and indigestion, or dyspepsia, as it was called, could actually be even more painful than menstruation, she reasoned. Comparing menstruation to digestion helped Jacobi to normalize menstruation and its associated discomforts. In her view, menstruation was just another "rhythmic" process of the body, like the beating of the heart or secretions of the stomach.[33] She argued that both sexes experienced physiological rhythms and rejected the assertion that "'periodicity is the grand (i.e. exclusive) characteristic of the female sex.'"[34]

Jacobi made another important anatomical distinction, differentiating the influence of thoughts and emotions on women. While Clarke claimed that a masculine education hindered girls' menstrual health by stimulating the emotions, Jacobi insisted that excessive emotions were generated by a lack of brain stimulation that weakened cerebral nerves.[35] Thoughts were localized on cerebral hemispheres; emotions were located in the ganglia. In the ganglia, emotions could cause blood vessels to dilate (leading to pain and cramps), disturbances in circulation, and the obstruction of the body's nutrition. She concluded that emotions, not brain work, caused discomfort during menstruation and that the dominance of the ganglionic nerves emerged from an understimulated brain that created an imbalance. In this way, Jacobi set up a strategic relationship between the brain and the nerves so that they were related but functioned separately.[36] Her interpretation described a female system that privileged rational thought over emotion.

Throughout her career, Jacobi vocalized concern about good "hygiene" in education, particularly for girls, and even admitted that special attention should be paid to girls during adolescence. She advocated for clean, well-ventilated classrooms, healthy meals during school hours, physical activity, the reduction of unnecessary nervous strain, and, perhaps surprisingly, the separation of the sexes during adolescence.[37] Boys and girls should be educated together during childhood but separated during puberty because of physiological imperatives, she argued, sounding a bit like Clarke. However, her reasoning differed from Clarke's in that she said girls needed more physical activity than boys.[38] Because interaction between adolescent boys and girls sometimes stimulated the emotions and disturbed the nervous system, girls needed "more profound training" than they currently had, and they also deserved "a more intelligent view of the real character of intellectual life, and of the exercises required to develop it."[39] After adolescence, Jacobi said, the need for coeducation increased, so that girls could receive training of the highest quality, on an equal level.

Ultimately, this essay prepared her to conduct larger studies on menstruation in the following years. She directed the next phase of her work to an audience of physicians, trying to convince the medical community that Clarke's work had no merit. In the next phase, she went further, using the tools of her trade to offer an alternative view of menstruation that challenged the medical community to rethink sexual difference, and, thus, the social roles of women.

To Rest or Not to Rest: That Is the Question

Jacobi's now well-known study, *The Question of Rest for Women during Menstruation*, is both a systematic argument against Clarke's *Sex in Education* and a performance of her expertise. This study incorporated both statistical analysis and experimental methods to illustrate her arguments and establish her credentials in the field of women's health. She presented an alternative view of female physiology and menstruation, not based on her own physical experience as a woman, but based on what she observed and recorded empirically about her research subjects. It was a view that was also more favorable to an active and educated model of womanhood, and to the physiological equality of men and women.

The Boylston Prize Committee at Harvard University presented Jacobi with the perfect opportunity to refute Clarke, who had been a member of their own institution. As part of their annual essay contest, they proposed the following topical question for 1876: "Do women require mental and bodily rest during menstruation; and to what extent?" The committee, staffed by some of Harvard's most important medical men, including the surgeon Henry Jacob Bigelow, obstetrician David Humphreys Storer, and the practitioner and surgeon Morrill Wyman, added fuel to the fire that raged over women's health and higher education. This was no coincidence, as the committee knowingly opened up another line of medical debate on the topic, inviting physicians either to challenge or to affirm the principles of *Sex in Education*.

The committee questioned Clarke's work as a legitimate piece of medical writing. Morrill Wyman found the study "'weak, one-sided and not sufficiently supported by facts.'" In a private conversation at the home of C. Alice Baker, a Boston women's rights activist and educator, he revealed that he did not consider Clarke's book "a dignified or trustworthy exposition of the subject." Baker learned that other Harvard physicians distrusted Clarke's analysis and that they welcomed other studies that were done "dispassionately" and with "statistics" to support their assertions. She also heard that "one or two members of the Prize Committee had spoken with great cordiality of [Jacobi's] essay in Mrs. Brackett's book as being strong and sound in its physiology."[40] Finding Clarke's work unsound, Wyman and his colleagues were open to alternative views about menstruation.

With the advice of Baker, Jacobi submitted an essay, anonymously, in "a masculine handwriting." She signed it only with the Latin phrase "*Veritas poemate verior*" ("A truth truer than a poem"), in reference to the credibility of her study.[41] However, it is clear that her piece was not so anonymous; at least one member of the committee, Morrill Wyman, may have recognized Jacobi's submission, having previously read her Brackett essay, showing it "great respect."[42]

Jacobi submitted an essay designed to satisfy an audience of Harvard physicians who valued science above sentiment. She hoped that with the use of statistics, diagnostic laboratory tools, and the science of nutrition, her study would be more effective than moral arguments or outright advocacy for the rights of women. Yet it was clear that her submission was an orchestrated effort by Jacobi and the women's rights community to use science for political purposes and prove Clarke wrong.[43] Jacobi also understood that the menstruation question was not of abstract significance for women and higher education but could have an impact on the admission of women to Harvard Medical School.[44]

Women physicians, starting with Harriot Hunt in 1847, had long recognized the educational and symbolic rewards that a Harvard education presented. In 1867, physicians Susan Dimock and Sophia Jex-Blake both applied for admission but did not succeed. In the mid- and late 1870s, the Harvard administration, short of funds for building expansion, was forced again to consider coeducation. When Marion Hovey of Boston offered $10,000 to the school on the condition that it admit women, the medical faculty thoroughly debated the matter, deciding ultimately that women would have to wait.[45] With the Harvard question in the backdrop, Jacobi did her part to show that there was no physiological reason why women could not be educated like men.

Although the Harvard faculty refused to admit women, the Boylston Committee decided to award Jacobi the prize. Its decision was not simply a victory for women and higher education, although it certainly aided the cause. Rather, it reflected a profession and an institution grappling with the meanings of "scientific medicine." Clarke had brought a lot of attention to Harvard with a study that was based not on laboratory studies or experimentalism but on anecdotes and moral dictums. Although he was trained in a physiological tradition and believed in "rational therapeutics,"[46] the moral science of female physiology presented in *Sex in Education* did not satisfy his colleagues. While his arguments were designed for a broad audience, Jacobi directed her essay to specialists, providing data and composing her work in technical language, meeting the academic expectations of the committee. Members of the Boylston Committee cast their votes based more on her approach than on the study's implications for women and higher education.[47]

After receiving notification of the award, Jacobi conveyed her appreciation to the Boylston Committee, saying she was honored that it "willingly conferred their prize upon a woman." She displayed great modesty, admitting that the piece was but "an imperfect beginning of labor" and conveying plans to attach more experimental observations in her published work.[48] Now known as the winner of the Boylston Prize, Jacobi drew vast attention with her book *The Question of Rest for Women during Menstruation*, an extended version of her essay, published in 1877, again by G. P. Putnam's Sons.[49] But the Boylston Committee now faced a big dilemma. Jacobi neglected to include the required disclaimer in her book, that the committee did not "approv[e] the doctrines contained in any of the dissertations"; her overt attack on Clarke now bore the stamp of approval from the Boylston Committee — and Harvard. Committee member Richard M. Hodges wrote to Jacobi and alerted her to the mistake. Sidestepping conflict, he asked her to correct the error, "not because there is any expressed dissent on the part of the committee from your doctrines," he said, "but simply because the rule is deemed an important one to be followed."[50] Jacobi apologized, claiming to be "mortified" by her error. But the oversight worked to her advantage, for the contents of the book and her professional image became historically inseparable from the Harvard award.[51]

In her book, Jacobi stepped up her evidence and armed herself with extensive statistical and experimental data; she also distanced herself from Clarke's sentimental and literary style in both structure and tone. Although she used clinical anecdotes herself in other studies, she condemned Clarke for relying on clinical narratives and excluding statistical and experimental data. By contrast, Jacobi transformed her clinic into a laboratory, evaluating her patients to produce statistics, visual representations, and measurements of physiological processes. Jacobi and Clarke both believed they were scientific practitioners, but they used different methods of medical analysis and intervention.

Jacobi began her study by first formulating a questionnaire. After participants were asked their age, the duration of their education, their occupation, and their medical history, they were asked to describe their menstrual experiences and to indicate whether or not they had pain and, if they did, for how long. She then asked women to evaluate their strength during menstruation and to document their own physical activity. Although coeducation and women's higher education were middle-class causes, Jacobi's study surveyed women from a variety of occupations and backgrounds. While there is no complete profile of her 268 participants, the study does refer to women whose educations range from "common" to "higher," and whose occupations varied from the professional to the industrial to the domestic. The New York Infirmary provided easy access to a pool of subjects, who were mostly immigrant and working women. Several participants also worked in teaching and medicine. From her questionnaires, Jacobi produced tables and a detailed statistical analysis of her findings.[52]

Although 35 percent of participants had never suffered any pain, the remaining women reported having some type of discomfort during menstruation. But, of those who suffered, two-thirds had inherited "physical defects" that caused forms of uterine disease or weakened their constitutions; others had serious "organic defects" that rest could not cure. Based on her numbers, Jacobi believed that immunity from menstrual suffering did not depend on rest but, instead, on a healthy childhood, a sound family history, marriage at a "suitable" time, a steady occupation, exercise during school life, and "the thoroughness and extension of the mental education."[53] Jacobi concluded: "Rest during menstruation cannot be shown, from our present statistics, to exert any influence in preventing pain, since, when no pain existed, [rest] was rarely taken." In fact, she wrote, "in a large proportion of cases, [rest] has been quite superfluous."[54] Attuned to the labor conditions of working-class women, Jacobi said rest could be helpful for excessive pain or for overworked "industrial women," like some of the participants in her study. But rest for the most part was injurious rather than helpful for most menstruating women. She concluded: "There is nothing in the nature of menstruation to imply the necessity, or even the desirability, of rest, for women whose nutrition is really normal."[55]

Jacobi then argued that menstruation was a time of increased vitality by explaining that women had a "reserve of nourishment" in their bodies that was used for reproductive functions. This nourishment was derived mostly from reserves in the voluntary muscles, whereby the body diverted blood to the uterus in order to "increase its functional capacity." The diversion of forces for menstrual functions did not necessarily lead to weakness and debility because the body was "supplemented" by a reserve of force from elsewhere. "We have a certain number of facts," Jacobi argued, "which indicate that the period of menstruation may be one of increased vital energy and especially of increased mental force."[56] Jacobi used the concept of waves and the idea of nutritional surplus to rethink common understandings of menstruation and allow her to establish her own menstrual theory.[57]

To test her theory and corroborate the surveys, Jacobi mapped the physiological signs of her subjects in a chapter titled, "Experimental."[58] Emphasizing her use of laboratory techniques, she combined both physiological and chemical methods to measure the levels of nutrition in her subjects. To trace pulse rates, she used a sphygmograph, an early pulse writer developed in European physiology labs in the 1860s. Strapped to the wrists of patients, the sphygmograph created a visual representation of the pulse rate, as a small writing instrument drew wave lines on a rectangular board. The pulse waves illustrated the rise and fall of arterial tension.[59] In healthy patients, arterial tension was at its highest right before menstruation commenced; at menstruation, the tension of healthy patients reached a healthy minimum. A second test showed that patients produced more urea before and during menstruation. Urea, a substance in urine excreted by the kidney, was measured using Liebig's volumetric method to trace the depletion and replacement of the substances in muscular tissue. According to Jacobi, chemical analyses indicated an increase in the volume of urea, demonstrated an acceleration of the nutritive process, and showed that the week preceding menstruation was a period of increased vigor and "nervo-muscular strength."[60]

Jacobi tried to visually demonstrate this increase of strength with a dynamometer, a device designed to register muscular pressure, usually through recording the squeezing motion of the hand. She asked a small number of subjects to take part in the experiment: seven women had increased strength, seven had less strength, and one had the same strength during menstruation. These were not the definitive results that Jacobi had hoped for. Trying to compensate for these mixed findings, she blamed the inaccuracy of the instrument, saying it did not reflect muscular strength but rather the subject's skill at using the instrument.[61]

Building muscular strength was important, Jacobi insisted, for maintaining the necessary levels of nutrition needed for normal, painless menstruation. When a woman "breaks down," it was not due to the improper expenditure of nerve force, as Clarke and others argued. "Practically," Jacobi explained, "we find that the habit of disordered and painful menstruation is more frequently associated with habits of feeble muscular exercise than with any other one

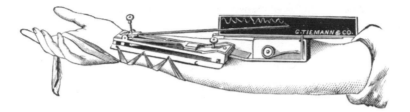

Sphygmograph on a woman's arm. From George Tiemann
and Co., *American Armamentarium Chirurgicum*, 1889.
Courtesy of the New York Academy of Medicine Library.

·✦·✦·✦·

circumstance."[62] In the years to come, Jacobi stood by her prescription for physical activity, and recommended specific calisthenics, sports, and even exercise machines to keep women healthy.

Mapping physiological signs showed that menstrual functions were not "periodic" but "rhythmic." Jacobi concluded: "Reproduction in the human female is not intermittent, but incessant, not periodical, but rhythmic, not dependent on the volitions of animal life, but as involuntary and inevitable as are all the phenomena of nutritive life."[63] By privileging nutrition, a constant process, she rejected the idea that menstruation was an illness. This was important because those physicians who called menstruation an infirmity "base[d] the epithet mainly upon the periodicity of the hemorrhage," she said. Periodicity in the mid-nineteenth century had "come to be considered as a mark of constantly recurring debility, a means of constantly recurring exhaustion demanding rest as decidedly as a fracture or a paralysis."[64] Connecting menstruation to a larger, continuous process allowed Jacobi to shift the focus of medical discourse away from therapeutic remedies designed to rehabilitate women during their week of weakness, and toward those that would strengthen women in their daily lives.

In her rejection of periodicity, Jacobi also questioned ovulation theory. Ovulation theory was the subject of debate in medical journals but stood as the most acceptable explanation for menstruation in the 1870s. According to physicians, the rupturing of the Graafian follicle and the disintegration of the ovules caused the menstrual flow.[65] Many physicians viewed this process, which occurred at intervals, as a great disruption, a "perturbation of the economy," and a "morbid circumstance." Ovulation theory, said Jacobi, "isolated menstruation from all other physiological processes, which rendered its ordinary course dangerous, its derangements fatal."[66] To challenge ovulation theory, she looked back to an earlier theory of menstruation, the "plethoric," and applied it to her own research on nutrition. The plethoric theory of menstruation, originating during the time of Hippocrates, equated the menstrual flux with other bodily evacuations. Such evacuations purified and balanced the system, ridding it of superfluous materials, consisting of excess nutrition, not physical depletion.[67] Equating menstruation with the evacuation of a nutritional surplus, Jacobi ironically reached far back to ancient concepts to offer a "new" interpretation of female physiology.

Jacobi rejected a second aspect of ovulation theory: the simultaneity of ovulation and menstruation, and its association with sexuality. Physicians developed ovulation theory from studies of estrus in dogs, not studies of women. Since dogs ovulate and bleed at the same time, many physicians believed that women must ovulate during menstruation. Nineteenth-century physicians associated the new theory of ovulation with estrus, linking nerve force, sexual arousal, and reproductive functions.[68]

The association between human ovulation, heat, and sexual arousal prompted Jacobi's rejection of ovulation theory. She stated, "All the processes concerned in menstruation converge, not towards the sexual sphere, but the nutritive, or to one department of it — the reproductive."[69] Jacobi reconceptualized menstruation in humans as a nutritional process, not a sexual one, and rejected new associations between heat and ovulation. To illustrate the centrality of nutrition, she made analogies between women and plants, not animals. "The woman buds as surely and as incessantly as the plant," she wrote, "continually generating not only the reproductive cell, but the nutritive material without which this would be useless." It was women's nutritional reserves, not menstruation, that signified their difference from men. By arguing that nutrition "constitutes the essential peculiarity of the female sex," Jacobi was able to distinguish between men and women in a way that emphasized their corresponding characteristics rather than their differences.[70] Rejecting an oppositional approach to sex differences, she focused on the physical commonalities between the male and female body, creating a biological model that supported a social model based on symmetrical gender roles.

As seen in the early medical writings of Mary Putnam Jacobi, the medical debates on the "woman question" were also disagreements over what constituted legitimate evidence and solid science. She purposefully engaged with this debate by differentiating between her work and that of Edward Clarke. By constructing her own work as scientific and demonstrating her expertise, Jacobi tried to undermine the legitimacy of medical men like Clarke. In the process, she drew attention to her research and her alternative views on menstruation.

Beyond the Boylston Prize, her study won praise from several members of the medical community. The *Medical Record*, for example, called *The Question of Rest* "masterly" and said "every page in the book gives evidence of great erudition."[71] *The Philadelphia Medical and Surgical Reporter* also offered high praise, noting the book's "wide range of observation, experiment, and new statistics."[72] In *The Nation*, Henry Pickering Bowditch of Harvard University said that "her successful competition for the Boylston prize, rendered her sex a far more important service than if she had directly advocated their claims."[73] Bowditch recognized the meaning of the prize, and how scientific discourse could have more persuasive power than direct calls for women's rights.

Jacobi's physiological theories were also generally well-received by physicians, many of whom appropriated her methods and sometimes reproduced her results. For example, many physicians approved of her challenge to ovulation theory, particularly as they began to question the notion that menstruation and ovulation occurred simultaneously.[74] Jacobi's work on the menstrual wave also garnered serious attention, and was cited and adopted by colleagues. In 1878, Dr. John Goodman published "The Cyclical Theory of Menstruation," arguing, as did Jacobi, that the vital activities of women, that is body temperature, blood pressure, and pulse, functioned in a wavelike pattern and correlated to the intermenstrual period.[75] Even George J. Engelmann, president of the American Society of Gynecologists, cited Jacobi for her study of menstrual waves. Like Goodman, he documented changes in the pulse, temperature, and blood pressure of girls during the span of a month. But Engelmann, as late as 1900, still contended that the premenstrual period, the height of the wave, produced "morbid nervous symptoms as characterized by the hystero-neuroses" and argued that mental influences generated pathology in American girls.[76] Physicians like Engelmann may have accepted her methodologies for "measuring" female physiology, but they still dismissed her conclusions about women's education.

Despite these acclamations, Jacobi believed her work had not been fully recognized by the medical community, due mostly to her gender. In 1882, William Stephenson published a medical paper discussing the phenomenon of nutritional waves and referenced Jacobi. Although he rejected her conclusions, he supported her basic concept and called for further study. Thereafter, it became known as "Stephenson's Wave," and Jacobi lost her identification with the wave theory.[77] Years later, she complained that she had not received

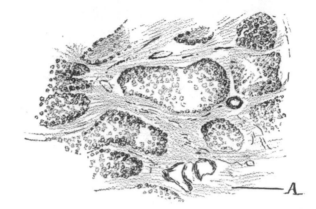

Representation of microscopic examination of uterine tissue in a patient with
metritis. Reproduced from Mary Putnam Jacobi, "Studies in Endometritis,"
1885. Courtesy of the New York Academy of Medicine Library.

·✦· ·✦· ·✦·

"credit where credit [was] due," particularly after winning the Boylston Prize.[78]
Jacobi was also very disappointed that a large body of her work, specifically
her subsequent articles on menstruation, had been ignored.

   In the mid-1880s, Jacobi continued her research on menstruation and reported her findings in her "Studies in Endometritis," a series of articles in the
American Journal of Obstetrics and Diseases of Women and Children. She tried to
disprove that menstruation was essentially a uterine disease, an idea popular
in gynecological literature.[79] "Studies in Endometritis" examined the uterus
and ovaries at the cellular level to contrast the normal growth and expulsion of
menstrual tissue with pathological inflammation. By conducting microscopic
examinations of uterine tissues or diseased ovaries removed from patients, she
produced images of both healthy and diseased tissue formations. While the
studies presented in *Question of Rest* measured physiological signs of nutrition,
these later studies provided visual representations of the tissues themselves.
With these images as evidence, she argued that the accumulation of blood
in the endometrial lining was not equivalent to congestion or engorgement
but rather was a normal nutritional process that either readied the uterus for
pregnancy or was evacuated at the end of the cycle.[80] Jacobi was uncertain
as to why inflammation occurred so often in the uterus and ovaries, but she
suggested some cases resulted from complications of either childbearing or
being childless; other cases emerged from diminished nutrition of the uterine-
ovarian nerves, explained by the direct connection between the reproductive

and nervous systems.[81] Jacobi's "Studies in Endometritis" brought her work on menstruation full circle, almost ten years after she began her research.

The Boylston Prize is cited as one of Jacobi's major achievements, for it was public recognition of her competence, and illustrated her ability to carry out a complex study, apply laboratory techniques, articulate her findings, and convince an audience of men to reconsider concepts of female physiology. Despite the impact and notoriety of her study, Harvard Medical School remained closed to women. A few years later, Jacobi took more direct action, writing to Morrill Wyman and zoologist Alexander Agassiz and calling for coeducation in support of Marion Hovey's offer. Then, in 1882, she joined Emily Blackwell and Marie Zakrzewska in raising another endowment, this time of $50,000, and offering it to Harvard on the condition that it accept women by 1891. Although financial difficulties forced college officials to consider the proposal, outraged faculty stepped in, and with threats of resignation, halted the women's efforts. Women did not enter Harvard Medical School until 1945.[82]

Despite the continuing barriers to coeducation, Jacobi and her feminist allies saw the Boylston Prize as the triumph of "truth" over prejudice. Jacobi's studies countered the volume of literature that equated women and illness. And yet, like her theoretical rivals, Jacobi could not escape her own views of gender and sexual equality; they were embedded in the very questions and methods of her research. Her work represented the intersection of experimental physiology, positivism, and women's rights as she used the tools of orthodox medicine to endorse unorthodox views about women and their bodies.

"Positively" Hysterical

Menstruation shared the Victorian medical stage with hysteria, the troubling nervous disease that seemed to plague so many women. A Greek term meaning literally a disturbance of the womb or uterus, hysteria had been associated with women since the ancient period.[83] Although post–World War I psychology described a male form of hysteria, before the twentieth century, hysteria was mainly a feminized condition. But the meaning, etiology, and treatment of hysteria was the subject of great debate; multiple interpretations of the disease surfaced in the late nineteenth century that reflected divergent ideas about womanhood itself. Medical men and female patients alike adopted hysteria as a diagnosis to explain particular behaviors and symptoms that seemed "disorderly" in Victorian life.[84]

Mary Putnam Jacobi contributed to the controversy over hysteria with her own research and writing that addressed the sources of disease, its many manifestations, and methods for restoring women to health.[85] Jacobi rejected common explanations for hysteria that attributed the condition to female nature or to physical decline resulting from women's attempts to step outside of their assigned sphere. Instead, Jacobi blamed hysteria on physiological and nutritional deficiencies that resulted from constraints on women's lives, and she again rejected rest as a legitimate therapy. Most suffering women needed stimulus rather than sedation to free themselves of hysterical symptoms. In arguing her position, Jacobi challenged another leading figure in the profession, S. Weir Mitchell of Philadelphia, America's expert on hysteria. To fight science with science, she built her expertise in neurology, and again employed positivist rhetoric to claim objectivity and authority over the country's most prominent neurologist. As she took on Mitchell, she turned hysteria into a disease that reflected not the weaknesses of women but the failure of society to produce gender equality.

Mitchell's writings on hysteria attracted large audiences of lay and professional readers as he tried to resolve the plague of "American nervousness" and explained nervous ailments as the outcome of modern, industrial life.[86] He wrote popular books on the problem of nervous disorders in American life, including one on the topic of anemia, called *Fat and Blood*, and one about nervous exhaustion, called *Wear and Tear*.[87] His diagnoses and prescriptions for rest appealed to urban Americans who were feeling pressured by modern notions of work and the stress of the urban world. They also appealed to men and women disconcerted by new forms of femininity; Mitchell's answer was to restore health through rest and maintaining traditional gender roles.

Like many of his contemporaries, Mitchell used hysteria as a rubric for describing a wide variety of nervous symptoms, particularly behaviors associated with women. Loss of speech, anorexia, choking, paralysis, feebleness, uncontrollable spasms, ovarian pain, and melancholy all fit into his conception of the hysterical disorder. Physicians of the period saw many forms of motor hysteria, involving either paralysis of the body, face, or vocal cords, or hysterical fits, characterized by fainting spells, thrashing, or trembling. Basing their claims on reflex theory, and the notion that "sensory stimulation [is converted] into muscular movement," they asserted that somatic symptoms resulted from a mental disturbance.[88] Experts pointed to multiple causes; Mitchell and his colleagues blamed hysteria on excessive mental stimulus during adolescence, both inhibited and excessive sexuality, emotional indulgence, moral weakness, a lack of willpower, and the transgression of domestic and maternal roles. Ultimately, all aspects seen as part of the feminine condition became integrated into the diagnosis of hysteria, a powerful cultural symbol of womanhood gone awry.

Irritated and impatient with invalidism, Mitchell found many cases impossible to cure. He treated mostly women of leisure, who he said became "pests" of the household with their annoying behavior and trifling concerns: "I meet a yet larger number of women of the upper classes, where the disease is caused by unhappy love affairs, losses of money, and the daily fret and wearisomeness of lives which, passing out of maidenhood, lack those distinct purposes and aims." Of the many cases physicians had to deal with, he added, "none [were] more annoying, and none more dreaded than those of hysteria." "What shall we do with them?" he asked.[89]

Mitchell's therapeutic solution was famously known as "the rest cure," or, as he described it, the "absence of all possible use of brain and body."[90] Developed as a treatment for injured Civil War soldiers, his regimen soon became associated with the treatment of women.[91] The rest cure involved an intense program of sleep and relaxation with little physical movement. Women, and sometimes men, undergoing the treatment remained in full seclusion from sources of excitement and irritation, including "indulgent friends and sympathetic relatives," who, according to Mitchell, only seemed to encourage chronic invalidism. Mitchell prohibited reading and writing to facilitate mental inactivity and complete repose. In this condition, patients "pass[ed] into an atmosphere of quiet, of orderly control," where nurses and doctors used different methods to restore physical strength. Medical attendants fed hysterics big meals to restore strength to their bodies; they massaged patients, "substitut[ing] passive exercise for exertion." Physicians also applied electric current on all areas of the body to contract muscles.[92] Patients were first immobilized only to be rejuvenated, not by their own will, but by their doctor.

Although Mitchell was not a misogynist, as modern feminists once described him, he did believe women were destined solely for domesticity and motherhood; they were not fit for public life, higher education, and certainly not for careers in medicine.[93] He truly believed that the rest cure not only worked but was appropriate for women invalids. Some female patients appreciated his guidance and used rest to cope with their personal struggles and discomfort with social change. Some educated women, and even some supporters of women's rights, claimed to benefit from his treatment.[94] Many women, particularly those calling for a radical reversal of gender roles, disagreed with Mitchell, but his loyal patients, though sometimes writers and feminists themselves, did not, for the most part, challenge the dominant paradigm of femininity.

Despite their many differences, Jacobi and Mitchell did share some similar assumptions about women's health. Jacobi admitted that women suffered more than men from hysteria, agreeing with Mitchell that there was a "wide diffusion of the 'hysterical temperament' in women."[95] They also agreed on reflex theory, and that the nervous and reproductive systems were interconnected, and they both believed that uterine and ovarian disease could be related to nervous maladies. Jacobi and Mitchell concurred that hysteria resulted from hindered nutrition, which caused tissue depletion, a loss of muscle mass, and a reduction of nerve force. But the two physicians disagreed on the cause of hysteria in women. Mitchell believed that thin blood was partially to blame for female nervousness, but he focused more on how women inappropriately drained themselves of energy, exacerbated their symptoms, and clung to invalidism. By contrast, Jacobi blamed hysteria on inactivity; she also said that hysteria resulted from the dominance of the emotions, or the sensory function, over the motor function.[96] Women had unique physiological constraints, Jacobi admitted, due to their "generally lesser capacity for the storage of force" and their "physiological limits."[97] Therefore, building force and strength was an important prophylactic measure against nervous disease.

However, the etiology and nature of hysteria remained elusive for most medical experts, as interpretations changed over time. In the 1880s, physicians slowly began to see hysteria as an organic disease affecting brain tissue and the result of nervous irritation, inherited constitutional weakness, or a diseased central nervous system. They also associated nervousness with worn and weakened nerve centers, which had been damaged by the stress of modern life, calling it neurasthenia. By the end of the century, psychological models rose to prominence, linking hysteria to the mind and emotions rather than to physical defects of the brain and nerves, paving the way for studies of psychogenesis and the unconscious.[98]

Jacobi's views both reflected and refined these interpretations. While she attributed some forms of hysteria to the depletion of nerve force and some on brain lesions, she also attributed others to utero-ovarian diseases. Many of the women she diagnosed with hysteria had prolapsed uteri, which she treated with cup pessaries. She, too, would rethink "reflex irritation," but she continued to believe in a neurological/utero-ovarian connection: "nervous or even mental disorders . . . are the direct expression of cerebral disease or cerebral malnutrition, which also causes the vaso-motor paresis [slight paralysis] in the vascular territory of the ovaries."[99] Later in her career, she began to explore questions of mind and matter, the relationship between neurology and psychology. But for most cases of hysteria, Jacobi studied them as somatic disease and took a physiological and neurological approach. She aimed to restore motor strength and nerve force in her patients through stimulus.[100]

Jacobi addressed female nervousness most comprehensively in her volume *Essays on Hysteria* (1888), a series of papers read before the Neurological Section of the New York Academy of Medicine.[101] She located the disease in the nutritional inadequacies that caused women's systems to become weak. The process of nutrition created a finite quantity of force to be divided among a number of activities, including digestion, the maintenance of heat, and muscular and mental effort.[102] Hysteria, then, was the "congenital or acquired deficiency in the power of nerve-elements to effect the storage of force in nerve-tissues."[103] This deficiency, she continued, could only be overcome by "increasing the amount of stimulus to which these elements are subjected," thereby increasing their ability to store nerve force effectively. Influenced by the Viennese neuropathologist Theodor Meynert, whose theories she called "bold and ingenious," Jacobi was extremely interested in the mechanisms for building and storing nerve force. She looked to Meynert's theories on stimulus, such as the "innervation sensation," to better understand how mental and motor actions left impressions on cells to store force for future use.[104]

To prevent and treat hysteria, she argued, social conditions for women must be positive and their intellect normally active; lack of activity led to physiological and nutritional breakdowns, for it sapped women of their vitality and creativity. For reinforcement, she quoted German neurologist Albert Eulenberg:

> The predominance of hysteria among women depends, ultimately,
> far more upon the social conditions to which they are subjected, than
> upon uterine catarrhs and erosions. These conditions combine to arrest
> energy of will and independence of thought in women; to suppress
> impartial comparison of their own individuality with external objects;
> to restrain or suspiciously supervise all impulses to free action; and
> especially to obstruct and oppose any attempt at emancipation from the
> limits of a narrow and trivial existence. To these circumstances are due
> precisely the most severe, extended, and incurable cases of hysteria.[105]

For Jacobi, then, the etiology of hysteria combined physiological problems with social and economic constraints. She critiqued the "triviality" of middle-

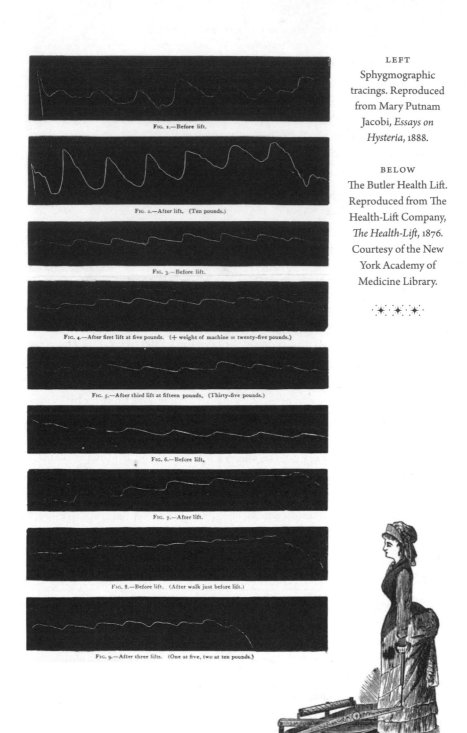

FIG. 1.—Before lift.

FIG. 2.—After lift. (Ten pounds.)

FIG. 3.—Before lift.

FIG. 4.—After first lift at five pounds. (+ weight of machine = twenty-five pounds.)

FIG. 5.—After third lift at fifteen pounds. (Thirty-five pounds.)

FIG. 6.—Before lift.

FIG. 7.—After lift.

FIG. 8.—Before lift. (After walk just before lift.)

FIG. 9.—After three lifts. (One at five, two at ten pounds.)

LEFT
Sphygmographic
tracings. Reproduced
from Mary Putnam
Jacobi, *Essays on
Hysteria*, 1888.

BELOW
The Butler Health Lift.
Reproduced from The
Health-Lift Company,
The Health-Lift, 1876.
Courtesy of the New
York Academy of
Medicine Library.

✣ ✦ ✣

class life for women and its social limitations. To remedy women's conditions, Jacobi recommended a change of scenery to distract patients from emotional sorrow and a change in occupation to stimulate motor activity.

Jacobi insisted that physical exercise was essential for treating patients with hysteria. She advocated that hysteric patients use the Butler Health Lift, a type of weight-lifting system.[106] She cited three cases in which exercise with the machine helped her patients feel "immensely better." Apparently cured of their general pain and digestive problems, these women also menstruated after long periods of amenorrhea. To prove the efficacy of the health lift, she again took sphygmographic tracings of several patients to demonstrate rising pulse rates.[107] These tracings showed that physical exertion caused greater arterial tension, which in turn, caused increased motor function, promoted nutrition, and helped restore her patients to health.

Other women physicians and educators subscribed to the same approach, recommending exercise regimens to young women. As part of the health reform movement, educators at Wellesley College in the late nineteenth century integrated physical training into the college curriculum. Middle-class health reformers viewed physical activity as a crucial antidote to the pathologies that plagued modern life.[108] Although the rest cure remained the favored treatment among Mitchell's followers, it had little appeal among these educators, who called it damaging. Jacobi offered reformers the scientific evidence they needed to justify their prescriptions for physical activity.

Jacobi also recommended faradization and galvanization to treat hysteria. This was not "shock therapy" but mild doses of current applied to the neck, the abdomen, and sometimes the uterus, causing contraction of the muscles, tingling, or a warming sensation.[109] As Rachel Maines has argued, some electrical treatments produced "hysterical paroxysms," or female orgasms.[110] While some patients described "feeling splendidly" after their treatments, Jacobi did not describe or explain electrical therapy in sexual terms.[111] Most often, she recommended electrical therapy to reduce pain, to generate nerve force, and as an alternative to gynecological surgery. She and other gynecologists, including George Engelmann, looked to electrical therapies developed by French physician Georges Apostoli for treating uterine fibroids and pelvic inflammation.[112] Jacobi said surgery was sometimes necessary, but electricity should be the first step in relieving hysterical pain. But faradization could also be used to produce nerve force. Electrical current did not replace nerve force, Jacobi explained; rather, it involved the "liberation or discharge of energies." Overall, she asserted, there was "no hysterical symptom" that could not be helped with faradizations.[113] Although electricity was effective, Jacobi reminded readers that physical exercise was the most beneficial way to produce force.

In some cases of hysteria, Jacobi supported gynecological surgery and removal of the ovaries, which was still a controversial and risky treatment.[114] If there was evidence of ovarian cysts in a patient, and she endured severe pain for an extended period, Jacobi recommended removal of the ovaries with Battey's Operation, a method introduced by Georgia physician Robert Battey.[115] She was more hesitant to endorse ovariotomy for hysterical cases but did so when a case "resisted all other means of treatment." Battey's Operation could relieve "an immense train of morbid symptoms," and cut off the transmission of impressions from the ovaries to the "cerebral sensory centres" that caused "hyperexcitability."[116] In other words, removing the ovaries would stop the nervousness resulting from problems in the reproductive system. But while Jacobi was open to ovariotomy, she did have concerns about the efficacy of the procedure, finding its success rate to be inconsistent. In some cases, pain and hysterical symptoms even seemed to increase. She also worried about the potential for abuse.[117] And yet in 1892 she defended the surgical practices of Dr. Mary Dixon Jones, who was on trial in Brooklyn for manslaughter and libel for her failed operations. Jacobi had been Jones's preceptor for three months in 1873 and continued to consult with her about surgical procedures in the years that followed. She and Jones agreed that female reproductive organs could be removed because they did not constitute womanhood itself.[118]

Treating anemia, a condition often closely related to hysteria, was another source of friction between Jacobi and Mitchell. Physicians believed that anemia, also diagnosed as chlorosis, resulted from the stress of female adolescence.[119] Jacobi and Mitchell agreed that massage therapy could help anemics by facilitating nutrition. But while Mitchell insisted on rest for anemia, Jacobi found that "rest was of the least consequence" in her cases. She preferred to use cold packs, enveloping patients in wet sheets and then covering them with blankets; muscular massage therapy followed. She then took urine and blood samples, and measured urea and hemoglobin levels.[120] Her laboratory analyses showed that this therapy produced higher levels of urea and rising levels of hemoglobin, both demonstrating that increased stimulation of body tissues resulted in increased nutrition. She concluded sharply, "These considerations have been entirely overlooked by Mitchell, in the popular essay already referred to, perhaps because in that essay *no scientific accuracy* was aimed at, but only certain rough, practical results. In this particular case, however, the theoretical *inaccuracy* constantly tends to defeat the practical benefit."[121] Jacobi pointed to the "scientific" and "theoretical" limitations of Mitchell's work to bolster her own research and treatment of anemia.

Mitchell had achieved wide public recognition for work Jacobi considered to be inadequate. She resented his fame and believed prejudices against women doctors limited her own recognition. She insisted that her research predated his and that her research methodology was superior. In a bold letter to Mitchell, she argued that her work was more sophisticated than his: "A year before the appearance of your little book on Fat and Blood, I published in Seguin's *Archives* an essay on the cold pack and massage in anemia, embodying a good many precise researches, and containing many suggestions, which proved to be quite identical with many of yours. . . . My essay appeared in book form about a year later, and a little after the publication of 'Fat and Blood.' It is not necessary to comment upon the extraordinary success of your little book, while mine, which was experimental as well as theoretical, has scarcely ever been heard of."[122] Unlike his "little book," Jacobi claimed her work was scientific and "experimental." Calling his science inferior, she tried not only to earn credit for her work but also to lend credence to her ideas, particularly those that favored active womanhood. Jacobi tried to out-science Mitchell, accusing him of being inaccurate and antiquated.

Within the growing New York neurological community, Jacobi built her knowledge and expertise. She was a member of the New York Neurological Society, acting as its corresponding secretary, and in the Neurological Section of the New York Academy of Medicine after her admission in 1885, eventually becoming the academy's section chair.[123] Her work fit in well with the approach of other New York neurologists because she attributed most nervous diseases to somatic causes and cited physical problems as a source of psychological distress.[124] Offering concrete answers to concerned patients, neurologists promoted their own professional status. Although she disagreed with the Neurological Society's famous president, William A. Hammond, on matters of women and invalidism, Jacobi earned the respect of many male colleagues. Ironically, she also earned the praise of S. Weir Mitchell, who wrote to her from Philadelphia: "Thanks for your book. . . . I envy you two things — your strong logical use of facts [and] theory. The essay on Hysteria is a wonder of this kind of brain work and most interesting."[125] While the two physicians held divergent opinions on the nature of women, they agreed on many neurological matters.

Despite Mitchell's praise for Jacobi, he did not approve of women doctors. Mitchell publicized his disapproval in a fictional series titled "Characteristics," which featured a physician who discouraged a young woman from pursuing medicine on the basis that the profession made women masculine and stripped them of all their feminine qualities.[126] Jacobi wrote to Mitchell in protest and chastised him for attributing hysteria to healthy women studying medicine. She asked: "Do you not almost inevitably get into the habit of extending to the whole sex the estimate which you justly form of the multitudes of them which absorb your professional attention?"[127] She then defended women physicians and lamented their limited opportunities for work. For Jacobi, challenging Mitchell was a matter of correcting "bad science," claiming credit for her work, and contesting his position on the "woman question."

Jacobi's long-term frustrations with Mitchell informed her treatment of his most famous patient, Charlotte Perkins Gilman.[128] Gilman's story *The Yellow Wallpaper* (1892) has become a feminist allegory and a treatise against the problems of nineteenth-century medical practice. Gilman's novella reflected her own experience under Mitchell's care and described the road to insanity traveled by a woman undergoing the rest cure. Confined to her room and deprived of stimulation, including talking, reading, and writing, the narrator is drawn deeper into mental illness by her seclusion and what she considers the sinister patterns of the yellow wallpaper that surround her. While Mitchell's name has become synonymous with the rest cure, Gilman's name has become associated with protest against it. Her indictment of medical men like Mitchell stands in opposition to her reverence of women physicians. Whether as fictional characters or real practitioners, women doctors were heroic feminist figures in Gilman's writing and personal life.[129] In many ways, Jacobi was a more than logical choice to take over as Gilman's physician.

In 1901, Jacobi offered to treat Gilman for her "brain trouble," years after she fled the care of S. Weir Mitchell and almost a decade after the publication of *The Yellow Wallpaper*. In December of that year, Gilman noted in her diary, "Call on Dr. Jacobi & state my case. She is to undertake it — her own proposition."[130] Jacobi was eager to help Gilman because this was no ordinary case; her treatment had symbolic power, considering her very public critique of Mitchell and the rest cure. They were also "interested in the same things," both medically and politically, sharing deep concerns about the mental health of American women and the social restrictions that caused and exacerbated them.[131] They both operated professionally from feminist standpoints, and believed in the power of work to liberate women from economic dependency on men. Influenced by socialism, they shared an organic view of society, seeing it as a collective project where all members, including women, contributed to the broader good through their work and education. The two women were also interested in the science and social implications of evolution on American civilization, particularly the vitality of (white) women for the future of the race.[132]

Jacobi prescribed to Gilman a graduated therapeutic regimen of mental and physical training. She began with electric therapy, applying electricity to the solar plexus, a large nerve center in the abdominal cavity. To promote digestion, assimilation, and nutrition, she had Gilman drink a mixture of phosphoglycerates in wine.[133] To "set that inert brain to work," Jacobi assigned her mental and tactile exercises that gradually increased in their complexity to "reestablish the capacity for action."[134] Gilman started off by working with kindergarten blocks, "just building things," to regenerate her cerebral activity. She quickly moved to reading more complex books and scientific texts such as E. B. Wilson's *The Cell*, a text on cell theory, evolution, and inheritance.[135] Gilman followed Jacobi's advice and returned to writing her book *Human Work* (1904), a book that reflected her organic vision of society.[136] Soon after, Gilman began a program of physical exercise, joining a woman's basketball team and playing at Barnard College in New York. True to form, Jacobi's treatment of Gilman rested on a regimen of increased mental and physical stimulation.

Gilman's gradually more intense mental exercises were reminiscent of Jacobi's earlier work on intelligence training. In *Physiological Notes on Primary Education and the Study of Language* (1889), Jacobi explicated methods for training young people, especially girls, to build "perception and memory." Jacobi wrote, "The existence of a larger class of actively educated women must increase their demand for a larger share in that part of the world's work which requires *trained intelligence*." She studied how children best acquired language facilities and argued that it is far more important to learn the meaning of objects before learning modes of expression. Rather than "talking fluently without having any thing to say," Jacobi believed, children should grasp concepts and then cultivate skills of expression. With this study she attempted to link her physiological knowledge to research in human perception and thought processes. She also developed new ways to cultivate female intellectual skills, believing this type of early education could "develop more vigorous mental force" and "increase power, . . . a real means for attaining real ends."[137]

Jacobi's mental exercises with Gilman, particularly their reading assignments, reflected their mutual interests in evolution. With her graduated program and intelligence training, Jacobi expanded on the ideas of Herbert Spencer. She built on the idea that the mind, though a product of inherited traits, could also be trained, improved, and adapted over time with proper education that progressed from the most basic to the most complex lessons.[138] Wilson's *The Cell* focused on cellular evolution and inheritance, issues of great interest to Gilman, who applied evolution to her political writings on women and labor. While the two women shared hope for gender equality, they also shared prejudices of race and class. Their writings implied that white, educated women of privilege were fundamental to racial progress. Women, in fact, would lead "the race" into the future with their vital contributions.[139] In advocating building women's education and economic worth, they tried to push women up the evolutionary ladder, to stand on an equal plane with men, no longer between men and other races. Jacobi's treatment of Gilman reflected the intersection not simply of feminism and therapeutics but of feminism, socialism, and evolutionary biology.[140] Jacobi's rhetoric on race, womanhood, and progress intensified in the 1890s, particularly when she became active in suffrage and Progressive Era causes.

Although Jacobi directed Gilman's therapy, their relationship was also a collaboration between peers. In the final years of her career, Jacobi had a relationship with a patient that was personal, cooperative, and interactive, contradicting her earlier advice to women physicians that they remain emotionally distant from patients. Of Jacobi Gilman recalled, "[She was the] most patient physician I had ever known," who "seemed to enter into the mind of the sufferer and know what was going on there."[141] Gilman realized her treatments were experimental, but she was happy to oblige: "[Dr. Jacobi] said she had originated a system of treatment which she desired to try for that ailment, and nobody would allow her to do so. I said I was perfectly willing to let her try it on me, and we formed a compact. She proceeded to develop with me the original system, and the result was admirable. I worked under her for some months, going to her office every day, and she put me through a course of most remarkable performances."[142] Happy with the results, Gilman was, at once, Jacobi's patient, experimental subject, and friend. Jacobi offered what Mitchell did not: a partnership. Ironically, Jacobi had prided herself on being more scientific than Mitchell, not more "sympathetic."

Jacobi strongly believed she was offering a more accurate reading of the body than S. Weir Mitchell's. But her claims to expertise are more significant than whether she was, in fact, more scientifically rigorous than her opponent. For their disagreements show how science could be employed to argue both for and against the expansion of women's rights, and how knowledge reflected the social position of the knower.

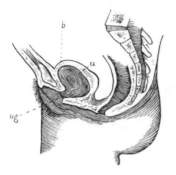

Illustration from Mary Putnam Jacobi, "Case of Absent Uterus," 1895. The caption with the original image reads: "Case of absence of the uterus with persistence of urogenital sinus (*ug*), which combines the urethra and vagina." Courtesy of the New York Academy of Medicine Library.

∹✦ ✦ ✦∺

"Every Individual Is Hermaphrodite"

In 1895, Mary Putnam Jacobi reported a "Case of Absent Uterus" to the *American Journal of Obstetrics*. She had treated a seventeen-year-old patient, known only by her initials, "B. M.," whose sister consulted her, worried because the girl had experienced monthly pelvic pains and paroxysms, and had never menstruated. Jacobi first assumed that the patient suffered from chlorosis, a common form of girlhood anemia, because she appeared thin and weak, so she prescribed an iron treatment. The patient's sister was extremely persistent and demanded further investigation. Jacobi did a physical examination. Then a colleague used an endoscope to examine the patient under ether, an exam that "failed to discover the least trace of uterus or ovaries."[143] Because this was so unusual, B. M. became the object of a very intimate and prolonged surveillance as doctors, nurses, and family members watched and waited for her to menstruate. Under observation for eight to ten weeks, seven of them at the New York Infirmary, B. M. showed no signs of vaginal bleeding. Missing reproductive organs and unable to reproduce, B. M. had "anomalous" and "ambiguous" sex characteristics, which at the time, pathologically classified her as a "hermaphrodite."[144]

Coming to Jacobi well within the third decade of her career, this case was the culmination of her career-long focus on the science of sex differentiation and its relationship to women's health. Although she was not a specialist on hermaphroditism, she used the condition to address broader problems of gender and to illustrate both the differences and commonalities between men and women. The case of the absent uterus provided her with an opportunity to argue against the absence of women in science, using hermaphroditism as a vehicle to promote the full inclusion and interaction of both men and women in science and society. Ultimately, Jacobi's writing on hermaphroditism was less about sexual anomalies and "malformations" and more about the "normality" of shared male and female traits and its consequences for advancing the rights of women.

With the case of B. M., Jacobi joined a cadre of American and European physicians in the late nineteenth century studying genital "malformation" and sexual identity. Ambiguous bodies provoked great interest because they not only presented physical anomalies but also provided physicians with an opportunity to assert definitions of what they considered "normal" and "pathological" sex development. In the backdrop stood theories of evolutionary biology, articulated by Charles Darwin, Herbert Spencer, and G. Stanley Hall, maintaining that humans, as the most highly evolved species, displayed the most extensive differences between male and female. Some theorists also suggested that women were less evolved than men, which explained their smaller size and physical frailty, and that they were designed by nature strictly for motherhood.[145] In the 1890s, Jacobi applied her ideas about nutrition to new knowledge on embryology, evolutionary biology, force, and metabolism to argue against oppositional sex differences.

Most physicians in the period subscribed to a binary, two-sex model.[146] Although a patient might exhibit signs of both male and femaleness, specialists denied the possibility of "real" hermaphroditism, that is, they argued that all individuals had to be only one sex, either male or female. The true test of a patient's sex hinged on the presence of either ovarian or testicular tissue. If an examination of this tissue did not prove conclusive, physicians looked to aesthetic appearance and social behavior for answers. Their work mirrored a broader body of scientific literature on evolution and sex differences, and reflected the Victorian cultural imperative to clearly separate masculine and feminine.

Jacobi also believed that physical hermaphroditism in adults amounted to pathology, as did a variety of anatomical malformations and sexual ambiguities; mixed and missing sex organs produced serious physical problems and often "psychic" complications. However, she distinguished between the abnormal "disassociation of sex attribute[s]," as seen in "B. M.," and "normal" combinations of masculine and feminine characteristics, as seen in ordinary people.[147] Men and women both possessed certain qualities of the opposite sex, she argued, especially when it came to mental powers. She used the case of B. M. and her missing uterus to challenge strict gender dichotomies and deployed biological evidence to show that women had the same intellectual capacity as men.

We do not know much about the patient B. M., but we can unpack Jacobi's case narrative for clues. B. M. was a "moderately-sized, rather thin, ill-developed" frail young "girl" who she seemed to be missing female sex organs.[148] Jacobi described B. M. as a silent, cooperative patient, with one possible exception: the patient, either voluntarily or involuntarily, urinated in Jacobi's hand during an examination, and Jacobi was forced to abruptly end it. Confined to the hospital for almost two months, B. M. was expected to demonstrate that she was a woman by menstruating, but she never did. It was the lack of menstruation that most disturbed the girl's married sister, who was insistent that something was gravely wrong. The sister was very worried about B. M.'s chances at marriage and her inability to have children.

In the late nineteenth century, with endocrinology in its infancy, most physicians blamed hermaphroditism on failed embryological development. According to germ-layer theory, human embryos were androgynous, or sexually neutral, possessing "primitive" urogenital organs that were neither male or female.[149] In the course of what was deemed normal sexual development, physicians believed, the embryo grew in three segments: the deep segment, where neutral "genital ridges" would evolve into either testicles or ovaries; the middle segment, where male ducts atrophied and females ducts would develop into fallopian tubes, uterus, and vagina; and the external segment, where the "genital tubercle and furrows" would develop into either penis or clitoris. Hermaphroditism occurred when one segment's development was arrested or when segments did not follow one clear-cut line of sexual development. Jacobi explained that when the cells of opposite sexes combine at conception, a "nutritive conflict" emerged until eventually one sex overrode the other to become the dominant force in the body.[150] An imperfect blending of characteristics could result in missing organs or double sets of organs, double physiological processes, or a double "sexual instinct." Also, it could result in "moral hermaphroditism"—a behavioral category—which was viewed as a form of psychic degeneration.[151]

According to Jacobi's observations, B. M.'s development had been arrested, and consequently, her sex organs were "embryonic." While she did have urinary organs, her genital organs were absent. She did have what was called a "urogenital sinus," believed to be an intermediate organ between vagina and urethra, in the embryological state.[152] Her case showed that the three segments did not always develop in coordination, meaning her middle segment atrophied as it would in a male, but did not develop as in a female, and yet the patient had the outer physical appearance of a woman. Although a postmortem exam may have told a different story, observations of the living body revealed an "abnormal combination" of organs, which led physicians to conclude that in such cases, it was "quite impossible . . . to infer with certainty the sex of the individual." As Jacobi demonstrated, B. M.'s was one of many of a broad spectrum of cases of "sexual confusion."[153]

Jacobi described the gradations of mixed physical and behavioral characteristics found in hermaphrodites. B. M.'s case appeared less extreme than other cases on the spectrum, for B. M. was missing organs but had the outward appearance of a woman. In other cases, Jacobi noted, sex combinations were more notable. For example, a twenty-seven-year-old Russian, Elizabeth Wulfert, had been brought up a girl but reportedly had both a "rudimentary vagina" and testicular glands, a feminine voice and a masculine larynx, and a sexual attraction for men and women.[154] Jacobi cited another famous case, the French hermaphrodite Alexina B., also known as Herculine Barbin, who was raised a girl but at the age of twenty-two was discovered to have male genitals. (A court pronounced her a man, and she later committed suicide.)[155] By illustrating the differences between B. M. and Alexina, Jacobi described a range of abnormal development and blended sex characteristics.

Jacobi's spectrum is significant because it was not simply a pathological continuum; it was a spectrum of both the normal and the abnormal mixing of sex characteristics in which *all* people could be situated. She distinguished between pathological and normal mixtures of masculine and feminine: "Too equable blending of opposite sex characters neutralizes each to the point of sterility, constitutes perversion, malformation, degeneracy. But from this level of organic disaster there is a steady gradation, through insensible degrees of variation, toward an organic perfection, where the blending of germ cells has secured the advantages of complex organization, an organization of both physical and psychical sex complexity, yet has evaded the dangers of sexual neutralization."[156] Some balance of both male and female attributes in an individual was normal and, in fact, desirable, Jacobi argued. And some qualities, particularly mental and emotional ones, were so neutral in origin that they did not belong exclusively to either sex. Both men and women possessed certain qualities of the opposite sex, she argued, especially when it came to mental powers. Jacobi used B. M. to discuss a range of physical developments that pathologized some forms of hermaphroditism but normalized some shared characteristics between men and women.

Discussing hermaphroditism through the case of B. M. gave Jacobi an opportunity to present another argument for the physiological symmetry between men and women. Jacobi used the biology of conception to argue for less sexual differentiation, and tapped into embryological theories of "primitive bisexuality." Many experts believed that all embryos originated with the morphing of male and female cells; individuals were therefore "compounds" of both sexes, although one sex eventually dominated and one was "latent."[157] According to this theory, males and females were not physiological opposites, she said, because each sex contained attributes of the other. Quoting French pathologist Paul Le Gendre, Jacobi agreed that *"chaque individu est hermaprhodite, non seulement dans ses organes sexuels, mais dans toute sa constitution"* (every individual is hermaphrodite, not only in his sexual organs [i.e., originally], but in his entire constitution).[158]

Jacobi also took up the issues of force and metabolism, challenging the ideas of Patrick Geddes and J. Arthur Thomson, authors of the famous *Evolution of Sex* (1889). They argued that men were more katabolic and women more anabolic, meaning men had a more destructive metabolism and produced more energy, and women had a more constructive metabolism and less body force. Geddes and Thomson used this argument to explain why men were physically larger and more mentally active than women. Jacobi argued that males and females had equal amounts of force but that they directed that force in different ways. Females had smaller skeletons, muscles, and nerve centers because they directed body force to reproductive functions, whereas males directed this energy toward simply sustaining themselves.[159] "On the whole it would appear that sex differentiation does not concern the quantity of nutritive force, but only its direction," she concluded.[160]

While many of her contemporaries focused on sex organs as the main identifiers of sex, Jacobi continually returned to nutrition. Sex organs were certainly a major health concern as the apparatus for reproduction and the locales of life-threatening disease. But in her view, they did not govern the body. Rejecting the primacy of the ovaries or uterus in determining womanhood, she argued, *"The sex is not due to any one character nor to the existence of any one organ, but to a consensus between many. The elements of the organism meet and combine into unity, but wherever the unifying power may be it does not reside in any one of these elements."*[161] In essence, Jacobi redefined womanhood so that it did not solely rest on reproduction but rather on multiple factors.

Jacobi used hermaphroditism to unsex the brain and, therefore, deny the fact that men, because of their natural design, were destined for mental work while women were not. Mental characteristics, she insisted, were not determined by sex but by social conditions.[162] The problem, said Jacobi, was that physicians connected sex organs to the brain, physical sex to psychic sex. In this assertion, she directly challenged Geddes and Thomson's argument that female physiology, characterized by anabolism, made women more passive, patient, and full of feeling. Challenging a great cultural convention, she wrote, "There is no proof that 'women feel more than men.'"[163] "It is a futile task to attempt to determine the masculine or feminine character of the brain or its mental activities from the sex of the individual to which it belongs," she declared. "This sex is only the expression of a predominance of organic attribute; it is relative not an absolute distinction."[164] In many ways, then, Jacobi reinvigorated the seventeenth-century Cartesian principle: "the mind has no sex."[165]

Jacobi's efforts to disconnect sex from the brain also constituted an effort to disconnect reproduction and sexuality from the brain as well. Although she believed in a physiological/nutritional connection between body and mind, she rejected the idea that sex organs alone determined mental activity or ability and that mental aptitude was simply a matter of sex. Women made fewer professional and intellectual achievements, not because they were anatomically female, but because they had not been privy to the same opportunities as men.

By establishing that women had the same mental capacity as men, Jacobi maintained that women could also perform the same work. She asked, "Have we not had enough of the dictum, 'Women cannot do men's work?'"[166] Of course, this had great relevance for her own experiences in the fields of science and medicine — in which women continued to struggle for admission, acceptance, and respect. With the proper training, women could do "men's work" because medicine did not inherently belong to men, she claimed, although some medical men tried eagerly to define it in that way.

If the brain had no defining sex, then one could argue males and females were both capable of the same work in the sciences. Jacobi again challenged the idea that women's minds worked in unique ways, arguing that when it came to scientific work, the mental qualities involved belonged to both sexes. For example, women were viewed as essentially more patient, and passive, according to Patrick Geddes. Even if that were true, Jacobi reasoned, women had a "tenacity of purpose" and an "appreciation for subtle details" which, she insisted, were actually "the basis of scientific investigation."[167] Geddes's characterizations of the sexes were futile, she insisted, because men and women, given the same education, were both capable of studying science.

Employing her own version of biological determinism, Jacobi argued that physical and mental similarities between men and women required social and political equality. Using a positivist rationale, she argued that there were physiological mandates requiring expanded roles for women. The social organism, in which males and females actively participated, was not entirely masculine or feminine in its character, but a mixture of both. Ultimately for Jacobi, hermaphroditism was not simply a vehicle with which to revise biological and social relationships between men and women; it was a metaphor for a society that embodied gender equality as well.

We do not know exactly what happened to the patient B. M. We can surmise, however, that Jacobi and her colleagues tried to restore her poor health, possibly treating her for anemia, and then discharged her back to her family. Despite the silence on the outcome of the case, we do know that B. M. offered Jacobi a platform for reasserting her ideas about sex differences to her colleagues in obstetrics and gynecology, particularly medical men intent on using female sex organs to delineate difference.

✳ WRITING ABOUT HERMAPHRODITISM, Jacobi observed that genital malformations provoked a "romantic interest" because they "threaten[ed] the fundamental basis of individuality." She understood that personal identity centered on the need to describe oneself as man or woman. A strict sexual division was overemphasized, she said, and female reproductive roles received too much attention, for the "individual is neither all father or all mother, but only more or less of each."[168] This was a radical notion for the Victorian era. If the physical and emotional differences between mothers and fathers were actually quite minimal, then nature did not mandate separate spheres for men and women. Rather, nature called for the greater blending of parental roles. Both parents could engage in both the caregiving and the breadwinning of the household; mother and father were capable of emotional and intellectual expression, and they were equally fit to both comfort and discipline children. Jacobi's conception of fluid gender and familial roles was ideological and political but also highly personal, for it played out in her own life, in both harmony and discord.

A MEDICAL MARRIAGE

Back in 1871, at the age of twenty-nine, Mary Putnam met Abraham Jacobi, a forty-one-year-old widower, at a meeting of the Medical Society of the County of New York. At the time, he was president of the organization, and, according to her own account, she gained admission at his "suggestion."[1] The two doctors proceeded to carry out what most Victorians probably considered an unusual courtship. At meetings of the medical society, they developed a relationship over graphic medical discussions, one of which included Mary Putnam's report of neurological experimentation and vivisection on a live rabbit. Together, they examined pathological specimens, some removed from patients or cadavers at their respective clinics. When they did not intersect professionally in the city, they wrote to each other on a daily basis, corresponding in Jacobi's native German. Mary described their "romantic" exchanges to her mother: "My 'Herr Doctor' writes to me every day in German and I reply in the same *Deutsche Sprache*."[2]

Married by William Frederick Havemeyer in a civil ceremony at New York's City Hall in 1873, they spent their honeymoon at Lake George, where they reportedly *worked*. The Jacobis collaborated on revising Abraham's manual on pediatric health and nutrition, *Infant Diet*.[3] During their first days as husband and wife they were immersed in discussions of cholera infantum, the nutritional value of breast milk, and infant hygiene. For the Jacobis, this was an ideal honeymoon.

Brought together by shared intellectual and political interests, the Jacobis had much in common. They bonded over a mutual conviction that science, through the revelation of absolute and accurate knowledge, had the power to correct social ills. In 1848 and 1871 Abraham and Mary were engaged with movements against the tyrannical authorities of European monarchies. They both embraced science rather than religion as their main authority and rejected the reigning power structures of Europe. Frustrated with bourgeois culture and individualism, they saw republicanism as a basis for the rights of the citizen and socialism as a model for a state created to provide for the people. Connecting science and socialism, they both viewed society as a living organism, parts of which were interconnected and interdependent.

But Mary Putnam Jacobi and Abraham Jacobi also disagreed on political priorities and how to integrate science in medicine. Their relationship was a metaphor for tensions in nineteenth-century medicine and cultural life and was a microcosm for disputes over what constituted "good science" at the end of the nineteenth century. Comparison of the two Jacobis shows that a wide spectrum of ideas, emotions, and intentions existed among men and women practitioners. The comparison shows the multiple understandings of science at the time and challenges the notion that to be "more scientific" was essentially to be "masculine." Their commonalities and differences undermined gendered codes of behavior and dismantled assumptions about what it meant to be a man or woman in medicine.

Personal Politics

The Jacobi marriage was not a model of nineteenth-century romantic love but an ideological and political union, forged by two people who, in thought and practice, shared the belief that medicine had the power to promote and create greater social equality.[4] They were attracted to each other first by their common ties to European radicalism and their mutual interests in medicine and politics. They found a sense of comfort and familiarity in each other, reminiscent of past relationships, but were also inspired by new hopes for the future. And yet the two doctors had significant personal and professional differences that intensified over the years, forming cracks in their relationship that broke open in the face of personal tragedy.

Although Abraham Jacobi was in some ways an appropriate intellectual partner for an ambitious female doctor, he was an unusual choice for a Putnam, given Mary's Protestant background and colonial lineage. Born in Prussia in 1830, Abraham was the son of Eleasar Jacobi, a cattle trader, and Julie [Abel] Jacobi, a shopkeeper in the village of Hartum, near Minden, Westphalia. Of Jewish descent, the family was quite secular, following the pattern of other Jews who assimilated into German society in the early nineteenth century.[5] In midcentury Germany, the approximately 200 Jews in Minden were relatively integrated and financially successful, but they still experienced economic and social isolation. Education offered a way to bypass some social strictures.[6]

As a young man, Abraham Jacobi received a secular education that reflected principles of the German Enlightenment, and the pursuit of *Bildung*. Studying in the Minden Gymnasium, he was influenced by the dynamic rise of radical politics in the *Vormärz*, the years leading up to the 1848 revolutions. Liberal-minded teachers exposed him to leftist politics and formed the intellectual circle of students who were fundamental to the politicization of his youth. Fellow students included Fanny Meyer, who became his first wife, and her sister, Sophie Meyer. After departing for the German universities, Minden and the Meyer sisters remained his home base as he pursued both his education and his political activities.[7]

During the revolutionary period of March 1848 to November 1849, Jacobi began his university education and simultaneously became absorbed in the struggle for liberal reforms against the German aristocracy. In a movement with socialist and pro-democracy elements, he joined the radical activists, who were intent on overthrowing autocratic rule and empowering the German people through revolutionary means. Leaving Minden in 1848, he first went to the University of Greifswald and tried to organize students and disseminate the writings of French socialists and banned German radicals. He moved on to Göttingen University and began his scientific education, spending two semesters studying pathological anatomy. Stopped by imperial troops from joining the Baden uprisings of 1849, Jacobi moved again, this time to the university in Bonn, where he began his clinical studies in medicine. In this more radically active locale, he joined the underground Communist League of Karl Marx and Friedrich Engels in nearby Cologne. It was in Bonn that he also met lifelong friend Carl Schurz, who was then plotting to free his mentor, the democratic activist Gottfried Kinkel, from the Spandau Prison. Until he received his medical degree in 1851, Jacobi continued to organize students and distribute radical materials at the university.[8]

As a student, Jacobi developed a radical philosophy that merged science and politics. Although he was interested early on in a variety of socialist thought, Jacobi became a committed Marxist, in that he was dedicated to the idea that a proletarian revolution could bring social and economic equality.[9] For Jacobi, the abolition of class differences went hand in hand with the downfall of the monarchy, and "democracy meant the total opposition to absolutism."[10] He supported a democratic, social revolution against both the Prussian monarchs, the Hohenzollerns, and the Catholic Church, which he believed oppressed the German peoples.[11] Anticlerical and against church power, Jacobi was also ideologically opposed to religious teachings and metaphysical thought. He valued materialism rather than spiritualism, and human beings over the mythical and invisible. Much like the young Mary Putnam, Abraham did not identify with his family's faith and believed in humanity over a deity, and building faith in a natural world that could be viewed and studied using the tools of science. He revealed these views in his medical thesis, *Cogitationes de vita rerum naturalium* (Thoughts on the Life of Natural Things).[12] Like many socialists, Jacobi also believed science was the best way to understand both the social and the natural worlds.

The teachings of Rudolf Virchow, the famed cellular pathologist and physician/reformer, instructed Jacobi in the inseparability of medical practice and social reform, and how medicine could eliminate social inequalities. Virchow famously declared, "Medicine is a social science, and politics nothing else but medicine on a larger scale." He also asserted that "physicians are the natural attorneys of the poor" or, in other words, physicians should lead social change and reform society based on physiological knowledge.[13] Using his research on cellular pathology, Virchow described the physiological body as a reflection of the social body. A response to humoralism and French empiricism, Virchow's research in cellular pathology centered on analyzing the malfunction of cells, and locating physical, not invisible, manifestations and etiologies of disease. This view imagined cells as equal components in a free system, like equal peoples in a democratic state.[14] Virchow said that a lack of freedom and prosperity, the absence of democracy and poor living conditions, produced unhealthy populations. He took part in a broad German medical reform movement that aimed to protect the medical profession from control by the absolutist state and to ensure "the right of each citizen to a healthful existence."[15] These goals merged with the revolutions of 1848, as Virchow connected the need for change to broader democratic agitation. As a result, he became a voice for the revolution, and his articles expressed growing dissatisfaction with both social and political conditions. His views inspired many young physicians, including the young Abraham Jacobi, who would see his role as a physician as essentially political.[16]

In April of 1851, Jacobi traveled to Berlin to take his state medical exam and to meet with a political comrade from Cologne. His colleague never arrived because he had been arrested in Leipzig. Jacobi himself was confronted by the Prussian police and arrested for radical activities. The police then searched

Jacobi's room in Berlin, his family home, and the home of the Meyer sisters and found banned materials, along with letters implicating several other activists. He and his colleagues were indicted for treason at the Cologne Communist Trial. Jacobi, specifically, was accused of distributing revolutionary literature, aiding fellow radicals, and plotting to overthrow the monarchy. He was ultimately acquitted on most counts but was found guilty of conspiring against the monarchy. Ultimately, he spent almost two years in prison, first in Cologne and then in Minden.[17]

When it appeared that he would be charged again, Jacobi fled from the Minden prison to England, following many other political activists who left Germany in search of a safe haven after 1848. There, he met Karl Marx and Friedrich Engels, expecting assistance from the now famous authors and fellow exiles. Although Jacobi managed to impress Marx with his medical thesis, Engels was irritated by the "little man," finding him ignorant, inexperienced, and intrusive for arriving at his home at 4 A.M. in need of lodging.[18] "This warlike Westphalian way of behaving" truly annoyed Engels, as did "the doltishness of [Jacobi] spending a whole week in London and then choosing a train that arrives in the middle of the night and, on the pretext of not knowing what's what, turning a man's house upside down and imposing himself."[19] Engels apparently "took the good party martyr by the collar" and sent him away to new lodgings.[20] The twenty-three-year-old then looked for ways to establish a medical practice in Manchester but found few opportunities in a town already heavily populated with doctors and German exiles. With reluctant support from Engels, who called him a "helpless sort of creature," Jacobi immigrated to the United States in 1853.[21] Fanny Meyer soon followed.

After a brief stay in Boston, Abraham Jacobi moved to New York and settled in the German district on the lower east side of Manhattan, known as *Kleindeutschland*, or "Little Germany." In the 1850s, it was a rapidly growing neighborhood that in the next three decades would house the third largest population of German-speaking peoples, after Berlin and Vienna.[22] A majority of these immigrants left central Europe as a result of economic stress caused by industrialization. Fleeing high land and food prices, artisans and farmers dominated the population of immigrants hoping to find better conditions in New York City. Some immigrants were able to continue to practice their skilled trades while others began to fill factory positions struggling at the bottom of the economic ladder. The wave of immigration also included "Forty-Eighters," like Jacobi and Schurz, who fled the German states after the revolutions in search of more friendly political and economic environs.[23]

In America, Jacobi continued his involvement in socialist politics. He joined workers associations, wrote for *Die Reform*, and continued to correspond with Marx and Engels. He took part in the creation of the New York Kommunisten Klub, or Communist Club, and the effort to mobilize German workers. Simultaneously, he set the groundwork for a unique and important career in medicine, believing that providing medical care to all classes was one path to creating a classless society.[24]

To serve the needy members of Kleindeutschland, in 1857 Jacobi and his colleagues established the German Dispensary of the City of New York at 132 Canal Street. Here, they fulfilled the medical reform agenda that had gone unrealized in midcentury Germany. But rather than plotting a political revolution, they initiated a revolution in medical care, one that encapsulated Virchow's teachings on social medicine and cellular pathology.[25] Jacobi, along with his colleagues, most importantly Emil Noeggerath and Ernst Krackowizer, both radical émigrés, used the German Dispensary as a mechanism for delivering medical care to the urban "sick and poor." Starting with 2,372 patients in the first year, their clientele grew steadily: by 1881, over 350,000 people had been served. The Dispensary was also able to employ physicians of German origins who had been excluded by the elites of the profession. They used the institution to build reputations, form community, and learn clinical medicine.[26] The Dispensary brought together a broad demographic of German immigrants that reflected the growing population in lower Manhattan.

In New York, Abraham Jacobi played a fundamental role in the development of pediatric medicine. His experience working with poor children inspired him to focus on the youngest of patients. He, like many Americans and Europeans, professional and bourgeois, began to believe that children deserved special treatment in the family and in society, and, therefore, in medicine. The new attitude toward children, who were becoming "economically useless and emotionally priceless," was inspired by Enlightenment philosophy, fueled by Victorian sentimental culture, and driven by industrialization and consumerism.[27] Rather than seeing children as sources of labor or animalistic, the nineteenth-century middle class now believed children were born as blank slates that needed to be protected, educated, and nurtured. These beliefs no doubt influenced the rise of pediatrics and had an impact on Abraham Jacobi. Shaped by his Virchovian ideology, he believed that all children entered the world as physiological equals and, with proper care and healthy living arrangements, could mature into equal citizens. He used his work at the Dispensary as a way to apply this philosophy to the immigrant population of Kleindeutschland.

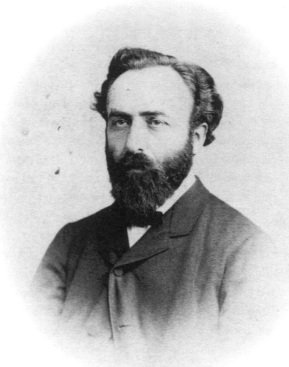

Abraham Jacobi, c. 1869. Courtesy of the
New York Academy of Medicine Library.

✦ ✦ ✦

He also used the institution to create a specialized knowledge about children, a science of pediatrics, as Russell Viner has shown.[28]

By the early 1870s, Abraham Jacobi had transformed himself from a struggling immigrant physician to a leading figure in the New York medical community. He led the movement to create a specific body of knowledge on children's diseases and therapeutic remedies aimed at young patients. As a consequence, he had a long career working and directing programs at a number of the city's institutions. He received his first faculty appointment as professor of Infantile Pathology and Therapeutics at the New York Medical College (1860–64) as the first chair of diseases of children in the United States. Jacobi then moved to the University of the City of New York (1865–70). But it was during his long career at Columbia University's College of Physicians and Surgeons as professor of the diseases of children from 1870 to 1902 that he was most productive in building a foundation for his specialty. During this period he also served on the staff at several New York hospitals, including the German Hospital (Lenox Hill), Mount Sinai Hospital, where he was a founder of the Department of Pediatrics, the Nursery and Child's Hospital, and Roosevelt Hospital.[29]

When they met in 1871, Mary Putnam had just returned from Paris as a witness to the Commune. She not only admired but romanticized Abraham Jacobi, whose reputation as a Forty-Eighter was well known. He was older, wiser, and influential in New York medical circles. His European origins, radical past, imprisonment, and exile made him intriguing if not a little mysterious to Putnam. Looking back, she said she was drawn to him because of his "individual and youthful tendency, to revolutionary innovation, [a] tendency which attracted me, and to which my own innate tendencies affiliated." She was clearly enticed by his radical spirit, "more so . . . than he ever understood," she added.[30] Abraham had many of the qualities of her former fiancés. Like her first, Ferdinand Mayer, Abraham was a man of science, an immigrant, and a Jewish intellectual. Like her second, Monsieur M. in France, Abraham was a physician and active in European radical politics. For Mary, Abraham surpassed these other men in both experience and status, and through him she could strongly connect her European past and her American future.

Before meeting Abraham, Mary Putnam spent years wondering if she wanted to become a wife, and mother, at all. One year into her Paris sojourn, she told her mother, "I have no particular desire to marry at any time."[31] And in a letter to her sister Edith she said of her little brothers, they "are all the children I ever expect to have."[32] But, she conceded, if "I should ever come across a physician, intelligent, refined, more enthusiastic for his science than me . . . I think I would marry such a person if he asked me, and would leave me full liberty to exercise my profession."[33] Putnam realized that her personal life needed to accommodate her public role as a doctor, and that marrying another physician was the best way to preserve her professional autonomy. Not unlike the character of Professor Fritz Bhaer, Jo's German mentor and love interest in Louisa May Alcott's *Little Women*, all signs indicated that Abraham would be Mary's intellectual partner, both a critic and a confidant in her professional life.

Mary Putnam also desired a marriage that reflected her own gender politics, that is, one based on equality between the sexes. She had been impressed with the intellectual and egalitarian marriages of the Reclus brothers in Paris. In this, she shared the marriage ideal of many nineteenth-century feminists, who called for uniting private and public life through harmonious unions based on sexual, intellectual, and economic equality.[34] Although she claimed to want to marry her "superior," someone of greater intelligence and accomplishments who could challenge and guide her, she insisted that men and women should be equally free to pursue their professional work.[35]

A surprising number of women physicians in the nineteenth century — 25–35 percent — were married, a high percentage compared to the marriage rates for women in other professions. Historians explain this pattern in a number of ways. Some scholars point to the greater flexibility of medical work, in that women could be self-employed or establish a home office that connected professional and private life. Some reason that men in the medical and scientific communities were more accepting of women in professional roles. Finally, by marrying, women doctors found a way to form a strong connection between professional and community life.[36]

Mary Putnam Jacobi contended that medicine had a particular "adaptability" that made it possible to combine marriage, family, and professional pursuits. According to her, medicine was a lifelong commitment, an endeavor that needed to be maintained throughout one's life. A woman trained in medicine could have children during her first years of practice, when she had fewer clients and lighter demands. After a woman had children, her career could thrive, for, Jacobi believed, "the organic vigor of women is naturally destined to be increased by child-bearing." In addition, "modern industries" contributed to the reduction in household work, freeing up women to conduct their professional work, she explained.[37] In her own household, a team of four to six servants made her professional life possible. For example, at one point the Jacobi family had three servants, a cook, an office maid, and a chambermaid.[38]

However, as Mary Putnam Jacobi knew full well, marriage and medicine did not always coexist without conflict. She warned her students in 1880 that marriage, "which complicates everything else in the life of women, cannot fail to complicate their professional life." But, she asserted, problems could be alleviated with "more complete intellectual development," for "more perfect training enables the woman to cope with the peculiar difficulties inherent in her destiny."[39] Again, education and training could resolve even the most personal conflicts in a woman's life.

While marriage could be challenging for a woman doctor, it was absolutely desirable for men like Abraham Jacobi, who preferred spousal companionship and was married three times. His first wife, Fanny Meyer, was a young woman in the village of Minden who was in Jacobi's socialist-revolutionary circle. While we know little about their life together, we do know that the couple occupied two homes in New York, the first on Forsythe Street and the second on Christie Street, both on the southwest end of Kleindeutschland.[40] As Abraham began his work at the German Dispensary and confronted the suffering of immigrant children, he faced personal pain of his own. In 1855, he and Fanny lost their one-day-old son, Julius, who died from meningitis. The following year, Fanny died at the young age of twenty-three from "phlebitis," likely a blood clot resulting from another pregnancy.[41] Despite this loss, Jacobi stayed connected to the Meyer family through a friendship with Fanny's sister, Sophie Meyer Boas, and by forming a bond with Sophie's son, Franz. Over the years, as "Onkel Jacobi," Abraham provided financial and professional support, as well as personal advice on marriage and moving to the United States, to his nephew, who eventually became a founder of modern anthropology.[42]

Abraham's second marriage was to the nineteen-year-old Kate Rosalie, who was more of a domestic partner than a political comrade. The daughter of immigrants (her father from Ireland and her mother from France), she was originally from the South, most likely born in Georgia.[43] The couple first lived on Amity Street, west of and outside the parameters of Little Germany, and then they moved to a larger home on West 34th Street.[44] With two servants and a cook, Kate oversaw the domestic sphere.[45] But for most of their marriage, she was extremely ill. Mary described Abraham's second wife as "a sickly patient of his own, whom he was unable to rescue from eight years of wretched invalidism."[46] His life with Kate was consumed by the loss of four infant children and the dangers of her failed pregnancies. Kate had two stillborn children in 1863, one in January and another in September.[47] The next baby, coincidentally named "Mary," lived one day and died of a "debility," according to Abraham, the attending physician.[48] A "male infant" also succumbed to a "general debility" and "premature birth" in 1868.[49] Pregnant for at least the fifth time, Kate died in 1871 from "acute nephritis" resulting from a miscarriage at seven weeks.[50] Coinciding with his growing activity and leadership in the field of pediatrics, Abraham Jacobi's personal bereavement moved him to take action against infant mortality in the city.

By the time he met Mary Putnam, Abraham had suffered tremendous personal loss, experiencing the death of two wives and five infants, not counting the known and unknown number of miscarriages. Twelve years his junior, Mary Putnam was not only intellectually compatible, but she seemed ready to bear children. She was in good health and extremely knowledgeable about obstetrics and pediatric medicine. Although Mary rejected the notion that women were destined solely for motherhood, she believed reproduction was a healthy process of nutrition in the female body.[51] Ultimately, she embraced the idea of giving her husband the family that had eluded him for so many years.

But Mary also worried about the survival of their children, and rightly so. Just eight months after they married, the couple lost their first child. Abraham Jacobi attended the birth of "a female child" that lived one day and died in their home on West 34th Street. The infant succumbed to what was then known as "Atelectasis pulmonum (from intrauterine respiration)," a congenital disease of the lungs observed mostly in newborns and infants.[52] When the lungs failed to expand, portions of the pulmonary tissue did not fill with air. The baby would have arrived without crying, or possibly with only a whimper; she would have been extremely pale and with little muscular movement. As her parents watched, the child would have breathed more and more slowly, or went into sharp convulsions, until death. Although Mary and Abraham searched for a clinical explanation, the cause of the disease was uncertain. Physicians believed the condition could form in utero due to poor fetal development or the ill health of the mother; it could also emerge at delivery, due to poor hygiene or a rushed labor in which the placenta was released too early. Lastly, a child's air passages could be obstructed with mucus.[53] Disappointed yet still hopeful, Mary told her brother Bishop, "I always felt that my first baby would not live, — I can scarcely know why, except that a great misfortune so often precedes a great happiness."[54]

One year later, Mary was pregnant again. In the early summer of 1875, with her due date approaching, the couple debated whether they should take their annual summer leave to Lake George for the delivery. Mary's colleagues, doctors Emily Blackwell and Isaac Adler, as well as her brother Haven, all urged her to remain in the city. But Mary and Abraham decided to travel upstate and deliver in their summer home, believing there was no advantage to staying in Manhattan, since there were no other physicians in the city who knew more about obstetrics than they did. The couple also knew that they could call on a local doctor for assistance. Despite their professional self-confidence, in the days approaching the delivery, both doctors were full of anxiety. Mary worried about the pressure on Abraham to successfully attend the birth, believing he was "too *excitable* about what *touches him* nearly."[55] As she told her mother, "My Doctor is in a most exalted state of mind. If everything goes right, he will be in the 7th heaven. But, what an *if*."[56]

The journey to Lake George was long and tiring, particularly for an expectant mother. The Jacobis first boarded a train in Manhattan, headed north along

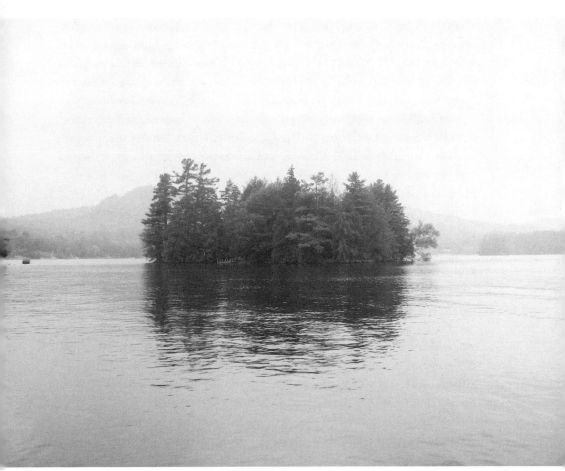

Hiawatha Island, Lake George, N.Y., 2007. Photograph by the author.
Printed with permission of Mary Martialay and Judy Martialay.

·✦· ·✦· ·✦·

the Hudson River to Fort Edward, and changed trains to Glens Falls; they then took a coach for ten miles on a plank road to the foot of Lake George near Fort William Henry. There, they boarded the *Minnehaha*, a paddleboat that transported them up the lake to Bolton Landing. At that point, they took a rowboat to Hiawatha Island, which was tucked into Huddle Bay on the western shore. Jacobi had purchased Hiawatha Island (named for the Native American legend and character in the poem by Henry Wadsworth Longfellow) in 1867 for fifty dollars, and it became his retreat from city life.[57] In 1875, he bought more property on the shores of Bolton Landing. Heavily wooded, the environs reminded him of his native Germany and the Black Forest.[58]

In the 1870s, Lake George was just emerging as a fashionable vacation spot for New Yorkers, the wealthy as well as the city's intelligentsia. The Jacobis were a part of this development, gathering with like-minded friends on what became known as Jacobi Point. Over the years, Abraham created a family compound, building a cottage for himself and his wife, one next door for the Schurz family, and eventually, a boathouse and a large home for his daughter, her children, and her husband. The Jacobi and Schurz families spent many summers together at Lake George, and while the children swam, canoed, and played, the adults wandered in the woods, talked politics, put on small plays, and wrote articles, letters, and their memoirs. They also visited Alma Farm, a 1,050-acre working farm and social meeting place established in 1875 by Theodore Meyer. Other guests included physician Ernst Krackowizer and Jacobi's nephews, physician Willy Meyer and anthropologist Franz Boas, who brought his wife and children. With several visitors of German origin, many connected to science, European radical politics, or both, Alma Farm formed an intellectual congress of liberal thinkers.[59] Much like a rural salon, Alma Farm guests engaged in lively discussions, often in German, reminisced about their youth in Europe, and talked politics. Mary Putnam Jacobi not only loved the environment of Lake George but easily immersed herself in this intellectual milieu, which was strongly reminiscent of the atmosphere at Vascoeuil, the French country retreat she frequented with the Reclus family.

Hiawatha Island would always have special meaning for Abraham Jacobi, since it was where his first child to survive infancy was born. On 3 August 1875, Mary began her labor in their dark and secluded island cabin. With just the light of candles or oil lamps, Abraham attended to his wife into the evening. According to family lore, at some point he decided to seek another doctor or midwife; but just as he stepped on to his rowboat, he heard the cries of a baby.[60] As the tale goes, Mary gave birth to Ernst on her own.

Named for their late friend, fellow physician, and Forty-Eighter Ernst Krackowizer, this infant son symbolized renewed hope for his father, who desperately wanted a child after so many losses. Mary told her mother: "The doctor's happiness in the baby, is so intense as to be touching and almost awful."[61] During a family voyage to Europe the following year, she wrote, "I know that few things would make the Doctor forego the pleasure of transcribing on the passenger list, 'Dr. Jacobi and family,' and details about the baby that would be considered a nuisance by so many, seem to furnish him with only additional interest and amusement."[62] Mary also showed great pleasure in her child, watching Abraham talking and singing to the baby in German, showering him with tremendous affection. But she was characteristically more reticent and analytical, even pensive, about the arrival of her first baby. Unable to separate medicine and maternity, her thoughts traveled between the sentimental and the academic, admiring her son's adorable qualities and then contemplating the science of breast-feeding and human evolution. She reflected on his innocence and the androgynous characteristics of infants: "A baby is not even a boy or a girl but just a baby, and that is really something wonderful."[63] She was most concerned with her child's survival, counting the days of Ernst's young life and hoping that the passage of time would secure his health and protect him from danger.[64]

Certainly, the Jacobi family was fragile, made clear by their first diphtheria scare in 1877. As Mary's mother, Victorine, told her daughter Amy: "We have had an anxiety about Minnie [Mary]. She had a sore throat with diphtheria patches, so she sent Ernst and Mary [Louise] over here to stay a day and night. But, the second day the patches disappeared under treatment, and the Doctor was as anxious about Ernst being out of his sight, that they recalled him, and Minnie was to exile herself from him. She is quite better now."[65] Mary showed signs of diphtheria, causing Abraham such fierce anxiety about the safety of his son that he brought Ernst home and banished his wife. In the course of their work, both parents certainly would have been exposed to the disease and have witnessed its havoc. The thought that Ernst would become a statistic, one of the increasing numbers of children ill with diphtheria, was unthinkable.

Soon after, Ernst came down with an "attack of pneumonia." The little boy's illness, again, scared the entire family but jarred Abraham to the core: "The Dr. of course is overcome with anxiety always at the least appearance of discomfort in the boy," Victorine observed.[66] "It was pitiful," she remarked, "to see the Dr.'s absorption in him. . . . It frightens me to think of the possibility of the dear child not living."[67] Undoubtedly, Ernst was Abraham's greatest joy and took precedence above all else. The child brought Mary happiness as well, but of a different kind, mainly, "the hope of seeing [him] grow up with a fundamental likeness to his father, in body and soul."[68] Although she scoffed at women who looked at their children as "compensation" for their husbands, Ernst brought her closer to Abraham and was now the glue in their marriage. Her mother realized that the baby now constituted the couple's fragile bond: "Ernst is a darling child. I tremble to think how much they depend upon him for their happiness. . . . One child is a terrible anxiety."[69] The boy overcame his pneumonia and while the doctors always remained concerned, they delighted in the birth of a second child, Marjorie, in 1878.

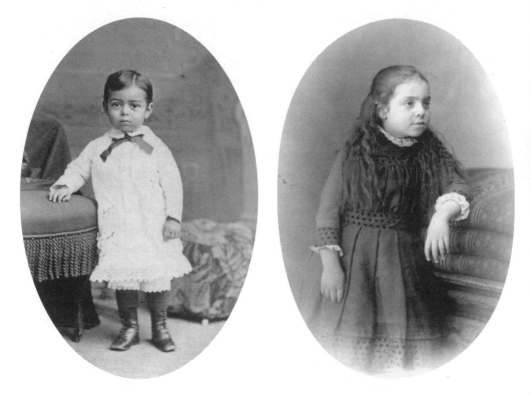

LEFT Ernst Jacobi. Courtesy of Prints and Photographs Division, Library of Congress.
RIGHT Marjorie Jacobi. Courtesy of Prints and Photographs Division, Library of Congress.

·✦·✦·✦·

The Jacobi marriage was now child-centered, just like Abraham's professional life. Ernst and Marjorie formed the heart of their home and emotional lives. As Mary said, "They are . . . our constant companions. . . [and] we never have any greater enjoyment than their companionship." The children were raised to reflect their parents' politics and values, as the couple worked intensely to shape them into good thinkers and citizens. Mary boasted of their effective parenting style to her second cousin, Mary Tyler Peabody Mann, wife of Horace Mann and sister of Elizabeth Palmer Peabody, all educators and reformers.[70] The doctors Jacobi were intensely didactic parents, constantly encouraging the children to study and learn a wide range of subjects. Abraham was determined to teach the children German, making it the dominant language in his home. Ernst and Marjorie responded well: "They think the acquisition of new knowledge or new ideas, the most delightful possible pursuit," Mary wrote. The couple had high expectations, wanting their children to have sharp and curious minds, acquire a wide range of knowledge, and share in their parents' lives and interests. Although they were allowed to play, play was edifying and practical; the children were exposed to "true" stories, not "fairy stories." Spiritually, the Jacobis taught them their own values: "They have never heard of religion, or even the name of God or the Bible: they therefore never ask who made them, nor who lives in the sky, nor where they would go if they died." Mary believed Ernst and Marjorie were "perfectly sympathetic to their parents" and to each other. She remarked that "the mutual sympathy, confidence, and pleasure is so great, that we have nothing to do but just live into their lives and allow them to live into ours."[71]

If the arrival of children nourished the Jacobi marriage, other factors weakened their bond, including their different temperaments. Extremely bold and eager to speak her mind, Mary was independent and determined to live life on her own terms. Although her husband was joyful around the children, Mary thought he was "unsocial" with adults and did not easily mix with new people; he was most comfortable in the company of old friends, preferring fellow physicians and activists, most importantly, Carl Schurz. A former Union army general who became a leading Republican as well as a journalist, orator, reformer, and the first German-born U.S. senator, Schurz shared Jacobi's political sensibility and memories of European radicalism. The two men were often described as "inseparable."[72] Over time, Abraham found intellectual inspiration more often in his male companions than in his wife. While she cared deeply for her children, she was not a model of nineteenth-century maternalism and did not relish their daily care. Abraham, by contrast, was more affectionate with the children, playing, cuddling, and singing them lullabies. Mary acknowledged their different parental relationships, predicting Ernst would adore his father and see her more as the disciplinarian and custodian.[73]

The two doctors disagreed on the gendered roles of parenthood, particularly how to manage the responsibilities of the household. Though Abraham felt personally attached to the children, he believed that overseeing their care ultimately stood with Mary. Although they employed a nurse and other household servants, Abraham expected that his wife would make the professional and personal sacrifices needed to raise a family. Their conflict over parental roles brewed for years, but it came to a head in the spring of 1883, following a birthday celebration for Carl Schurz. Both had been invited to the party, but Abraham believed that "some one had to stay at home with the children," and it should have been Mary, considering he was "*the* oldest friend of C.S." When she went to Schurz's on her own, Abraham refused to go. Following the incident, he confronted her over dinner about her behavior, prompting her to walk away from the table and leave the house, most likely to stay with Victoria White, a colleague and collaborator.[74] Abraham was angered by her disappearance and her mysterious whereabouts, although he suspected that she was in the city, "as on former occasions." Clearly, this was not the first time that Mary fled in anger from the expectations of marriage and motherhood.[75]

The couple had great difficulty working out a peaceful coexistence, or, as Abraham described it, "a quiet and rational modus vivendi." Mary insisted on living and working by her own decisions, and her husband grew more irritated with her actions. Believing in the similarities between men and women, or fathers and mothers, she saw no need to make serious concessions to her husband. Although progressive in his thinking, Abraham thought she was ungrateful for not acknowledging his support for her professional status. In a letter to Mary during her absence, he wrote, "If you had less temper, and more patience, and a less exaggerated conviction of what is due to you, you might have recognized the fact that I have done a great deal for you." But what Abraham saw as a "quiet and rational" existence, Mary saw as confinement.[76]

In the summer of 1883, not long after the squabble over Schurz's party, diphtheria spread throughout the city, and both Jacobi children fell ill from the disease. Marjorie survived, but Ernst died on 10 June.[77] Abraham was particularly devastated, especially because his only son died from a disease that he had spent years fighting, a disease that was supposed to kill the children of tenement-dwellers and recent immigrants, not of physicians. Abraham's grief was so severe that Mary could hardly think of her own, as she remarked to Toni and Sophie Boas: "The loss of this darling boy has been so overwhelmingly terrible to the doctor, that I have scarcely dared to think of myself. You could imagine what the loss of any son must be to him, — after he had waited so long for one."[78]

Marjorie, at five, felt her brother's absence intensely and while still recovering from diphtheria, she asked for him, continuously, which intensified the stress of her father and mother. Anguished and frustrated, Mary silenced her: "Do not ask for him anymore, he has left us and will not return."[79] But the pain of losing her constant companion stayed with Marjorie for years. Mary described how her daughter changed: "I seem to see her deprived of the halo with which she was formerly surrounded by Ernst's love for her, which was most exquisite. These two children lived in each other."[80] In the years to come, Marjorie, as their only surviving child, lived in the shadow of Ernst and embodied all remaining hope in the family.

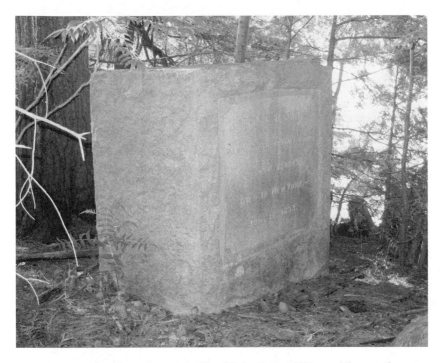

Ernst Jacobi Memorial, Hiawatha Island, Lake George, N.Y., 2007. Photograph by the author. Printed with permission of Mary Martialay and Judy Martialay.

⸱✦⸱ ⸱✦⸱ ⸱✦⸱

Mary handled the loss of Ernst by reliving the decisions made about his care. She punished herself for not being able to save him: "I feel sometimes as if the whole world must stand and hoot at me for my inability to retain this lovely child, when he had once been entrusted to me. — This rooted feeling of self contempt perhaps in one way helps me to bear this terrible grief, though in other ways it makes it worse."[81] During the next year, she found relief in being away from home and all the physical reminders of Ernst's death.

The Jacobis' mourning was profound and lengthy. The boy was buried, along with Abraham's other wives and children, near a large gravestone marked "The Babies" at Green-Wood Cemetery in Brooklyn. But Hiawatha Island, Ernst's place of birth, became the real shrine to his memory. Near the shore at the north end of the island Abraham erected a monument. The five-ton granite mass, still standing on the island today, reads: "ERNST JACOBI. BORN ON HIAWATHA ISLAND. AUGUST 3RD 1875. DIED IN NEW YORK. JUNE 10th 1883." Reportedly, Abraham visited the island and memorial every year on the anniversary of Ernst's death.[82] Mary, too, continued to mourn her son. In June

Calling card from Mary Putnam
Jacobi to Fanny Garrison Villard,
14 November 1890. Reproduced
with permission of the Houghton
Library, Harvard University.

❋·❋·❋

1890, she called upon her friend Fanny Garrison Villard, the only daughter of abolitionist William Lloyd Garrison, who had just lost her own son, Henry Hilgard, also at age seven. Fanny was either not home or too deep in mourning to receive guests, so Mary left a calling card, with a note: "Dear Mrs. Villard, It was on this same day, seven years ago that our dear boy also was snatched away from us. You may know then how we can feel for you."[83]

Mary Putnam Jacobi and Abraham Jacobi, two of New York's most prominent physicians, struggled for the rest of their lives over their inability to save Ernst. Years after his death, Mary reflected upon the loss of her son in a letter to her future son-in-law, George McAneny. She revealed some of the painful dynamics of her marriage at the time of Ernst's illness: "Dr. Jacobi . . . would not listen to my words of apprehension. And I having naturally a great confidence in his professional opinion and knowing his great love for our little son, did not sufficiently urge the different precautions about his health, which I now think might have sufficiently increased his power of resistance when the trial came, to have enabled him to escape as Marjorie did."[84] Mary had struck out the "k" in "know," suggesting that she "now" knew hers was the correct course of action. But at the time of Ernst's illness, she deferred to her husband regarding the management of diphtheria in the home. She had reservations about his handling of the situation but chose to stand back, knowing that Abraham would, ultimately, take charge of his son's health. Fifteen years later, she wished she had more strongly questioned her husband's authority. She also lamented that they had not taken protective measures and recognized that their children were not immune. In coping with their son's death, questions about the etiology and transmission of diphtheria became a fault line in the marriage.

The rift between the two physicians remained open for years. Family members recalled that the couple blamed each other for the death of Ernst and thereafter "carr[ied] on separately."[85] The two physicians, dedicated to saving the lives of other children, were unable to save their own child. For the Jacobis, this was tragic and unthinkable, considering they had the greatest authority and knowledge on pediatric illnesses, especially diphtheria. The loss of Ernst also tested their faith, for science could not save their son. The ambiguities and mysteries of diphtheria meant there was not a definite therapeutic or prophylactic solution but great uncertainty. In a marriage spanning over three decades, Ernst's death caused great stress, impacting their medical and political bonds, the very foundation of their union.

Medicine and Activism

Interested in promoting democracy through a unified social order, the Jacobis believed equal health and equal living conditions were the key ingredients to creating a just society. As medical activists, they believed in the power of science to create social unity and ameliorate human suffering. But while the physicians cared deeply about both the labor question and the woman question, they had different political priorities. Mary saw gender as the great divide in American society; Abraham believed class divisions stood as the largest barriers to true democracy. This played out theoretically, in their political philosophies, and in practice, as they promoted the health of children. Abraham hoped equal medical care for children would fundamentally undermine social hierarchies; Mary believed that educating women on physiology and good hygiene would produce healthier children and stronger mothers who could strive for equal treatment in the social organism. With different political emphases, the Jacobis also perceived gender and sex differences in unique ways. But they shared a faith in science and social reform.

Abraham Jacobi's political activism in the American context found its greatest expression in medicine, which he saw as the ultimate democratic project. Although Abraham remained conscious of the relationship between class and industrialization, he evolved from being a Marxist interested in revolution, to a socialist who believed in democracy and the power of the state to create social, economic, and material equality.[86] In the United States, already defined as a democracy, the goal was to fulfill the promises of that system, rather than to take it down. Though he would have identified as a Republican during the Civil War and in the Reconstruction era, he centered his activism on medicine and reform rather than on party politics.

According to Abraham Jacobi, providing medical care to all members of society was a state responsibility and a collective obligation. Reflecting his

Virchovian ideals and democratic socialism, he believed that society as a whole should provide for communities in need. Such action helped sustain the health of the social organism. He explained, "Society in general is benefited either by or suffering from its constituent parts, and therefore the care of the individual is a matter of common concern. If there is any meaning in the principle of general solidarity, it includes the right of every individual to a healthy body and a sound education."[87] Failure to help those in need unjustly hurt individuals, as well as the greater populace: "Society itself, the State, must be considered responsible for the life of every human being that can be saved. It is a duty, not good-will. It is good policy . . . to practise charity. Human society has committed both a blunder and a crime when a member that could be saved, physically, suffers death; when a member whose soul and heart might have been kept pure, will sin."[88] For Abraham Jacobi, in a true republican state, good health was a right that needed to be secured by government and the people. As did his wife, he believed, "The condition of every individual is intimately connected with the structure of society."[89]

Abraham Jacobi also argued that the profession of medicine itself, its members and its societies, should reflect democratic principles. In New York, medicine brought together physicians from around the world in common cause, and in its population of practitioners, the profession reflected the international character of the American commonwealth. He even acknowledged its role in harboring "fugitive republicans of Europe," like himself. In this idealistic vision, physicians of different national origins worked together, modeling greater social harmony, and in turn, "the unity of science may be but the precursor of the unity of mankind."[90]

While the Jacobis agreed on many political principles, Abraham's gender politics revolved around his vision of democratic socialism rather than a specific commitment to female equality. Rectifying economic and political inequalities via medicine was his main objective, and he saw women as part of a broader struggle to expand democratic rights to all people. Looking back, he recounted, "Personally I had no difficulty in settling the woman question in accordance with the principle of the Declaration of Independence of July 4th, 1776, which recognizes no distinction as to color, religion, or sex." In other words, he saw inequality as not a matter limited to women but a broader concern. Not willing to isolate or prioritize women's demands, he commented, "I never was a fanatic adherent of the woman movement, nor ever maliciously opposed to it, I have calmly looked on and watched conditions develop." He admitted that "only on rare occasions have I helped it along."[91]

Despite his reluctance to associate directly with the women's rights move-ment, Abraham Jacobi believed women should fully participate in the medical profession. He supported membership of both sexes because it was a matter of "justice or equity" and "giving every member of human society a chance to develop his or her faculties." It was the right choice, he said, to commit to "equal rights and universal solidarity, in a truly republican spirit." New York took the lead in welcoming women into the profession; it was a city where "differences of sex are not taken notice of" in medical circles, he said, perhaps too optimistically.[92] As president of the Medical Society of the County of New York in 1871, he boasted of recent changes in his own organization: "We have opened our doors to worthy members of the medical profession, male or female, white or colored, and thus granted reality to the gospel of American citizenship, the Declaration of Independence, according to which we are all free and equal." He asserted that the Society had "co-operated in solving the woman question in our department."[93]

Mary Putnam Jacobi agreed that her husband had been a significant ally of women in medicine. She openly acknowledged that he was especially impor-tant for promoting her own career. She attributed her smooth entrance into the New York Academy of Medicine and several medical societies, including the New York Pathological Society, the New York Neurological Society, and the Therapeutical Society of New York, to his assistance. In an essay on the history of women in medicine, she spoke of herself in the third person and described his role: "The facile admission of Dr. Putnam to these various privileges, in New York, at a time that the propriety of female 'recognition' was still being so hotly disputed in other cities, was due partly to the previously acquired honor of the Paris diploma; partly to the influence of Dr. Jacobi."[94] Despite his strong influence in most medical circles, Abraham Jacobi had little sway over the New York Obstetrical Society, from which she was denied access by "means of blackballs" in 1878.[95] Society records show that after she received endorsements from several physicians, her "application was voted upon and passed." However, two months later, in another round of voting, she was turned town with ten votes for and thirteen against. Abraham voiced some protest, asking to speak at the next meeting to "consider the treatment by the society of the last 3 candidates for fellowship." He was not present at the following meeting, however, and Mary Putnam Jacobi's application was subsequently dropped.[96]

The Jacobis also had divergent opinions about gender and the meaning of womanhood. Unlike Mary, who believed in sex similarities and equality in parenting, Abraham believed women had special characteristics that suited them for unique roles. For example, at first he hesitated to support coeducation, particularly in medicine. He did rethink this stance and eventually supported coeducation for the good of the "public" and to create a universal standard of medical training. He also said that women would have a "stimulating and ennobling influence upon the male youth. [The men] will not make so much noise, have fewer duels, be more gentlemanly, and will do better work."[97] In other words, Abraham backed coeducation for the safety of patients and because women had a civilizing influence, not because they deserved an equal education. In another example, he described the moral obligation for women to care for children: "All the working powers of an entire woman are necessary for forming brave men out of little children." Abraham called working women who were well-to-do "immoral," unless, that is, they worked in medical institutions for the poor.[98] But, regrettably, women physicians who left their children needed to hire help. While Mary's employment at the infirmary fit his moral schema, tension over managing work and family certainly existed in their home.

The Jacobis did agree to support common political causes at the intersection of labor and women's health. While Mary worked in the Consumer's League, seeking better working conditions for women in the city, Abraham spoke in favor of protective legislation for female workers who spent their days toiling in factories or doing painstaking work at home. In his experience as a physician, "Hundreds of them pass before my mind's eye. Hundreds of cases of misery I remember that lasted through decades, and scores I have seen die in their young years."[99] Deplorable working conditions, illness, and deprivation resulted from industrial capitalism, he said. "I know of only one prescription; that is a different configuration of human society, with less individualism, more solidarity, and more sense of responsibility on the part of society and state."[100] Socialism and solidarity would inspire change, he promised, through reform and legislation, not revolution, as he thought years earlier in Europe. Both Mary and Abraham used their voices as physicians to speak out on behalf of working women struggling in the city.

Inspired by radical movements against tyranny in Europe, the Jacobis both altered their social agendas in the United States, believing in reform rather than revolt, evolution rather than revolution. They ideologically remained "socialists," reflecting and refracting their ideas into the American context. Abraham continued to call himself a "Social-Democrat," while Mary identified as a socialist, "not in the sense of being a Communist or an Anarchist or a single-tax fanatic," she said, but as one who believed in the unbreakable unity, interdependence, and cooperation of the social organism.[101] By the end of the century, they had both turned to Progressive types of activism, believing society would gradually cure the diseases caused by industrialization and eventually that the complete rights of all citizens would be secured. In their medical practice, in the dispensaries and clinics of Manhattan, pediatrics served them not merely as a field of specialized knowledge but as a movement aimed at rectifying physical and social ills.[102] While the two doctors shared in this political project, their views on the applications of science in medicine often diverged.

Good Science?

Although Mary Putnam Jacobi and Abraham Jacobi shared a deep faith in science, differences emerged in their approach to pediatric medicine, as well as how they defined "good science." They had unique views because of their medical training and sources of influence. Educated in the 1850s, Abraham brought to his practice mid-nineteenth-century German knowledge, the strong influence of Virchow and cellular pathology, and a professional interest in the power of the pediatric physician. Trained almost two decades later, Mary shared an interest in pathology but was influenced more by the climate of Paris medicine in the late 1860s and the age of Claude Bernard. While both physicians treated and researched childhood disease, Abraham was the "pediatrician" and the "father" of the field, winning great honors and accolades as a man of medicine. Mary, on the other hand, though a practitioner and advocate for women and children, resisted identification with pediatrics and obstetrics. She preferred to be known as a generalist, rather than a woman practitioner who treated only mothers and babies. Working together and independently, they tried to integrate scientific practices into the clinic, and particularly, into the treatment of children. However, the two doctors disagreed on how science should be applied, and they focused their energies on childhood medicine in distinct ways.

In post–Civil War America, physicians transformed pediatric medicine into a specialty, and the Jacobis were central figures in this process. The medical movement toward specialization and the efforts to make medicine more "scientific" combined to promote a field of study focused on children. As a consequence, the management of children's health moved from the home to the hospital, from the control of mothers to the oversight of experts. But the emergence of "child-centeredness" in American culture also supported the creation of pediatric medicine.[103] Infant and childhood mortality remained high, about 20 percent in the middle years of the nineteenth century, and more and more middle-class parents sought out expert advice and treatment for their children.[104]

Reformers believed that urban working-class and poor families, who were hit hard by childhood disease, required extensive medical attention as well. In the cities, childhood illness was increasingly visible, and physicians pointed to its sources: poverty, lack of sanitation, poor housing, and, above all, malnutrition. For reformers, both the religious and medically minded, addressing the problem of needy and dependent children became a high priority. But rather than promoting religious institutions, physicians like Mary Putnam Jacobi and Abraham Jacobi argued that the future health of children rested on science.

Abraham Jacobi believed that physicians were responsible for both ensuring children's health and upholding republican political ideals. Later, reflecting on the role of children's medicine in society, he wrote: "Pedology is the science of the young. The young are the future makers and owners of the world. Their physical, intellectual and moral condition will decide whether the globe will be more Cossack or more Republican, more criminal or more righteous. For their education and training and capabilities, the physician, mainly the pediatrist, as the representative of medical science and art, should become responsible."[105] Jacobi envisioned a world where the pediatric specialist, or "pediatrist," occupied policymaking roles in all social and legal arenas, including schools, legislatures, and courtrooms. The pediatrician, in other words, would serve as the ultimate leader of social reform within a democratic state.

Infant nutrition emerged as a major issue in the new field of pediatrics, reflecting the medicalization of infant feeding and high infant mortality rates due to malnutrition and poor hygiene. In 1879, Abraham Jacobi noted that 40 percent of all infant deaths were caused by diseases of the digestive organs, marked by severe diarrhea and dysentery, often related to summer complaint, or cholera infantum (now called E. coli or salmonella). Viral and bacterial infections transmitted by unclean hands, linen, bottles, or contaminated food, milk, or water were largely responsible, though some children suffered directly from malnutrition and dehydration as well as food allergies.[106] Expert advice on feeding abounded with the increasing threat of childhood death from a variety of nutritional failures.[107] Physicians now directed mothers in how to properly feed children, extending their scientific expertise into the family domain.

Abraham Jacobi first addressed the nutrition issue in 1868, when he gave the New York Board of Health a list of recommendations for the systematic improvement of infant health, titled "Rules for Feeding Babies." In 1873, he published the "Rules" as *Infant Diet*, the first American treatise on feeding and a directive to public health officials for solving the child health crisis in the tenements.[108] Jacobi stated that mother's milk was most appropriate for infants but also recommended that some amount of wheat, oatmeal, and barley be included in infant diets. In the summer, he explained, heat inhibited proper nutrition and children died "from the heat [that] has weakened the digestion, reduced nervous force, and thus paved the way for gastro-intestinal catarrh and cholera infantum."[109] He also warned against overfeeding and of the poor effects of foul air, recommending cool baths in the summer, moderate proportions of food, and additional dietary supplements, including drops of whiskey. His recommendations incorporated medical information and "physiological facts," yet they were deliberately "simple" so they could be followed by an audience of any class or educational level.

Always politically minded in pediatrics, Abraham Jacobi saw his model for infant feeding as a vehicle for promoting human solidarity. His recommendations required little money and little expertise and therefore were open to all mothers. "It appears that, in our times of vast class differences amongst the nations of the earth," he commented "there is some sort of equality, at least at a certain period of life: equal laws and equal conditions."[110] By promoting mother's milk and pure barley over cow's milk and commercial food, he equated "natural" food with social equality. While some manufactured food had been helpful, he admitted, it was synthetic and tainted by economic interests. He insisted that "unvarying truth is in nature only; and that trade, or money, has no soul nor conscience."[111] Though he favored natural feeding methods, he constructed a particular version of the natural, one that privileged breast milk but allowed for several additions, including alcohol, grains, sugar, and baking soda. He privileged medical knowledge over maternal knowledge and wanted his public health audience in New York to know that science was the key to understanding the needs of infants, and to producing equality via infant feeding.

The Jacobis collaborated on a second version of *Infant Diet*, composed on their honeymoon and then published in 1874.[112] The new edition, "revised, enlarged, and adapted to popular use" by Mary Putnam Jacobi, contained similar feeding recommendations but, as part of the popular series "Putnam's Handy Book Series of Things Worth Knowing," had a different emphasis and audience. Directed mostly toward mothers rather than public health officials or tenement dwellers, the second edition communicated medical information with the intention of not only promoting children's health but also teaching women the science of feeding. Rejecting the idea that scientific theories should be avoided in books for the public, Mary argued that "the theory of a fact . . . concern[s] every intelligent person who is interested in its application." She expressed surprise at how "few women seem to be aware of the insult implied in the assertion 'that the theory is of no importance to them.'" She set out to teach the "scientific relations" of "vital phenomena to the physiological laws of the body in which they occur."[113] While Abraham's version of *Infant Diet* suggested that good feeding could eliminate class distinctions on both physiological and social levels, Mary's version added a gender dimension, targeting women in order to close the scientific information gap between the sexes.

Mary Putnam Jacobi's revision of *Infant Diet*, aimed largely at women, described the "chemical reactions" in the "infant economy" that characterized the process of nutrition.[114] She began by outlining the impact of maternal health on infant feeding, and explained how nervousness, menstruation, and diseases such as consumption, syphilis, and epilepsy could alter a mother's ability to feed naturally.[115] She also discussed the chemical components of breast milk and recommended that nursing women avoid dyspeptic foods, drink water, and eat salt and butter in moderation.[116] She also insisted on exercise, maintaining that it "accelerates the process of nutrition and denutrition, and hence makes room for more material to be taken up into the system, and utilized not only in the formation of solid tissues, but of such liquid tissues as the milk."[117] Cold bathing, massage, and the consumption of nutrients (to produce heat) also promoted good nutrition in the mother and the child.[118] Her focus on exercise and the "nutrition" of the mother and the infant are not surprising, considering her future professional studies on female physiology.

In the second half of the book, the emphasis shifts from the mother to the child, and the book stays true to Abraham Jacobi's original version, focused on the special needs of infants. The message is clear: children are essentially different from adults, so their diets should be different as well. While nervous ailments, such as fatigue and anxiety, caused disease in adults, a lack of nutrition caused disease in children, who were at the mercy of their mothers to be properly fed and cared for.[119] Error in diet could be fatal, and "intelligent mothers should be prepared to detect in their babies early signs of disordered nutrition, so that medical skill may be invoked before it is too late," the book warned.[120] Hot weather exacerbated illness in the summer, so the Jacobis recommended ways to lower temperature.[121] The book ended with a reiteration of Abraham's

"rules on the feeding of infants," redirected to the original "tenement population," who needed basic instructions, in common language, for how to nurse
babies, feed children, and avoid summer complaint. In this version of *Infant
Diet*, the Jacobis wove together a text directed toward a mixed audience of
"intelligent" mothers, public health workers, and tenement dwellers, reflecting
their attention to gender, class, and the role of the state — all components of
the social organism.

Mary continued to transmit technical knowledge to nonmedical women
throughout her career, so that by 1891, she was addressing experts and lay-
people together in one text. As the editor of Julius Uffelmann's *Manual of the
Domestic Hygiene of the Child*, she added explanatory notes so that the same
scientific reference could be of use to both "intelligent mothers" and physicians, as she saw it, "without emasculation."[122] Though some women insisted
on the power of maternal, instinctual knowledge, she believed women, under
the guidance of physicians, should use science to raise healthy children.

The Jacobis were theoretically in sync in the production of *Infant Diet*, but
this was their only collaborative publication. When they finished the book,
they continued their professional alliance, not through writing, but through
professional networks in New York hospitals and medical societies. Having
met at a medical society meeting, such organizations continued to be a common form of professional interaction for the couple, as they participated in
medical discussions and debates. And yet such public forums exposed their
professional disagreements and personal frustrations. As one colleague remembered, the Jacobis "would discuss and argue with each other over some
question or problem at the meeting[s]."[123] Despite this tension, they worked
in some of the same hospitals and pediatric clinics in the city. At the pediatric section of Mount Sinai, they likely saw some of the same patients, for
Abraham served the "in-door" department and Mary worked in the outpa-
tient dispensary, which she founded and managed with Dr. Anne A. Angel.[124]
At home, they exchanged information about cases, reported unusual symptoms, inquired about therapies, and discussed recent medical publications.
Medicine remained the primary topic of conversation, with some significant
disagreement.

Mary and Abraham also joined forces to rid medicine of homeopathic influences and to argue for the value of science in medicine by opposing reenactment
of the American Medical Association's Code of Ethics. A document originally
intended to restrict physicians from consulting with homeopaths, its regulation of practitioners was seen as obsolete and unnecessary; scientific principles

should direct practice, and the profession should police itself from homeo-pathic influences. The Jacobis believed that the A M A Code was a violation of the physician's independence and personal liberty. They joined the Association for Preventing the Re-Enactment in the State of New York of the Present Code of Ethics of the American Medical Association and hosted meetings at their home to organize and mobilize support.[125] Although they agreed that science was the foundation of medicine, they meant different things by "science."

Abraham Jacobi was part of a cohort of physicians who wanted to make clinical medicine a science. Influenced by the physiological and pathological studies conducted in German laboratories at midcentury, these physicians were reacting against the early-nineteenth-century model of French empiricism and wanted to bring knowledge from the laboratory into the clinic to rationalize and standardize disease diagnosis and treatment. They believed pathological knowledge could lead to universal therapeutic principles and disease specific-ity, so that symptoms could be grouped and understood as distinct maladies. For Abraham Jacobi, these concepts applied directly to children, who needed to be analyzed and studied separate from adults. Since his earliest years as a physician in New York, he worked tirelessly to convince fellow physicians that children had their own unique conditions, and that they should be understood via the sciences of physiology and pathology. For example, auscultation and percussion were considered scientific methods of diagnosing bronchitis and pneumonia and informed treatment.[126]

However, by the 1880s, the model of German laboratory medicine frag-mented, as physicians differed on what they meant by science itself. As John Harley Warner shows, although some American physicians promoted the Ger-man program of scientific medicine in the United States as a coherent model, the clinic-laboratory connection was "multifaceted" and could be interpreted in different ways.[127] Also, some physicians, like Abraham Jacobi, now wor-ried that the laboratory was out of control, for some new forms of therapeutic knowledge were based not on sound proof but on speculation, drawn not directly from humans but from specimens and animals in the laboratory.[128] Although he defended animal experimentation, he feared that too many phy-sicians made generalizations from the laboratory that did not hold up in the clinic. "Make your own diagnosis," he told physicians; select therapies based on experience with real human bodies; avoid unmediated research on rabbits or guinea pigs; use your own judgment, not the removed advice of "famous men who worked in the laboratory." Pay attention to the specific conditions and variations of illness in patients, he advised, since "the human organism is not a test tube in which the external circumstances are always uniform." Science was critical to modern medical practice, but laboratory testing could not replace the judgment of the clinician, he believed.[129]

Mary Putnam Jacobi had a different view. Certainly, she too was influenced by German laboratory medicine, engaged in pathological studies, and found inspiration in Virchow. However, trained almost two decades later, she saw the laboratory as an even more powerful force in directing medical practice than did the physicians who first rejected empiricism. Mary expressed an even greater faith in the experimental laboratory to deliver information needed to properly treat patients. Whereas Abraham Jacobi wanted to make pediatric medicine a science, Mary wanted to integrate experimental science into clinical care.

Mary Putnam Jacobi fused the pediatric clinic and the laboratory, using her patients to produce experimental data and informing their treatment with experiments on live animals. Her experiment with quinine to treat pneumonia serves as a prime example. In an article in the *New York Medical Journal*, she reported administering quinine to approximately fifty children with pneumonia ranging in age from three weeks to eight years old; her goal was to reduce fever, which she hoped would lead to *"the dissipation of pulmonary congestion."*[130] While some physicians believed quinine was helpful, they did not know why, unsure as to whether it worked as a sedative or as a tonic to accelerate the nervous system and heart.[131] She attempted to find out which by administering different amounts of quinine to frogs and rabbits and then performing cardiac tracings. The frog experiment amounted to vivisection: "A frog, previously quieted by a quarter of a milliagramme of woorara, was attached to the frog-plate and the heart exposed. A light lever ... reposed on the heart, and registered its movements on the revolving cylinder."[132] She tracked the stimulative qualities of quinine by administering it to a rabbit, with fatal results: "In a small rabbit to whom I gave hypodermically ten grains of quinine, the blood-vessels of the ears almost immediately dilated; in five minutes the animal had an epileptiform convulsion; five minutes later a second, which terminated fatally. In another rabbit the same sudden flushing of the ears occurred five minutes after a dose of 8 centigrammes, but in twenty minutes had began to subside. The animal died two hours later."[133] Her conclusion, based on these experiments, was that moderate doses of quinine were beneficial but that larger doses threatened heart failure, as seen in the rabbits.[134] Here, her experiments corroborated theories about the therapeutic qualities of quinine and the quantity to be administered to patients. Mary Putnam Jacobi defined scientific medicine in this way, making the clinic a laboratory, and the laboratory a direct informant of the clinic.[135]

Reflecting their different views on scientific medicine, the Jacobis disagreed on the value of bacteriology. Bacteriology represented a particular type of scientific medicine, one in which the laboratory was now determining and defining disease, sometimes at great distance from the patient. To a practitioner like Abraham Jacobi, the new science threatened to undermine the advances made by those who first initiated the call to make medicine more scientific. Although a subject of great debate, bacteriology appeared to represent the future direction in American medicine, and to a woman physician, being part of this new direction had its advantages.

Mary Putnam Jacobi also parted ways with some of her female colleagues on bacteriology, including Elizabeth Blackwell and Marie Zakrzewska. Blackwell resisted the theory because it contradicted her basic principles of health, hygiene, and morality. In her mind, disease resulted from a physiological imbalance, not a live agent. Zakrzewska, a physician who spent her medical career endorsing the value of science in therapeutics, began to question the value of the "new" laboratory science by the late 1880s, as Arleen Tuchman has shown. Zakrzewska, like Abraham Jacobi, worried about the bacteriology fervor, believing that it was ungrounded and created a gulf between laboratory and clinic.[136]

The Jacobis disagreed about new knowledge on the nature and transmission of diphtheria during and shortly after the death of their son. Mary accepted theories about diphtheria bacteriological agents more easily than her husband.[137] The couple's disagreement over the etiology of diphtheria caused severe tension as they tried to understand and rationalize Ernst's death as well as prevent the further spread of the disease in the city.

Tragically, Abraham Jacobi had been one of the nation's leading experts on diphtheria in the years preceding the infection of his own family. In the 1870s and 1880s, diphtheria posed a severe challenge to physicians and was extremely difficult to identify and diagnose, as Evelynn Hammonds shows, for it resembled other conditions, such as croup or even a severe cold.[138] Drawing on his vast clinical experience with the disease in children, Abraham Jacobi published the widely read *Treatise on Diphtheria* (1880), which focused on identification, prevention, and treatment.[139] Although the disease could produce a variety of symptoms, he said, it should be identified by the pseudomembrane, a lesion in the larynx, that obstructed breathing and eventually suffocated the patient. He also recognized that a poison infected the blood, which then spread and damaged organs.[140] To prevent the spread of the disease, he recommended the cleaning of nasal and oral cavities and the strict isolation of afflicted patients.[141] Treatments were limited and often ineffective, but he recommended that doctors move quickly to reduce fevers and, depending on the type of infection, administer stimulants or alcohol and prescribe steam inhalation. Only certain circumstances required more aggressive treatments, such as membrane removal, tracheotomies, or administering high levels of mercury.[142]

Abraham Jacobi believed that diphtheria was highly contagious, but he did not accept new theories that a bacteria was its sole cause. He acknowledged that the disease moved from person to person, and could manifest itself in dwellings, fabrics, and furniture. Therefore, maintaining cleanliness and removing filth were of utmost importance. Ultimately, Jacobi was more interested in pathological process than finding a specific agent.[143] He focused on how the disease formed and progressed, how the diphtheric spots and the pseudomembranes developed, and how the poison attacked certain parts of the body. He rejected the "no bacteria, no diphtheria" dictum, believing patients could show symptoms of the disease without having the bacteria in their systems.[144] His views placed great value in the physician, who observed firsthand how the disease formed and impacted patients; his approach to treating diphtheria privileged the pediatrician over the bacteriologist, and favored the science employed in a clinic over the disconnected science of a remote laboratory.

Abraham Jacobi's focus on pathology reflected the thinking of his generation and his medical training. He had been fighting the disease among children dating back to his first years in the United States at the German Dispensary.[145] At midcentury, physicians worked from the premise that diphtheria was a zymotic disease, meaning one generated by poisons. Similar to the miasma theory, the zymotic hypothesis linked the disease to a bad atmosphere generated by poverty and filth. By the 1880s, many physicians still believed that diphtheria resulted from squalid conditions, but they now acknowledged that it was transmitted by a parasite.[146] Rejecting this trend, Abraham Jacobi wrote emphatically against the overload of bacteriological theories, calling their growth an "epidemic" and their popularity a "calamity." He maintained that "the safest verdict of the sober critic is still: 'not proven.'"[147] Jacobi's focus on pathology over bacteriology also reflects his Virchovian approach to the science of medicine.[148] Although he would disagree with Virchow over how to identify diphtheria, Jacobi's concentration on disease process reflected the views of several German pathologists.[149] This generation of physicians had a hard time accepting the new science of bacteriology, led by the German physician Robert Koch, who became famous for isolating the tubercle bacillus.

At first, some physicians questioned the work of Koch's assistant, Friedrich Löffler, who claimed to identify the bacteriological agent of diphtheria. Löffler found a specific bacteria in the pseudomembranes of several patients who had died from the disease, but he admitted that further research was necessary because he also found the bacteria in the mouths of healthy people. Physicians debated whether his ambiguous findings were significant. New York practitioners were particularly divided.[150]

Abraham Jacobi made his feelings clear about Löffler and the growth of bacteriology, speaking as president of the New York Academy of Medicine in 1885. He warned members not to succumb to "bacteriomania," a craze in modern pathology marked by the abundance of hasty publications connecting bacteriological agents to disease.[151] These articles were full of false promises, he said, and then asked,

> Have we not had enough yet of the monthly instalments [sic] of new bacilli which are the invariably correct and positive sources of a disease, and replaced by the next man who comes along? Have we not yet enough of the statements, that, as for instance several bacilli are claimed each to be the only cause of diphtheria, by several observers, that there may be several distinct bacilli every one of which can produce the same scourge? Is it not just as safe to still presume, that, when several forms of bacilli are believed to be such sole causes, that the real cause is in neither?[152]

The new claims about bacterial agents were not just unfounded and exaggerated, Jacobi asserted, but they also symbolized an ominous new trend in scientific inquiry. Bacteriomania, Jacobi suggested, should be equated with the rise of "empire," particularly the German empire, and a new industrial culture of speculation and fortunate-seeking. Speculation was becoming equally common in science as in the markets. "Any young man can look through a microscope — perhaps he will draw the prize in the lottery of alleged science," he said, snidely referring to the ignorance of a younger generation.[153] For Abraham Jacobi, knowledge on infectious disease had as much to do with one's age and politics as it did with rigorous science.

Abraham Jacobi resisted universal bacteriological explanations, but he did believe that diphtheria could travel person to person. Although he was uncertain about the exact mode or agent of that transmission, he blamed filth and irresponsible disease carriers. The real "scourge of the community" were people with mild cases of diphtheria, or those who felt well enough to work and move about the city and ignored their symptoms or disregarded the danger they posed to others. "*There is as much diphtheria out of bed as in bed; nearly as much out of doors as indoors*," he asserted. "Many a mild case is walking the streets for weeks without caring or thinking that some of his victims have been wept over before he was quite well himself."[154] He accused domestic servants of posing the greatest threat. To prevent the spread of the disease, one should pay attention to the hygienic conditions of the house. He went further, advising families to physically inspect hired help, particularly nurses, and dismiss or not hire anyone with signs of infection.

To illustrate his point, he told the story of a physician's family that employed a nurse who had concealed her symptoms and exposed two children, a boy of seven and a girl of five. The children were ill for many years, until "the girl came near dying, and the boy died." Ultimately, the nurse was discharged, and "that was the end of the boy, and of diphtheria in that family."[155] The uncanny resemblance to his own tragedy was no coincidence. The story mirrored his struggle to save Ernst and Marjorie and his dismissal of their family nurse. One of the Jacobis' "trusted" nurses was blamed for bringing diphtheria into the family and was sent back to Germany. Abraham pointed the finger at either Emma Wedigan or Mary Deacks, both of whom were servants in the Jacobi household in the early 1880s, originally from Hanover.[156]

Abraham Jacobi, like most reformers of the age, was among the city's professional class and educated elite, so, despite his political principles and desire to help needy immigrant families, he assigned blame for disease transmission to "foreign" sources. Although an immigrant himself, by the 1870s and 1880s, Jacobi's foreign identity was based on his political fame, not his commonalities and personal association with newly arrived immigrants. This distancing was not unique to him, as seen with other immigrants-turned-reformers, such as Jacob Riis. Ironically, he located disease with "the other half," that is, the working-class and immigrant populations living in the city's crowded tenement houses and neighborhoods.

Abraham Jacobi refused to acknowledge his own potential for transmitting the disease, arguing that physicians have "a certain degree of both active and passive immunity."[157] Although it is clear that Mary had diphtheric "patches" on her throat years earlier, at the same time the children became sick, he refused to consider that he and his wife may have exposed them. Both doctors, and particularly Abraham, had spent years treating diphtheria cases. But

Abraham could not even consider that he may have contributed to the death of his only son by way of bacteria that recognized no boundaries of class and neighborhood. It was not until the mid-1890s, in fact, that Abraham Jacobi began to concede that the bacillus was responsible for the scores of childhood deaths in the city.[158]

Mary Putnam Jacobi more readily accepted bacteriological theories. She, too, had treated and studied diphtheria for years in the clinical setting, and wrote on methods for differentiating the disease from croup.[159] In the aftermath of losing Ernst, her interest in bacteriology grew, and she wrote to the wife of Dr. Edward Curtis, a pioneer in micropathological studies of diphtheria, about her deepening interest in his work: "[Bacteriology] is indeed a subject on which I have been reading all summer, and expect to devote myself to; it has a horrible fascination for me. I cannot get away from it. But I never should feel that any knowledge now gained, or even any lives saved, would be in any way a compensation for Ernst."[160] Learning about bacteriology may not have been compensation for Ernst's death, but it at least could lead to a scientific explanation for their sad family narrative. Looking back, she wished they had been more careful about protecting their children from exposure to the disease, by secluding them from all sources of contagion, whether it be nurses or themselves.

Unlike her husband, Mary Putnam Jacobi was very interested in Löffler's findings. At a meeting of the Clinical Society of the New York Post-Graduate Medical School, she presented a detailed outline of his claims about the bacteriological nature of diphtheria. While she pointed out faults, she thought his research showed great promise for improving knowledge on the disease: "It seemed as though Loeffler's experiments had approached nearer than any others to the solution of the preliminary question, What was the micro-organism which was the causal agent in diphtheria?"[161] Tensions rose when Mary publicly disagreed with her husband on Löffler in front of an audience of other physicians. By taking different sides, both physicians staked out their position on diphtheria and, by implication, who or what was to blame for the death of their son.

As the rupture in the Jacobi home played out in public, so did their disagreements about the uses of science in medicine. Their views show the ways in which men and women practitioners represented an array of views about the state of medical knowledge. Their actions and beliefs did not fit into neat categories of gender. As several medical men worked to describe science as masculine, Mary Putnam Jacobi opposed them, in her rhetoric, writings, and living example and was more eager than her husband to rely on the laboratory. In her family life, she challenged gender norms as well, as an unconventional Victorian mother who integrated work and family life. Mary and Abraham also challenged familial gender norms, as they performed atypical parenting roles in raising their daughter, now an only child.

"Meiner Lieben, Grete"

The Jacobi home was not the same after Ernst died in 1883. The couple, once connected through collaborations, drifted apart in their professional and personal lives. No correspondence between Mary and Abraham survives from this period, but fragments of evidence reveal the tension that remained between them. One source of information can be seen in their relationship with their daughter, Marjorie.

Mary Putnam Jacobi took the lead in overseeing her daughter's education and professional plans from a very young age. She concentrated on building Marjorie's intellectual talents and applied her hopes for expanding women's education to her own daughter. Treating her as both protégé and research subject, Mary gave her daughter daily lessons, teaching her language and object recognition through systemic exercises. It is also likely that she integrated Marjorie into her long-term study *Physiological Notes on Primary Education and the Study of Language* (1889), bringing her professional interests in the physiology of learning and memory into the home.[162] Calling her subject "little Marjorie Fleming," she worked intensely with this child in an "experiment in primary education," increasing her daughter's mental powers through training exercises in perception and memory. Her daughter grew tired of the systematic nature of their lessons, reportedly once complaining, "You make everything a lesson, Mama."[163]

Mary tried to balance her child's training with outings on Sunday afternoons to visit with friends. To Marjorie these trips seemed an effort "to satisfy some romantic mother-and-daughter picture in her [mother's] own mind," possibly of intellectual companionship, by exposing her to "stimulating talk" of science, literature, and politics.[164] Beyond academic lessons, she taught her daughter strength and bravery, as seen in 1889, when Mary, the usually robust doctor, fell extremely ill. Fearing her own death, she recorded parting words in a letter that was to be read only if she passed on, "[as] Ernst did." She told Marjorie to always be "absolutely truthful" and "gentle while strong" and to have an endless thirst for knowledge. Above all, "never . . . allow your liberty to be taken away from you by anyone."[165] Mary expressed her love to her young daughter through personal guidance and edification.

When Marjorie moved on to college, Mary stayed involved in her education at Barnard College. Mary had strong connections to the school and played a supportive role in its early years, serving as an associate member of the board of trustees, attending college administrative meetings, donating money, and lecturing to the students on matters of women's health.[166] As a member of the class of 1899, Marjorie was a very active student, writing for the yearbook, taking part in the bicycle club, and joining the Beta Epsilon Chapter of the Kappa Kappa Gamma Fraternity. Known by other students for her humor and "many-sided character," she was extremely social and, unlike her mother, interested in the latest fashions. But she also took interest in some of the social and political matters that were important to her parents, particularly labor reform. In her senior thesis, "Employer's Liability," she wrote about the need for legislation to protect the health and safety of workers, demonstrating knowledge of labor systems in both the United States and Europe.[167] In the 1890s, as Marjorie worked on her thesis, Mary increased her involvement in the Consumer's League, and was no doubt pleased that they shared a common interest.

Abraham's relationship with Marjorie was also intellectual, but it was cultivated independently of his wife and was a more personal and emotional bond. This can be seen in photos, as well as in a two-volume collection of Abraham's writings, assembled and published for his daughter on the occasion of her sixteenth birthday. He dedicated the book to "Meiner Lieben Grete" (my dear Grete), always preferring to use her German name.[168] Years earlier, he started a collection of his writings as a gift to Ernst but, after his son's death, decided to publish them for Marjorie. He wrote, "The memory of children, lovely Grete, for whom I took up the sword, leads me back now to my own child." He wanted to give her something that represented the many days and hours of his life spent caring for other children. He also wanted to give her something unique, saying she already had an abundance of possessions and mountains of affection, especially from her "uncles," Willy Meyer and Carl Schurz. Without a surviving son, Abraham gave his life work to his daughter, so she would know him better, and carry on his memory.[169]

Abraham was delighted in Marjorie's choice of a husband, New York reformer and politician, George McAneny. He was a close friend of Carl Schurz, who, McAneny said, "was a sort of Godfather of mine." While visiting Schurz at Lake George, McAneny met Marjorie and easily became integrated into the family circle. Ideologically, he had much in common with the Jacobis, believing

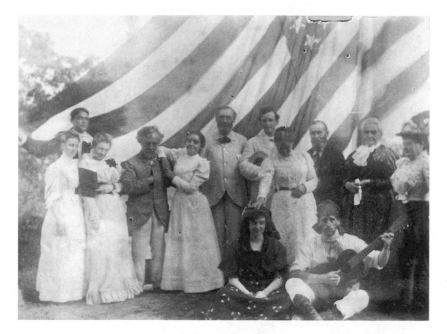

Jacobi and Schurz families, Lake George, N.Y. *Fourth from left*: Abraham Jacobi; *fifth from left*: Marjorie Jacobi; *fourth from right, standing/looking down*: Mary Putnam Jacobi. Reproduced with permission from the McAneny Family Collection.

·✦·✦·✦·

in the central role of the state in providing for the people. He is known for civil service reform, working against corruption, his leadership in the expansion of the subway system, and his role as Manhattan Borough president. He also had a utopian vision of the city, seeing New York as a place where all peoples could live, connected by mass transit. He worked to create a strong city bureaucracy and, like many progressives, sought to ameliorate the industrial chaos of the past century through reforming the city and its populations. McAneny became the son Abraham did not have, and his marriage to Marjorie strengthened the father-daughter bond.[170]

Mary Putnam Jacobi approved of George McAneny but was surprised by her daughter's personal choices. Unlike her parents, Marjorie had a bourgeois wedding. She wore a white dress, had bridesmaids, and was surrounded by college friends; the ceremony was in the chantry of Grace Church, "much to [her] father's disgust."[171] Marjorie also became a mother quickly and decided to not pursue a professional career. Over the years, she did take part in civil service reform and charity work, activities that reflected her role as the wife

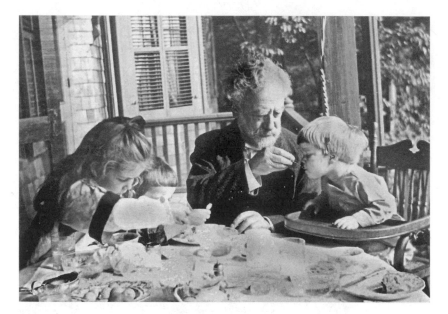

Abraham Jacobi with grandchildren, c. 1917. Reproduced
with permission from the McAneny Family Collection.

·✦· ·✦· ·✦·

of McAneny, but she chose a very different path than her mother, who put
medicine above all else.[172] Mary was pleased to have grandchildren and was
thankful for their good health, but Abraham Jacobi worshipped them, showering them with affection and attention. Although he never recovered from the
loss of his only son, his grandchildren eased that pain later in life.

It seems that Mary and Abraham Jacobi took the stress of losing Ernst to
their graves, for they are buried, literally, on opposite sides of the family plot.
At Green-Wood Cemetery, next to "The Babies," lie the graves of Abraham's
children and first wives. Mary's grave sits at the far left end; stones for Ernst and
Abraham sit at the far right end, with a large, open area in between. While it
was Victorian custom to be buried next to one's spouse, Abraham wanted to be
situated next to his son. In a letter to the staff at the cemetery, George McAneny
confirmed the intentions of his father-in-law: "The grave to be opened will be
at the *extreme* right front of the block, on the *opposite* side from the grave in
which his wife is buried, and next to the grave of his son, Ernst Jacobi."[173]

In the marriage of Mary Putnam and Abraham Jacobi, the lines between
private and public, professional and personal were deeply blurred. Both the
tension and the harmony in their relationship could be seen in their work and

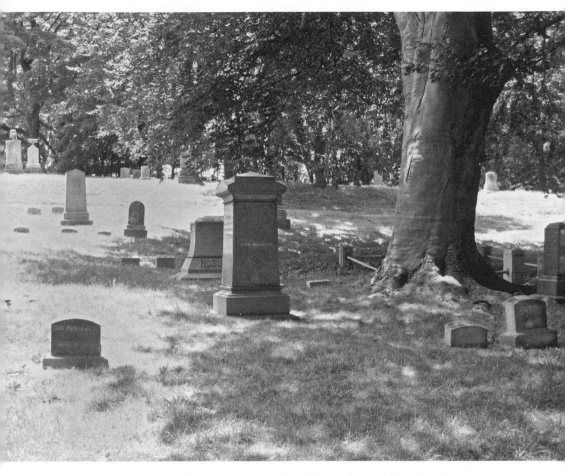

Jacobi gravesite, Green-Wood Cemetery, Brooklyn, N.Y. *Far left*: grave of Mary Putnam Jacobi; *center back*: grave marked "The Babies"; *far right*: graves of Ernst Jacobi and Abraham Jacobi. Photograph by the author. Printed with permission of Green-Wood Cemetery.

⋅✦⋅ ✦ ⋅✦⋅

in their home. Theoretical disagreements became intimate matters, and private issues had public consequences. Their differences and similarities as parents, physicians, and activists show the tensions over gender, work, family, and politics that animated late-nineteenth-century life. Inspired by radical politics, the couple challenged established gender roles, though not without conflict. And as they confronted new forms of scientific medicine, they defied categorizations as "male" and "female" practitioners. In this medical marriage, the politics of gender pervaded the examining room as well as the family home.

✶ 6 ✶

HIGHLY EVOLVED ORGANISMS

In 1897, at a meeting of the Mother's Congress of the City of New York, Mary Putnam Jacobi reminded her audience about the vital importance of exercise and education to young women's health. Now at the end of her third decade as a physician and activist, she returned to familiar themes, with new urgency. She told New York mothers that the health of their daughters had direct impact on the future of "the race," for "individual lives are attached to the main life of the race as branches are attached to a tree."[1] As Jacobi continued to argue for active girlhood, she more deeply wrapped her rhetoric in discourse about evolution and racial health, as she connected women's bodies to the fate of American civilization.

In her dual role as a physician and activist, Jacobi now placed greater emphasis on evolutionary concepts to justify the full incorporation of women into the social organism. Like other women's rights activists of her time, she made selective use of evolutionary theory, in her case highlighting the advancement of middle-class women and challenging the claims of Darwinian thinkers who constructed oppositional sex differences and placed men at the top of the evolutionary hierarchy.[2] She countered the notion that women were less evolved than men and closer to "lower animals" by emphasizing the great intellectual and economic strides made by women of her class since the early nineteenth century.

By now, much had changed about Jacobi's political activism. Once reluctant to support woman suffrage, Jacobi was now the leader of a growing and revitalized movement for women's right to vote. While she had long supported principles of socialism, she now expressed them through labor reform and improving conditions for working women. Historically opposed to female separatism in medicine, she now formed a stronger solidarity with groups of medical women to campaign for their rights in the profession. Jacobi extended her political agenda to incorporate some of the major causes of the Progressive Era, including sanitarian efforts, tenement reform, dress reform, and municipal reform against government corruption.[3] In doing so, she took part in a critical turning point for women's rights activism, away from its abolitionist and Quaker roots to Progressive politics, as activists in the "suffrage renaissance" linked their campaign to an urban reform agenda, and garnered support through inter-organizational cooperation and the well-established women's club culture.[4] At once a physician, suffragist, and labor activist, she also legitimized the growing field of social science, and the total incorporation of scientific methods and social reform.

Jacobi continued to champion experimentalism as fundamental to medical practice, taking her endorsement beyond women's medical education to the national level. There, she engaged in a heated disagreement over vivisection that intersected with the most pressing women's rights issues of the day. She entered a storm of gender politics that forced her to articulate how science and rationalism, suffrage and reform, were complementary, not contradictory. She showed that women's ability to be scientific demonstrated their potential to be educated, to serve the public, and even to vote. And if women were capable of the rationality and intelligence needed for experimental practices, they had more in common with men than their animal relatives. Now highly "evolved," women even surpassed some men in their abilities and education. For Jacobi, still the positivist, seeing was believing, and experimenting, working, and voting were all visible performances of female competency. She treated acts of citizenship and science as part of the same effort to make gender equality "a matter of fact."[5]

"The Fate of Cats and Rabbits"

By the 1890s, Jacobi's medical career had grown tremendously since her first years of practice in New York. She was now an established figure in the medical community, as seen in her membership and leadership positions in several societies. Although she resigned from teaching at the Woman's Medical College in 1889, she continued her clinical work at the New York Infirmary until 1897 and was a visiting physician at St. Mark's Hospital until 1902. Neurological studies dominated her medical research, as did her ongoing study of sex differences. She also continued to conduct and promote laboratory work, making the support and defense of vivisection a top priority in her political agenda.

"No physiological doctrine has ever been established without vivisection," Jacobi wrote definitively to the editor of *The Century* in 1890.[6] Her belief in the value of live-subject experiments had not waned as the debate over vivisection intensified in the profession and the nation at large. Equating vivisection with medical expertise, Jacobi continued to defend the practice as "good medicine" and a necessary act of scientific investigation. She privileged the social organism over the animal organism, humans over animals, and stood by animal vivisection as fundamental for human survival. The practice of vivisection could both demonstrate the similarities between men and women as they worked side by side in the laboratory and reinforce the distance between humans and animals. If both sexes could manipulate and control animal life, women could show they had little biologically in common with the animal kingdom. To connect science with the advancement of women, Jacobi tried to undo constructions of vivisection as a brutal masculine activity.

Many animal welfare activists rejected the notion that live-subject experimentation would help women, or medicine for that matter, believing that vivisection represented unnecessary acts of human cruelty against the natural world. Politicized and mobilized, these activists provided a strong challenge to Jacobi and those who saw "progress" through the microscope and on the dissecting table. From different angles, antivivisectionists defined animal experimentation as unnecessary and used their gender identity to claim moral authority on the issue. Women, especially, claimed to know right from wrong, humane from inhumane. Projecting feminine ideals and moral superiority, they placed themselves in opposition to many men of medicine, who they claimed were willing to be brutal for the sake of scientific knowledge. From this perspective, Jacobi and other female experimenters were unwelcome anomalies who defied nature through acts of cruelty that violated Victorian notions of morality and womanhood.

The debates over vivisection highlight the tensions brewing over gender and science in American culture. Diverse configurations of medicine and gender coexisted and competed in this period, so that an individual's stance on vivisection could not be easily categorized merely by gender or profession but by one's gender identity, politics, and notions of professionalism. Multiple feminisms and multiple feminine and masculine identities coexisted within the same movements and institutions. The suffrage movement, in particular, split over vivisection. Debates within the women's rights community and beyond show how the politics of pain and cruelty extended beyond the laboratory, to the walls of Congress, and even to the voting booth.

In the "Age of Innocence," reformers and concerned middle-class citizens often expressed deep sympathy for those who were unable to protect or defend themselves, especially children and animals, who were transformed by industrial forces from sources of labor to sources of affection. Middle-class Americans were viewing certain animals more as pets than as pests. Darwin and his theories of evolution had forced members of the urban middle class to develop a new relationship with animals, as reformers claimed animals needed to be protected against pain, suffering, and the instruments of science.[7] Jacobi took a different position, believing that human kinship with the natural world reaffirmed the viability of animals as reliable research subjects to inform therapeutics.

As animal experimentation grew in medical significance, so did opposition to the practice, spawning efforts to regulate and control it, especially in the late 1880s and throughout the 1890s. Vivisection critics charged physicians with mistreating animals with unnecessary, uncontrolled experiments. They also forecast that humans would be the next victims. As historian Susan Lederer has shown, critics uniformly believed that uncontrolled animal experiments would evolve into the abuse of human subjects.[8] Concerns about animal suffering coincided with a societal occupation with physical pain. Historians have explained the Victorian revulsion for pain as a product of both medicalization and secularization. The effectiveness and widespread use of nineteenth-century anesthetics, such as ether, chloroform, and morphine, eased pain and at the same time made it less tolerable when it did occur. The fear of pain was also a byproduct of a secular culture focused on alleviating human suffering, not accepting it as God's will.[9] These concerns about human welfare translated directly into concerns about animal welfare.

Leading the effort to regulate animal vivisection was physician Albert T. Leffingwell of Aurora, New York. A practitioner, reformer, and physiology instructor, Leffingwell founded the American Society for the Regulation of Vivisection and served as the organization's secretary. Leffingwell sought to limit animal suffering and prevent the widespread use of human subjects in the lab. Although Leffingwell did not want to outlaw all forms of experimentation, he worked tirelessly for regulation, including legislative restriction.[10] He worried most about the unbridled use of vivisection for physiological instruction in American medical schools, the needless pain inflicted upon animals, and the general insignificance of vivisection for therapeutics. On this final matter, he said, "Now I venture to assert that, during the last quarter of a century, infliction of intense torture upon unknown myriads of sentient, living creatures, *has not resulted in the discovery of a single remedy of acknowledged and generally accepted value in the cure of disease.*" He admitted that the "majority of men belonging to the medical profession" viewed vivisection as "wholly a scientific question" and often favored "professional privilege against sentiment."[11] Thus, Leffingwell realized the weight of his own role, as a man inside the profession, to oppose a practice he deemed overused and unnecessary.

Leffingwell received support from other medical men who advocated either restriction or prohibition. Surgeon Henry Jacob Bigelow of Harvard University was known to oppose vivisection, especially as a method for teaching impressionable medical students. Matthew C. Woods of Philadelphia, president of the Pennsylvania Society for the Prevention of Cruelty to Animals, said some of the best medical minds were lost "following the false trail of vivisection." The British surgeon (Robert) Lawson Tait had a voice in the American debate and spoke strongly against vivisection at home and abroad, claiming that vivisection played no part in advancing human surgery. While some medical men focused their opposition on needless animal pain and suffering, others framed their complaints about vivisection by outlining how little the practice had contributed to scientific progress.[12] In this way, they did not forego their identification with science, just the type of medical science that condoned live-animal experiments.

Men of letters outside of medicine also voiced opposition to vivisection. Mark Twain, for example, criticized the practice. John C. Kimball, a Unitarian minister from Hartford, Connecticut, condemned vivisection, saying it was "cowardly and unmanly to inflict pain on weaker, innocent creatures, deprived of all power to resist us, for the sake of saving ourselves from pain."[13] While some physicians tried to link manhood and science, men like Kimball associated their manhood with the protection of animals rather than the advances of the laboratory. The views of men inside and outside of medicine reveal that rival notions of masculinity accompanied debates over experimentation.

Competing notions of femininity can also be seen in the vivisection debate. Although some men condemned vivisection, the antivivisection movement became publicly recognized as a woman's cause and the rank and file of the movement consisted largely of female participants.[14] Organizations like the American Humane Association (AHA), the American Anti-Vivisection Society (AAVS), and the Woman's Christian Temperance Union (WCTU) campaigned to modify and end such experimentation. Women dominated these societies and linked their efforts to protect animals and vulnerable patients to their broader crusades for the protection of innocent women and children.[15] Inspired by their evangelical faith, many of these activists worked in the name of Christian mercy, hoping to eradicate needless cruelty against all of God's creatures. In the process, they created a gender identity for themselves as mothers and moral crusaders, working for the good of humanity. Poised as righteous, pious women, they fought vivisection as they resisted other masculine-coded improprieties, such as alcohol and violence. Like their British counterparts, female antivivisectionists in the United States connected their activities to an array of political and social reform work.[16]

The feminized nature of the movement can be seen in the pages of *Anti-Vivisection*, a journal "opposed to experimentation of live animals, and every other phase of cruelty in the world."[17] With graphic textual and pictorial representations of live animal experimentation, the journal tried to expose the brutality of American and European men of science. The journal published lists of physicians who they believed committed the worst acts of violence against animals. These compilations of medical offenses were accompanied by images of bound and dismembered animals taken from physiology textbooks and medical journals. Other hand-drawn tableaus juxtaposed idyllic scenes of kind women petting animals with images of cruel men equipped with saws and scissors, ready to sacrifice helpless animals.[18] The writers also attacked women practitioners, like Frances Emily White, who taught at the Woman's Medical College of Pennsylvania. The journal accused White of vivisecting rabbits without anesthesia, much to the disgust and fear of her students, noting, "The vivisecting mania is constant proof of how man's (and woman's) natural instincts may be perverted to gruesome monomania."[19] Female vivisectors, like White and Jacobi, were especially offensive to activists who linked their devotion to protecting animals to their own identity as women.

American suffragists, especially the old guard of the American women's rights movement, formed a robust strain of opposition to animal experimentation. Suffragists associated with Lucy Stone's American Woman Suffrage Association were especially vocal. These activists had strong roots in abolitionism and advocating for the civil rights of African Americans. They developed a critique of vivisection that denounced the practice, but they remained faithful to the mass of women in the medical profession who practiced "sympathetic" medicine. Alice Stone Blackwell, editor of *The Woman's Journal* and daughter of Lucy Stone, stood firmly against the practice. In the pages of her newspaper, she labeled women "the sex most sensitive to moral and humane considerations" and called upon them to voice their opposition to vivisection. Linking suffrage to antivivisection, she asserted that if women had the right to vote, they could be the decisive force behind outlawing such cruel practices.[20] With the vote, she believed, women would "clean house," putting an end not only to political corruption, illegal business practices, and widespread poverty and vice but also to animal torture. Here, Stone Blackwell promised that women voters would modify and moralize science for the good of all.

Live-animal experiments and demonstrations, now part of the curriculum at the Woman's Medical College of the New York Infirmary, sparked outrage, especially among dedicated friends of women in medicine, who believed vivisection was incompatible with the femininity that was at the heart of sympathetic medical practice. To these critics, women could be doctors but not experimenters; they could sacrifice their lives to caring and curing in medicine, but they could not sacrifice animals. In essence, they were qualified for the clinic but not meant for the laboratory, the site so central to Jacobi's definition of good medicine. Men who were sympathetic to the women's rights movement weighed in on the subject. John C. Kimball, minister and supporter of the Woman's Medical College, expressed his outrage over female vivisectionists. He fully supported women physicians but opposed the violation of their "natural instincts" via vivisection. It not only went against women's "gentler manners and higher ideals," but it also worked against their political struggle. Women have resisted their own moral, legal, and social "vivisection," or oppression, he argued, so women should extend their efforts to other sufferers, applying their goals for fair treatment to animals. "The animal's cause is woman's cause; the securing of their rights is one of the ways of securing her rights," he declared.[21] Suffragists and their supporters tied the two issues together, using sympathy for innocent animals to the advantage of the women's rights cause.

Jacobi, of course, did not see vivisection as a violation of women's nature or a barrier to women's rights, but rather an important tool in scientific education and a key to women's acceptance and authority within medicine. She also believed the antivivisection movement only hurt the cause of women's rights by reifying women's alliance with sentimentalism. Jacobi argued that vivisection did not corrupt, but reinforced, women's ability to practice medicine. Vivisection was mandatory for both genders, she believed, as a prerequisite for making therapeutics an exact science.

In the pages of *The Century*, Jacobi publicly defended vivisection by connecting it to another controversial practice, ovariotomy, drawing parallels between vivisection and human surgery.[22] She argued in 1891 that the tools and techniques used in vivisections were often applied to humans, under the knife, in order to save lives. To the inexperienced eye, surgical procedures could appear just as invasive, violent, and bloody as vivisection. But like life-enhancing surgeries, vivisection was necessary, she claimed. With this strategy, Jacobi may not have won over many readers. Although she condoned ovariotomy when it was necessary, she addressed a general reading public that was divided over the benefits, dangers, and problems of risky gynecological surgery.[23]

In 1900, Jacobi took her endorsement of vivisection to the nation's capital. She testified before a congressional committee in opposition to Senate Bill 34 for the Further Prevention of Cruelty to Animals in the District of Columbia.[24] The bill was designed to stop vivisection at a local level; it had emerged as a response to the instructional use of vivisection in Washington, D.C., elementary and secondary school biology courses and in government laboratories. But the impact of the hearing was not limited to the District of Columbia; it had national consequences due to the growing debate over animal welfare. Supporters of the bill claimed to be seeking the regulation, not abolition, of vivisection. They asked Congress to impose strict controls on the practice by requiring licenses, outlawing it in public schools, eliminating procedures painful to animals, and verifying that all experiments actually contributed to the advancement of scientific knowledge.

Opponents of the bill saw it differently, believing the legislation threatened the scientific use of the practice and blocked medical advancement. Animal experimentation provided the basis for research in several fields, they argued, citing bacteriological, pharmacological, and physiological studies. In 1900, when skepticism and criticism of bacteriology were still alive and well, the hearings provided an opportunity for supporters of experimentation to articulate and demonstrate the contributions of science to medical knowledge.[25] While they began the hearings in a defensive posture, opponents of the bill ultimately carried out their testimony in an offensive mode, using the debate to secure a central role for science in medicine in the next century.[26]

The Senate hearing was significant for Jacobi because it provided her with a national forum to argue in defense of vivisection and to identify herself as a woman of science. It also formally associated her with a team of the most prominent medical men in the United States: William Williams Keen, surgeon and president of the American Medical Association (1899–1900); Henry P. Bowditch of Boston; William Welch, dean of the Johns Hopkins University School of Medicine; and William Osler, the eminent Hopkins clinician. Alongside these men, Jacobi invoked the expertise of medical scientists and criticized the incompetence of her opponents.

In her testimony, Jacobi claimed that "ignorance" was the true "vice" of the legislation in question. She directly attacked Albert Leffingwell, one sponsor of the bill, targeting his disregard for all of the medical advances made by way of experimentalism. Citing medical efforts to reduce pain, she maintained that experimenters often used anesthesia on their animal subjects. Antivivisectionists, blinded by their fanatic opposition and focus on medical brutality, she charged, did not differentiate between the many types of pain, or between different types of animals and their ability to endure physical discomfort. Physicians were in a "strenuous warfare with misery," Jacobi insisted, and animal suffering was an unfortunate outcome in the battle against human suffering. Opponents of vivisection also seemed to focus on the most insignificant modes of investigation, she recalled: "I remember being severely denounced myself because during some weeks I administered cod-liver oil to a kitten."[27] Jacobi discredited any proposed government oversight of the practice. A longtime believer that religion had no place in science, Jacobi now insisted that the government was in no position to intervene. "Has not the supreme Government of the United States more urgent problems to discuss than the fate of cats and rabbits?" she asked.[28] In her view, physiologists and other medical experts should regulate from within the field, not take direction from laypersons.

Jacobi's testimony was useful to her male peers, not only because of its pointed language, but because she was the only woman to speak against the bill and only one of four women in the chamber during testimony.[29] Jacobi provided welcome help from what William Welch called the "humane sex."[30] The Welch camp clearly tried to capitalize on their female ally, hoping she would put a moral face on their brand of medicine. But they also hoped she would put a rational, feminine face on experimentation, providing a contrast to the sympathetic and "emotional" women antivivisectionists, from whom she consciously separated herself. Jacobi also strategically drew a stark line between scientific physicians, like herself, and misguided men like Leffingwell. Focusing on her "ignorant" opponent, Jacobi publicly critiqued him before the U.S. Senate for his lack of scientific enthusiasm and his disregard for truth. Coming from a woman, such accusations against a medical man were stinging, as Jacobi knew full well.

While Welch, Keen, Osler, and others welcomed her testimony, opponents singled her out at the hearings as a woman with an unnatural stance. Matthew C. Woods associated vivisection with the "hardening of human hearts" and was disturbed that Jacobi "manifests both in her life and writings that even women ought to vivisect."[31] Leffingwell presented the most severe critique, a scathing rebuttal aimed squarely at Jacobi. He claimed she had "carelessness and inaccuracy . . . stamped upon nearly every sentence of her statement." This was outrageous coming from Jacobi, "one who loves science and who believes that we can render her no greater homage than by speaking the truth in all that concerns her."[32] He also accused her of deliberately ignoring the severity and brutality of the particular experiments, which "a lady with the acquaintance which Dr. Jacobi has of vivisection must know."[33] What she described as "an experiment on artificial respiration," he described as the extraction of canine hearts, involving up to forty dogs and other creatures. Leffingwell also brought up Lawson Tait, a physician whom Jacobi criticized for opposing vivisection, claiming his innumerable operations on female patients amounted to human vivisection. By contrast, Leffingwell described Tait as a devoted physician who successfully completed difficult operations on women and did not deserve to be "calumniated by one of the sex for whom he did so much."[34] Trying to use gender to his own advantage, Leffingwell attacked Jacobi for both her medical opinions and her unconventional gender position, emphasizing that she was a woman who advocated unthinkable acts.

Despite criticism, Jacobi stood by her science and against many representatives of her sex. She attacked women in the antivivisection movement for taking up "excited crusades" against the physiological experiment.[35] Here, she used the same tactics as men in her camp to challenge her opponents. She formulated a rebuttal that cited female ignorance of science and distanced herself from women antivivisectionists, chiming in with male colleagues who criticized their misdirected feminine sympathies. Jacobi condemned a particular type of femininity, one that she constructed as overzealous and irrational with misdirected empathy. But while some men defined scientific medicine as a "man's practice," she continued to see vivisection as a genderless practice, open to women who were willing to abandon sentimentality and embrace the experimental life.[36]

Jacobi and her allies viewed the bill's ultimate failure as a victory for science in medicine. In the years to come, vivisection played a significant role in medical research, despite persistent criticism from opponents. Research institutions eventually began to self-regulate and heed some of the new guidelines for experimentation distributed by the American Medical Association. Despite these efforts, debates over the scientific use of animals continued and became more closely tied to questions about the use of human subjects. In the decades to come, human subjects occupied the most prominent place in debates over experimentation as the clinic and the laboratory grew even more enmeshed.[37]

In the end, although Jacobi attacked women antivivisectionists, she did not blame them for being politically misguided. Instead, she blamed their subordination and status as second-class citizens. If women had political rights, she asserted, they would not have to be "meddling" in these trifling matters but would turn their attention to more meaningful public issues than the sentimental defense of animals.[38] While some women defined antivivisection as a central cause of social reform, Jacobi saw it only as a hindrance to women, and an impediment to science. She believed that woman suffrage held out the promise that it would redirect women's activism away from trivial subjects toward matters of greater importance. In other words, women's enfranchisement would not only liberate women as human beings, but it could even liberate science.

"Fit" for Voting?

For many years, Mary Putnam Jacobi was "theoretically opposed" to woman suffrage. She had stood quietly against it for several years, not publicly denouncing it, but not endorsing it either. Women's education and work in the professions were bigger priorities because they could provide the true means for gender equality, she believed. With the woman suffrage movement split and struggling in the 1870s and early 1880s and the failure of Reconstruction to secure black male suffrage and citizenship, Jacobi did not see the vote as a pressing need for women. Her scientific faith determined her priorities, so that early on, conducting medical experiments was more important than casting votes. But by the last stage of her career, science and suffrage had become related, if not inseparable, causes.

In 1885, she publicly vowed her support for women's political enfranchisement. In a short article in *The Woman's Journal*, the suffrage newspaper of Lucy Stone and Henry Blackwell, she announced, "Please count me henceforth among those who believe in woman suffrage."[39] In the years that followed, Jacobi became deeply involved in the resurgent suffrage movement, so that by 1894 she was the leading voice for the New York City campaign. Explaining her commitment to the cause, she told Agatha Schurz, daughter of Carl Schurz, "My great reason for desiring Equal Suffrage, is as a formal recognition of the equality of the sexes, — and because such recognition as a matter of theory is essential to securing equality as a *matter of fact*."[40] Late in her life, she came to see suffrage as the most important right of citizenship and, consequently, that it represented the actualization of gender equality.

Jacobi initially opposed woman suffrage as a matter of strategy and priorities but also because she opposed universal suffrage, in general. She believed it granted the vote to the uneducated and, in her eyes, the undeserving. Showing both her scientific sensibility and class position, Jacobi held that voters should be intellectually agile and properly trained to comprehend complex questions and analyze data. She explained her position: "Persons habituated to technical pursuits are . . . always inclined to distrust the action of masses in relation to subjects about which they must be inadequately informed."[41] For years Jacobi questioned the ability of the male "masses" to vote with integrity; she also questioned whether women were intellectually prepared and ready for the vote. Frustrated with the spotty educational opportunities for women early in her career, she at first was reluctant to support woman suffrage. But by the mid-1880s, she believed that women had evolved and were ready and capable of enfranchisement. They were no longer a political liability but an asset in the promotion of social justice and the struggle to end corruption. Jacobi now echoed fellow women advocates who celebrated women's "progress" as a justification for female enfranchisement.

Philosophically, Jacobi also changed her mind because she had come to see woman suffrage as compatible with her positivist views on women's health and the social organism. She believed that "the real basis of democracy, republicanism and justice is the physiological equality or equivalence of human beings." Society could be a healthy body when all of its elements contributed to the larger whole, and this meant the full inclusion of women in political activity. When women were denied the vote and full political participation, they were prohibited from being complete living organisms, and the social organism failed to function to its most healthful capacity. She believed this denial explained a "large share of . . . the physical ill health of women, not to speak of [their] moral unhappiness."[42] Again, Jacobi used her identity as a woman physician to blame female illnesses, as well as social ills, on women's second-class status.

If a healthy society was, indeed, like a healthy body, then all people needed to contribute to the health of the state, especially well-qualified women. In her *Woman's Journal* announcement, Jacobi told readers that although she still distrusted the voting masses, her views had "nevertheless been singularly modified by recent reading of a famous passage in one of the most famous of Plato's dialogues — the *Protagoras*." She relayed an allegorical conversation between Hermes and Zeus in which Zeus explains that the survival of states requires that the virtues of justice and reverence be distributed among all members of the citizenry. Quoting and revising Plato, she argued that the survival of the state required the complete participation of "every man," or, as she amended it, "*every one*."[43] Declaring "Plato for Woman Suffrage," her announcement, ironically, claimed support from a major critic of democracy in ancient Greece.

Professional and personal considerations may have also altered her view on suffrage. By 1885, Jacobi was an established physician who had garnered respect from men and women physicians alike. She could now afford to be associated with an aggressive women's rights stance because there was less risk of alienating male colleagues and jeopardizing her position in the medical community. She found a new generation of suffrage allies, other educated, "accomplished" women interested in using their education and professional positions to advance the cause. Her turn to suffrage activism also followed the death of her son. As tensions strained her partnership at home, she found other political comrades in a family of women activists.

And yet Jacobi still did not always see eye to eye with the suffrage leadership. She had long rejected the sentimentality and "sympathetic" views of the old guard of the women's rights movement. She also opposed them on some key political issues, such as the prohibition of alcohol and the connection between suffrage and temperance reform. She engaged in a heated debate with Alice Stone Blackwell in the pages of *The Woman's Journal*. Temperance, Jacobi wrote, "imperil[ed] the logic of woman suffrage" by making it seem that women were interested only in "passionate and emotional" issues, rather than real political matters. Women activists who attacked men and tried to reform individual behavior made more enemies than allies. It was more "rational" to fight the abuse, rather than the use, of alcohol and to be realistic about the impossibility of enforcing prohibition in a political system with a male majority. Suffragists needed to be guided by logic, not emotion, pragmatism, not moralism. Stone Blackwell ardently disagreed, believing prohibition laws were viable, and that drinking and criminality were inseparable. Validating the right of minority opinions against majority rule, she argued that woman suffragists, for the most part, sided with prohibition because when it came to politics, "moral or humanitarian interest needs to be involved, to interest the majority of women." Stone Blackwell argued that passion and emotion fueled all politics and suggested that suffrage benefited from its links to moral causes; women wanted the vote to extend their positive feminine influence. Jacobi disagreed with other women's rights activists on the issue of prohibition as well and challenged their notions of what it meant to be a woman and a viable female political actor.[44]

During the winter of 1893–94, Jacobi became a major leader in the suffrage movement centered in New York City. With a large population of educated and wealthy women, New York offered suffragists a strong pool of potential supporters with financial means and social influence. She joined an activist cohort of other educated women in the city, such as writer Lillie Devereux Blake, reformer Josephine Shaw Lowell, missionary and evangelist Adele M. Field, and philanthropist Olivia Slocum (Mrs. Russell) Sage. But distinct from this group, she was a physician who brought the erudition and clout of knowing and doing science. Considering her profession, the Putnam family history, and her marriage to a leading specialist in pediatrics, Jacobi was well-positioned to be seen and heard among the city's elite. She hosted suffrage meetings and recruited support from middle- and upper-class women, inviting them into her comfortable midtown home near Herald Square, which one journalist said "deserves to be called a mansion in the richness of its furnishing and appointments."[45]

Jacobi's activism highlights the class dynamics of the movement, as she both mobilized the city's elite and wove working women's concerns into arguments for woman suffrage. The leaders of the 1894 movement connected the need for industrial reform to the suffrage cause and emphasized the benefits of enfranchisement for working women; they tried to legitimize them as potential voters by calling attention to their economic value and widespread industrial contributions. The suffrage leadership's overtures to working-class women signified a turn toward a reform agenda that incorporated the interests of women beyond their own social class. Nevertheless, campaign leaders did not include trade unions, labor activists, and wage-earning women into their organizational activities, as Harriot Stanton Blatch did a decade later. As historian Ellen Carol DuBois suggests, leaders of the 1894 campaign spoke on behalf of working women, rather than with them.[46] In doing so, they reinforced class hierarchies, even though they theoretically stood for alleviating the struggles of the working class.

In the 1890s, Jacobi also played a significant role in making New York City a center of suffrage activism, as suffrage leaders tried to build its power in the city, the state's economic and cultural center. They also knew that the New York State Constitutional Convention in the summer of 1894 provided an opportunity to connect suffrage to larger urban issues, for the convention's agenda focused on resolving political corruption in Manhattan. The convention also presented a chance to revise state voting laws to include women.[47]

As political reform activity in New York shifted downstate, women's rights activists initiated plans to expand the suffrage campaign in the city.[48] Leaders disagreed, however, about how to reach such a dense population of potential supporters. Susan B. Anthony devised a plan to launch a massive door-to-door petition campaign in New York City and asked Jacobi to take the lead. The doctor chose an alternative strategy. Rather than simply gathering signatures, Jacobi believed women of standing needed to gather together in the homes of other influential women to learn about the cause and spread the word.[49] Using this strategy, starting in 1894, "parlor meetings became the order of the day everywhere," transforming a seemingly innocent domestic space into a powerful arena for political discussion and mobilization.[50]

For the first time, a large contingent of elite women in the city showed interest in the suffrage cause, and, as a result, the movement reflected their customs and values. *The Woman's Journal* reported that, among the upper classes, suffrage "is becoming the theme of the hour. Fashionable women are taking it up, and one set of ladies of wealth and position have taken headquarters at Sherry's, the fashionable caterer's apartments on Fifth Avenue and Thirty-Seventh St."[51] One observer described Sherry's as a haven for women with high tastes: "There, at a table decorated in white and gold, surrounded by soft lounges, sits a lady in charge of the petition book. A sign on one of the cases filled with bon-bons called attention to the petition for woman suffrage."[52] While some women may have been drawn to the bon-bons, others became engaged with politics and attended meetings at Sherry's and the Cooper Institute to hear Elizabeth Cady Stanton speak. Stanton later acknowledged Jacobi's vital organizational role in expanding their base of support: "Dr. Mary Putnam Jacobi endeavored to rouse a new class of men and women to action in favor of an amendment granting to women the right to vote."[53]

In 1894, New York City suffragists followed Jacobi's lead, taking up the "society plan," which became a fundamental recruiting tactic in the new suffrage era.[54] The plan was first employed in 1893, when Lucy Stone and Carrie Chapman Catt encouraged suffragists in Colorado to seek support for a state suffrage referendum from Denver's wealthy women. Thereafter, the National American Woman Suffrage Association (NAWSA) tried to convert large numbers of wealthy women, already active in social clubs, civic organizations, and charities, into suffrage supporters. Suffragists now asked affluent women, with financial means and social connections, to redirect some of their money and free time to a woman-worthy cause. Support from women of standing broadened the suffrage umbrella and deemphasized the radical nature of demanding legal and political recognition of gender equality.

Jacobi also enrolled the city's most educated women into the movement and used them as a justification for woman suffrage.[55] In *The Woman's Journal* in 1893, she wrote, "It is absurd to give a girl the mental training of a man, and then refuse the suffrage." She then called on "college-bred women [to] lead the van in the movement for the political emancipation of their sex." The upcoming constitutional convention was a "great opportunity for educated women to demand that their education be allowed to count for at least as much as the ignorance of thousands of men voters."[56] Educated women voters would balance out the "ignorant vote," which would benefit the entire populace, she promised.

Despite her own conflicted history with suffrage, Jacobi now had no patience for women who opposed it, particularly the New York "Antis," a group of elite women who denounced suffrage, formulated petitions, and collected signatures at the Waldorf Hotel. These women contended that woman suffrage would undermine womanhood by tearing women away from motherly and wifely duties and jeopardize American democracy by enfranchising poor and uneducated working women. At parlor meetings, Jacobi accused the Antis of being traitors, equating them with "Copperheads," northern Democrats who opposed the Civil War. Annoyed with this breach of political camaraderie among women, she asked, "How is it possible not to expect a . . . concert and alliance among those belonging to the greatest class ever established in society, and submitted for centuries to the most profound, and most extensive, the most humiliating disabilities ever imposed on human beings — I mean the women?"[57] Jacobi tried to undermine the arguments of the Antis by reminding women of the many historical injustices faced by their "class" and the political potential suffrage presented for advancing the interests of accomplished women. Meanwhile, New York newspapers publicized and sensationalized disagreements among women on the suffrage issue. Extracting from her speech at a meeting, the *New York Times* dubbed Jacobi "a suffragist on the warpath."[58]

In the spring of 1894, with the state constitutional convention fast approaching, New York City suffragists rallied their efforts. In February, Susan B. Anthony had worried about the city contingent, with its "poor little showing of only *20,000* petitioners — to its near 400,000 voters . . . New York & Brooklyn gave the smallest ratio of signatures of any section of the State."[59] But activists stepped up their efforts in the following months, holding sometimes three and four parlor meetings a day and collecting as many signatures as possible. At the end of May, suffragists from the city gathered together on a train and traveled upstate to Albany, where the hearings commenced on May 24 with a speech by Anthony. The New York City hearing followed on May 31, when Jacobi led the arguments for woman suffrage and was first to address the assembly chamber.[60]

Jacobi gave a lengthy, "logical and able exposition" of women's progress in public life and declared that women now deserved suffrage.[61] She told listeners that the enfranchisement of women would be "momentous" but "no sudden shock or overturning of established order." Rather, it would be part of the "orderly evolution" of modern society, the natural outcome of changes in the condition of women.[62] Jacobi embodied the ideal female voter she described in her speech; she was an exemplar of the educated and accomplished woman, a model of female progress. She had fit herself into a largely male-dominated profession, without great disruption to the profession itself, showing how voting women would not unravel the social order. Speaking as a scientist and rational thinker, she performed logic and reason to convince listeners that women could and should vote.

In her speech, Jacobi provided evidence of women's progress in the industrial, legal, and educational spheres. She described women's need for political participation due to their economic contributions, in both professional and industrial work. She spoke on behalf of working women who contributed to the wealth of the state but were helpless, with no political voice. She described the plight of "poor and weak women" who were "defenceless" and "require[d] the status of a definite representation."[63] Jacobi spoke of the three thousand female teachers in New York City who deserved representation, especially on school-related issues. In the legal realm, women were now "distinct individuals" who controlled their earnings, held property, paid taxes, inherited and bequeathed money, and represented themselves in court. Though they now existed independently under the law, they had no individual voice in politics, which was a great injustice. Finally, incredible strides had been made in education. The expansion of high schools for girls, coeducation at Cornell University, and the graduation of Elizabeth Blackwell from Geneva Medical College all proved that New York surpassed most other states in granting women educational opportunities. This led naturally, she added, to the great number of professional women in New York pursuing teaching, law, social work, and medicine. Their growing public influence, as seen in their expanded roles in labor and the professions, should lead to their political equality.[64]

In these prosuffrage arguments, Jacobi adjusted her statements on sex differences to please her more conservative audience of lawmakers. Despite her medical stance on sex similarities, and her personal antipathy toward Victorian femininity, she relented that enfranchised women would have "special influence" on society. She maintained that men and women had the same abilities to analyze and reason, but she promised lawmakers that women would not be unsexed if they received the same political rights as men. "It is not in order to be men that [women] now desire to vote," she told the assembly chamber. "It is because they are — and are fully satisfied to be — women."[65] She and her colleagues argued, in the vein of "municipal housekeeping," that women voters would not threaten social stability or topple the American family but strengthen society by using feminine qualities to reform American political life.

Jacobi tried to redirect the suffrage question from one based on sex to one based on political intelligence and social standing. In fact, she argued that many accomplished women of New York out-qualified the majority of voting men. With other members of her activist cohort, she tried to reformulate the debate by highlighting differences in class, family origins, and race: "For the first time, all political right, privilege, and power reposes undisguisedly on the one brutal fact of sex. . . . For the first time, all women, no matter how well born, how well educated, how intelligent, how rich, how serviceable to the State, have been rendered the political inferiors of men, no matter how base-born, how poverty-stricken, how ignorant, how vicious, how brutal."[66] Former slaves and illiterate and poor men, criminals and beggars, immigrants and "tramps" all had the right to vote, but the women who served as teachers, managed almshouses, or worked on behalf of the needy had no political rights. While New York allowed illiterate men to vote, Jacobi protested, "the [women] writers, journalists, physicians, teachers, the wives and daughters and the companions of the best educated men in the State, are left in silence; blotted out, swamped, obliterated behind this cloud of often besotted ignorance."[67] Jacobi addressed the fears of middle-class New Yorkers and the concerns of the legislators who gathered in Albany in 1894. Problems of political corruption associated with party machines and the masses of immigrant and working-class voters topped the agenda of the constitutional convention. Arguing that educated women would solve the problem of the "ignorant vote," Jacobi merged suffrage with the convention's goals of political reform. Women could relieve "the vulgarization of the conception of political life which has crept over America with the advent of universal manhood suffrage," she clarified.[68]

At the end of their sessions in Albany, New York suffragists hoped they had gained support from several legislators at the convention. Although the women claimed to be nonpartisan, they anticipated support from Republicans, in particular. But the suffrage amendment failed in a vote of ninety-seven to fifty-eight, and party politics worked against them.[69] As Jacobi put it in a letter to Carl Schurz, who opposed woman suffrage: "The desire of the Republicans to retain the prestige of the Convention, . . . to keep their grip on the State, introduces calculations inimical to the women's claim."[70] Many senators obviously agreed with Francis M. Scott of New York, who proclaimed to the chamber: "'I vote, not because I am intelligent, not because I am moral, but solely and simply because I am a man.'"[71] Many New York politicians believed that when it came to the vote, sex superseded all other considerations.

The failure of the suffrage amendment at the convention did not dissuade activists from continuing their campaign. Returning to the city that fall, Jacobi decided to further disseminate her arguments and expand her convention speech into a treatise, *"Common Sense" Applied to Woman Suffrage* (1894), the most important text produced by the campaign, ultimately with lasting significance.[72] Intended for a middle-class audience, G. P. Putnam's Sons published the book and sold it widely in its "Questions of the Day" series. The title "Common Sense" came from Thomas Paine's revolutionary pamphlet, and it connected the cause to the founding fathers, a common tactic utilized by men and women alike in nineteenth-century political discourse. Jacobi's book pointed to the important role played by American women in the development of the nation, including the Revolution. The title "Common Sense" reflected the book's main purpose: to explain what seemed obvious to Jacobi, that suffrage was the logical outcome of women's legal, intellectual, and industrial emancipation in the nineteenth century. Jacobi's *"Common Sense"* was also a reversal of Paine, who maintained that the distinction of king and subject was unnatural but that "male and female [were] distinctions of nature."[73] She, on the other hand, asserted that commonalities between the sexes were natural and most distinctions were manufactured barriers that could be overcome through the education of women and changes to the social order.

In *"Common Sense,"* Jacobi illustrated women's "fitness" for voting through the concept of "evolution." In a section titled "The Evolution of the Status of Women since 1848," she demonstrated the natural progression of women in the professions, industry, education, and legal sphere since midcentury.[74] Women had earned greater financial independence, contributed to the welfare of the family, controlled part of their own wages, and forged a reciprocal relationship with the social organism through their labors.[75] Jacobi also employed the concept of evolution to distance qualified women from unqualified men and to justify woman suffrage by placing them on a higher step of the Darwinian ladder. At the same time that there was a "rise [in the] capacity of women," she asserted, there was a "fall of political dignity of men," marked by corruption and rights granted to "unworthy" voters.[76] Noting that all men — even the "half civilized hordes" of immigrants, Indians, and "the negro on the cotton plantation"— received the right to vote, Jacobi used racialized terms to criticize universal suffrage. She complained that "the white woman of purest blood, ... who, in her own person, or that of mother or grandmother, has helped to sustain the courage of the Revolutionary war[,] to fight the heroic battle of abolition and to dress the wounds of the Rebellion, — this woman must keep silen[t]."[77] Employing rhetoric of race and class common to the suffrage campaign in this era, she cited women's "evolution" and progression in contrast to the regression of the nation's male masses.[78]

Jacobi applied principles of positivism and nutrition to the suffrage question. While she called for the full inclusion of all members of society, she implied that women played a special role in securing the vitality of the social body. "Our American State ... it is a vast, real, living organism, with most complex functions, most subtle yet mighty vital processes, most glorious of vital powers." These powers, she argued, rested on the inclusion of all its members, including women: "This organism cannot be constructed like a brick wall, in segments of caste or class, adjacent, superposed according to long traditions of place or etiquette of precedence. Its elements must be individual cells, grouping themselves into organs according to their individual affinities and capacities — the microscopic function of each, ennobled by its relationship to the whole; the healthful activity of the whole, insured by the punctual action of these parts."[79] Again, Jacobi used the body as a metaphor for government and characterized women as the vital cells that insured the health of the organism. In this conception, "women also are brought into direct relations with the State, independent of their 'mates' or their 'brood.'"[80]

"Common Sense" had great appeal among women's rights activists and readers who sympathized with her cause. It incorporated the major arguments of the revived late-nineteenth-century movement, combining themes of female progress, political reform, evolution, and positivism, and making historical references to the founding of the nation. A reviewer in New York's popular Home Journal praised her work as an excellent exposition on the subject that promised, undoubtedly, to contribute "to the final triumph of the cause it so powerfully advocates."[81] In the years following the publication of her book, *The Woman's Journal* advertised and distributed the volume. As late as 1915, nine years after Jacobi's death and on the eve of another New York State Constitutional Convention, state suffragists memorialized her words with a new edition of *"Common Sense."*[82]

But Jacobi's suffrage treatise also received ample criticism. A reviewer in *The Critic* described the book as a bitter attack on men with "sweeping assertions unsupported by evidence."[83] A *New York Tribune* book review complained that *"Common Sense"* supported enfranchising lower-class women, who would further "degrade the quality of the popular vote."[84] Clearly, Jacobi was unable to persuade many readers that woman suffrage would solve rather than exacerbate the problem of an uninformed electorate.

Following the failure of the 1894 campaign, Jacobi proposed that the future of the suffrage movement focus on raising the political competency of women through education.[85] She and fellow suffragists founded the League for Political Education, a study group for women to discuss current political issues and readings on governmental institutions, history, and economics.[86] This "movement for self-education" transformed traditional women's clubs into venues for suffrage activism. The league forged ties with other women's organizations, urging them to see suffrage as part of their regular activities, whether they be charitable, reform-based, or social in character.[87] The Women's Municipal League and the League for Political Education doubled as anticorruption organizations, opposing Tammany corruption and, consequently, the electoral influence of Democratic Party machines over immigrant men. In these organizations, Jacobi built on her suffrage base and tried to rally women to speak out against Tammany and in favor of reform candidates. The leagues worked in conjunction with the larger anticorruption movement and groups such as the Civil Service Reform Association, staffed by Jacobi's son-in-law, George McAneny.[88] Reporting on a reform meeting at Madison Square Concert Hall in November of 1894, the *New York Times* expressed surprise that fashionable women were moved to action against corruption: "The social belles, debutantes, and matrons applauded [the overthrow of Tammany] with as much, if not more, energy than they usually do at the theatre or opera." By recruiting women of wealth, women's political clubs tied themselves to government reform movements in order to gain legitimacy as positive, ethical influences on electoral politics.[89]

As a leader of the League for Political Education, Jacobi tried to keep up the momentum of the suffrage renaissance in New York. She discussed the progress of American women with greater intensity while expressing deeper frustrations with women after the defeat of the Massachusetts suffrage referendum in 1895.[90] Still baffled by those who were against suffrage, Jacobi warned members not to capitulate to masculine domination in public life and used Western notions of superiority to argue that American women needed to move beyond domestic entrapments. After returning from a trip with her family to the Olympic Games in Greece in 1896, she reflected on the status of women in the East, particularly that of "Oriental" women she observed while traveling through Constantinople. The majority, she said, were passive participants in this "absolute masculine supremacy"; they were veiled, trapped in a harem, and housed in a "gilded cage" that was "no less a prison when it is most luxuriously a palace."[91] "From Massachusetts to Turkey," she wrote, there was "a sliding scale of feminine circumstances" that grew more degrading as one traveled east.[92] Trying to spark fear in antisuffragists, and affirm the pro-suffrage convictions of the league, she said that women who opposed the suffrage initiative in New England had a great deal in common with "Oriental" women, who accepted their degraded state.

Mary Putnam Jacobi's suffrage arguments combine some of the major intellectual trends of the Progressive Era, arguments that may seem contradictory today. For example, though she believed in the physiological similarities between the sexes, some of her suffrage speeches highlighted unique feminine virtues. While she championed "equality," she celebrated the superiority of women in her own class and cited the inferiority of the male masses as reason to enfranchise women. She worked on a daily basis providing health care to immigrant children and supported the social and political emancipation of African Americans, yet her rhetoric reinforced social hierarchies. Jacobi worked to improve conditions for working women, making the Consumers' League one of the main outlets for her activism in the last years of her career, yet she did not campaign for suffrage alongside working-class women. In the 1890s, anxieties about race, class, and gender were part of even the most "progressive" movements, and they surfaced in the most supposedly "common sense" discussion of political rights.

The Industrial Organism

Although Jacobi's suffrage circle did not include working-class leadership, the health and labor conditions of wage-earning women were a major source of concern for reformers. They made the struggling working-class woman into a symbol for the problems and failures of industrialism. In New York, the Working Women's Society, and later the Consumers' League, studied work environments, uncovered poor working conditions, and publicized their findings as a way to force change and advocate for workplace improvements. Complaints about the unfair labor practices of the Gilded Age punctuated discussions of working women, whom reformers described as most vulnerable. In these reform efforts, the body of the female wage-earner became a political cause, as activists used health concerns to persuade elite New Yorkers to take part in a movement to change the power dynamics of industrial capitalism.

Using her expertise in science and medicine, Jacobi backed the social science of labor investigations and applied her knowledge of women's health to the labor question. As we have seen, she had long recognized that poor working conditions placed industrial women at greater risk for physical illness. In her 1877 study, *The Question of Rest for Women during Menstruation*, she conceded that some rest may be required by women "engaged in industrial pursuits."[93] In the late 1880s, she became a leading medical voice for labor reform and testified to the negative impact of industrialism on the health of American women. For the next decade, she played a large role in the Consumers' League of New York City, first as a founding member, then as a vice president in 1891, a member of the governing board in 1895, and finally honorary vice president in 1898 and 1899.[94] She also participated in charities for unemployed working women, such as the Women's Conference of the Society for Ethical Culture, which set up "relief workshops" that hired unemployed women to sew clothes that were then distributed to those in need. Providing a fair wage, free lunch, and eight-hour days, relief workshops modeled good working conditions that contrasted with those existing in New York industry.[95] Activists like Jacobi were advocates of workers' rights and collectivism but were not direct participants in trade unionism or strikes. Jacobi joined concerns about women's health with a blunt critique of industrial capitalism, translating her socialism into efforts on behalf of women wage-earners.

In *"Common Sense,"* Mary Putnam Jacobi drew a direct connection between women's work, the vote, and the health of society. Women's labor nourished the social organism: "The productive forces of the community [labor] occupied the same relation to the life of the State, as the nutritive forces of the bodily organism to the individual life."[96] Jacobi had long advocated women's economic independence, an idea taken further by her patient and fellow feminist Charlotte Perkins Gilman in *Women and Economics* (1898).[97] Gilman used evolutionary theory to argue that the current sexual division of labor, that is, the domestic existence and limitations of white middle-class women, had hindered their evolution. Placed in a "primitive" condition, women now needed to evolve to an equal place to advance "the race," Gilman argued. Jacobi agreed that women's work advanced their evolution and thus earned them both personal autonomy and the right to vote. Women's labor was not an isolated endeavor; it supported society and the state, and to nourish the state, the body of the female laborer needed to be strong and healthy.

The Working Women's Society initiated female labor reform efforts in New York City. Led by Alice Woodbridge, a former wage-earner herself, the society examined the city's department stores and reported that clerks were paid low wages and subjected to long hours without overtime pay, poor sanitary conditions, and unjustified dismissals. "In all our inquiries in regard to sanitary conditions and long hours of standing and the effect upon the health," Woodbridge concluded, "the invariable reply is that, after two years, the strongest suffer injury."[98] Josephine Shaw Lowell, a leader in the scientific charity movement, showed Jacobi the Woodbridge Report, hoping she would join forces with the Working Women's Society.[99] Jacobi agreed to become the medical voice of the society and teamed up with Lowell to further publicize the report's findings.[100]

To rouse the sympathies of New Yorkers, the Society held a mass meeting in May 1890 at Chickering Hall at Fifth Avenue and Eighteenth Street, where a "gratifyingly large" crowd gathered.[101] Many concerned women of the city attended, along with prominent lawyers and clergymen, to hear Woodbridge's emotional pleas on behalf of the city's working women, specifically those employed in retail stores. As a result, the Society gained new membership and moved forward to make formal requests to the board of health and the state legislature to improve conditions. The meeting also produced a resolution calling for an evaluation of city shopkeepers and a public listing of stores with healthy and fair practices. Following the assembly, activists decided to broaden their reach and create a formal organization, known henceforth as the Consumers' League, taking its name from a similar British organization.

Although concerned with several aspects of labor and female health, the New York Consumers' League decided to focus on working conditions for women in department stores. Arguing that shoppers "employed" workers because their purchases supplied the wages, the league encouraged its members and the city's elite to change their shopping habits.[102] In department stores, elite women had power through their pocketbooks. The league asked ladies to examine their shopping habits and rethink their own participation in a system of exploitation. Even if they could not be voters, women could voice their stance as consumers.

Following a systematic study of working conditions, the Consumers' League produced a "White List" of retail merchants who met the "Standard of a Fair House." These stores paid a decent living wage, required only daytime hours, 8 A.M. to 6 P.M., of their employees, supplied "retiring rooms" for sufficient breaks, and exhibited "humane and considerate behaviour toward employees."[103] The league asked merchants to sign an agreement promising to stick to these standards and to allow inspection of their premises in order to ensure adherence to health guidelines. The "White List" appeared in the daily papers and was mailed to four thousand people on the Social Register, an annual publication listing the city's most "prominent" families and their addresses. As Lowell remembered, "At the same time [the List] was placed, by permission of the managers of twenty of the largest hotels, in the ladies' parlors, in a neat cover, marked with the name of the League."[104] The "White List" became the main mechanism for raising awareness; it was also a shaming tool, created to instigate reform through public pressure.

The Consumers' League aimed to define itself and middle-class women as a political force in labor politics by defending vulnerable working women. Like other women's reform societies, including the Young Women's Christian Association, the league focused on "girl advocacy," and aimed to "rescue" young women from the abuses of industry and vices of urban life.[105] The women they helped were wage-earners who were hard working and who, without protection, they believed, could fall into poverty or turn to more degrading forms of work, like prostitution. Jacobi wrote to Agatha Schurz that women turned to prostitution out of desperation because of "the hard conditions of their industrial situation" and "the unequal conditions in which women are compelled to work."[106] Reformers viewed themselves as moral guardians who could exert pressure on employers and defend young, unmarried women who were vulnerable to employer abuse. As Lowell explained, "They are all women; and consequently usually timid and unaccustomed to associated action . . . without the wisdom, strength of character, or experience which would enable them to act in their own behalf."[107] Customers, across the counters from retail clerks, were part of the system that forced working women into poor conditions, and as the league maintained, the "purchasing public . . . have the power to secure just and humane conditions of labor if they would only use it."[108] However, as league members spoke on behalf of working-class women, they often reinforced the cultural and economic "counter space" between them.

Beyond her position as medical expert, Jacobi supported a radical refor-
mulation of labor relations by promoting the right of employees to acquire
"partial ownership" of industry. She spoke to the Consumers' League about
this idea to elucidate the need for a reconfiguration of the relationship between
workers and employers.[109] The employee had become a servant to the master
in the industrial complex, receiving no part of its acquired wealth; personal
relationships between employer and employees disappeared. Losing all power
and individuality, factory and shop workers were vulnerable to maltreatment
and inclined to feelings of alienation. Jacobi's arguments for a redistribution of
industrial wealth to employees rested on both democratic principles and socialist philosophy. She told the Consumers' League that business organizations
should reflect egalitarian political ideals: "No one questions today that the state
consists not of the king, but of the people. We should try as fast as possible to
bring about the régime where every business and industrial organism will also
be seen to consist not of a single man, but of all the people, men and women,
in it, each of whom has the right to speak, [and] the minimum right of a single
vote."[110] With such an arrangement, workers and employers would both have
decision-making power and a stake in the industry, much like citizens in a
democratic nation. And just as all people, men and women, had the right to a
political voice, so too did workers have a voice in American industry. An industrial enterprise "is a complex spiritual organism, whose constituent parts are
the vital actions of human beings."[111] With this approach, Jacobi joined other
socialists and intellectuals who formulated an organic image of industry that
was dependent on the contributions of its workers.

Throughout the 1890s, Jacobi remained active in supporting the expansion
of the Consumers' League. The league built up its membership, holding parlor meetings, enrolling more members, extending its White Label campaign,
and resisting complaints from merchants who opposed the public listings and
refused inspections. It also sought to permanently revise the shopping patterns of its middle-class constituency. Members were called to shop at off-peak
hours, especially during the holiday season, in order to reduce the stress on
store clerks. They were also encouraged to vocally protest their opposition to
labor conditions while shopping in the stores. The Consumers' League also
worked to revise labor laws by supplying data and testimony to the Rhinehart
Commission, a state committee designed to examine the conditions of New
York's working women. Success came in the spring of 1896, when the Mercantile Inspection Bill passed, limiting work hours and mandating that the board
of health examine shops.[112] In 1899, Florence Kelley led the formation of the

National Consumers' League, building the organization into a national force for labor reform and legislative action in the early twentieth century.[113]

As Florence Kelley later said, Mary Putnam Jacobi played an important role in drawing attention to "the relation of industry to disease and death."[114] She provided critical information and data to justify legislation to limit shop hours; her reputation provided strategic support to the league and early trade unions as they combated the health problems of the "dangerous trades."[115] Jacobi "was a pioneer among physicians in going among working women not merely to cure, but to help *them* to change industrial conditions which create the need for cure, to help *them* make conditions of work such that disease and death need not be forced upon them."[116] Despite the economic distance between activists and working women, Kelley believed that Jacobi actually empowered female wage-earners to take charge of their own health. As the scientific voice of the Consumers' League, she legitimized the health concerns of the organization.

Jacobi believed that the science of biological life was directly connected to the science of social life. For many women, like Kelley, social science — rather than laboratory science — provided a better way to unite systematic investigations, reform work, and political activism. Social science and social work became "feminized" professions. By the 1890s, though Jacobi was still committed to the complete integration of men and women in the medical profession, she observed how women's networks and the female solidarity characteristic of the feminized service professions could bring some real personal and political advantages.

"Building the Hive"

In the last decade of the nineteenth century, Jacobi's professional activism in medicine mirrored her expanded role in the organized suffrage and reform movements, in that she promoted gender solidarity among professional women. Because she believed that women suffered from an "imperfect cohesiveness" and a "deficient ability for collective action," which limited their ability to achieve political rights as well as professional goals,[117] she placed strategic emphasis on female networks and collaboration. Women should cooperate, she said, "to do this as the bees work, without any special reference to individual advancement, but the intention of contributing to the upbuilding of the hive."[118] In her leadership roles in women's medical associations and alumnae groups, she connected the professional interests of medical women directly to the women's rights movement.

By the 1890s, American women in medicine had experienced notable gains, growing in numbers and finding opportunities for education and practice, especially in women's institutions. But they still faced resistance and struggled for access to complete scientific instruction, coeducation, hospital work, and professional societies. They also had fewer opportunities for laboratory research, just as the role of science was elevated in the profession and experimentation was becoming a vital component of a doctor's repertoire. At this moment of both progress and frustration, women's medical societies served as critical networks of professional advocacy and promotion.[119]

Though she worried about female isolation in the profession, Jacobi long recognized the importance of women's medical societies. She was a founder of the Association for the Advancement of the Medical Education of Women, a sister organization to the Woman's Medical College of the New York Infirmary, and served as its president from 1874 to 1903.[120] She also served as president of the Alumnae Association of the Woman's Medical College of Pennsylvania, traveling to Philadelphia and leading its yearly meetings. Until women had the same access and resources as men, such societies were essential for fund-raising, creating professional alliances, and producing quality forums for research presentations and publications.

Not surprisingly, Jacobi's top priority was to encourage a scientific research agenda in the societies. She insisted, "The best way to ensure the multiplication of [medical] triumphs is to cultivate among young physicians the laboratory habit of mind."[121] She maintained that laboratory work should be the highest priority of women physicians and urged women's medical societies to formulate collective research initiatives. For example, in her New York association, she encouraged women physicians to take part in more bacteriological and hematological investigations, embryological studies on animals, and normal and pathological anatomy research on nervous tissues. She worked in a similar vein in the Alumnae Association of the Woman's Medical College of Pennsylvania. Despite her difficulties with the administration over her own graduation decades earlier, she occupied several leadership roles in the association, including president, vice president, and member of the board of censors.[122] Here, too, she encouraged women to engage in research and present their findings to colleagues at the annual alumnae gatherings. She hoped to expand its annual report into journal form, publishing research papers and transactions of the meetings and modeling the association after the male-dominated medical societies.[123] When other members moved to alter the order of business and decrease the time allotted for research presentations, Jacobi put her foot down:

"The object of this Association is to stimulate the flagging interest in the discussion of medical subjects among medical women . . . [and] to offer a reason to medical women for writing; to urge the members of this Association to write, or rather to study, some subject so thoroughly that they shall have something to say about it."[124] Jacobi tried to model her women's medical societies on the larger societies dominated by men. She worked with women so that they could eventually compete professionally, not just among themselves, but "with men." And they would outdo medical men not only in "moral considerations," but also in the intellectual and research arenas where men seemed to have greater advantages in education, research, and employment.[125] For women, then, to surpass men, despite their disadvantages, would be a powerful coup.

Jacobi took advantage of her broader political network to continue her agitation for coeducation in one of the nation's top institutions of science. In 1890, plans for a new medical school at Johns Hopkins University provided a window of opportunity for women to campaign for coeducation.[126] University officials had hoped to join its hospital with a school of medicine to create institutions at the forefront of medical research. When plans for the project stalled due to a lack of funding, a group of women, known as the Women's Fund Committee (WFC), stepped up and raised the needed money. Led by Baltimore philanthropist Mary Elizabeth Garrett and M. Carey Thomas of Bryn Mawr College, the WFC consisted of women activists who received support from local subcommittees in the nation's largest cities.[127] Jacobi, along with Emily Blackwell, physician and sister of Elizabeth, were among the leaders of the New York contingent. Women of wealth and the wives of medical men also joined, such as Mrs. Louis Agassiz, Mrs. William Osler, and surprisingly, Mrs. S. Weir Mitchell, whose husband had criticized women doctors. Within a year, the committee had acquired more than $100,000, but they made it available to the university under one condition: the Hopkins medical school must admit women.[128] They were turned down. Two years later, Garrett added pressure to the administration by offering to raise her own donation, totaling more than $350,000, and to secure the school's endowment.[129] Garrett and other professional and nonprofessional women of affluence acted in a concerted effort to exert their power monetarily and in the realm of public opinion.

Jacobi and M. Carey Thomas, two key spokeswomen in the Hopkins effort, developed a political alliance based on common criticisms of the American educational system for its exclusion of women. Thomas, who modeled Bryn Mawr on men's colleges, agreed with Jacobi that women should be educated in exactly the same way as men. As the two activists engaged in intellectual exchanges about their mutual concerns, Jacobi described for Thomas the contradictions in American medical education for women: "America is the only country that has promptly granted women a legal right to practice medicine, and where the public has promptly secured them a clientele — yet where they have been compelled to stumble along without any hospital advantages worthy of the name, and upon educational curricula, uncontrolled, unsupervised by any competent authority, and which therefore has been usually quite incompetent. The situation is scandalously anomalous."[130] Thomas respected Jacobi's opinions on education but found fault with her personally. Reporting on a dinner conversation, she told Mary Garrett that Jacobi was "such a talker and so prejudiced against women." She was long-winded and spoke about "women's med[ical] education in *no* measured terms with an [amount] of plain speaking that will serve me instead of my annual dose of Zola." Finding her knowledge limited to medicine, and ignorant of art and literature, Thomas was "disappointed" because Jacobi was "very clever in a very tedious way."[131] This may be why Thomas preferred "Miss Lyon" to head the New York branch of the WFC, even though Jacobi, as a physician, would have been an obvious choice.[132] While these two strong-willed women may have had personal differences, they both believed that educating women like men translated into real social power.

Jacobi campaigned on behalf of coeducation at Hopkins with the hope that the admission of women to the medical school would set a new precedent and revolutionize women's place in American medicine. Still insisting that women must be educated like men and with men, she asserted, "Unless all the opportunities, privileges, honors, and rewards of medical education and the medical profession are as accessible to women as to men, women physicians cannot fail to be regarded as a special and distinctly inferior class of practitioners."[133] Jacobi anticipated that coeducation at Hopkins would provide women with an unprecedented opportunity, for Hopkins was to become the model medical institution of the future, a place where teaching, research, and clinical care could be combined on a massive scale under one roof. Clearly, this is why the WFC proposal generated controversy in the medical world.

When voices of opposition emerged, Jacobi took them on in print. She protested against an editorial in New York's *Medical Record*, "The Temptation of Johns Hopkins," which suggested that the school was being bribed into admitting women. The anonymous author said that "the disillusioning propinquity of lady medicals" would drive men away while damaging the "prestige" and spoiling the "usefulness" of the institution.[134] Jacobi replied with anger to the accusation that women students would lower educational standards: "It will no longer be possible to absolutely deprive the best intellect in the one sex of the necessary opportunities which are freely accessible to the most mediocre capacities in the other." Few people ever questioned the stipulations of endowments made to Harvard and Cornell, she jabbed. These "ungenerous" attitudes of dissent would disappear, she concluded, once "women shall have had the freedom [to attend] universities for a century."[135]

Despite opposition from some faculty members at Johns Hopkins, the trustees ultimately accepted the women's money and the committee's provision.[136] The decision created tension in the medical community as medical men divided on the issue. At Hopkins, President Daniel C. Gilman and Dr. William Welch both initially opposed coeducation. William Osler and other faculty sympathetic to the women's cause and attuned to the economic needs of the medical school helped change their minds. Osler, an eminent physician and vocal advocate of scientific medicine, used his power of persuasion to influence a number of his colleagues. He stood by the trustees' decision, explaining: "If any woman feels that the medical profession is her vocation, no obstacles should be placed in the way of her obtaining the best possible education, and every facility should be offered, so that, as a practitioner, she should have a fair start in the race."[137] Osler sided with Jacobi, whom he had long admired, for both principled and pragmatic reasons: without the women's funds the institution could not materialize. But it was clear that coeducation would not top the Hopkins agenda. "The success of the laboratories of a university rests in great part upon the men in control, and the extent of the equipment," said Osler, who assured everyone that women would not dilute standards.[138] Ultimately, the WFC succeeded because they used their financial clout to take advantage of a critical moment in Johns Hopkins' history.

While the Hopkins decision was an important symbolic victory and opened the door for women to attain a prestigious scientific education alongside men, it did not automatically deliver revolutionary change. In fact, medical school admission became far more competitive and resistant to women. As women entered the twentieth century, they faced a new set of gender barriers to acquiring a medical education.[139] Efforts to close unworthy medical schools, extend the length of medical education, and institute laboratory and scientific training in the profession placed greater constraints on women physicians and women's medical colleges. Financial problems led to the closing of several women's medical schools, leaving the Woman's Medical College of Pennsylvania as one of the only institutions still standing in the early twentieth century. Laboratories and hospitals were less accessible to women with the decline of single-sex institutions. The greater emphasis on laboratory science in medicine proved less attractive to many women, who found social work and the social sciences more appealing and socially relevant. Ironically, the move toward coeducation, standardization, and experimentation in American medical education did not deliver equality for women, as Jacobi predicted.

✦ IN THE 1890s, Jacobi combined medicine and politics through the convergence of science and suffrage, education and experimentalism, labor and women's health. She formed alliances with both women reformers and the nation's leading medical men. She stood by principles that were unpopular in some women's rights circles, defending vivisection, opposing the prohibition of alcohol, and believing that men and women were similar in mind and body. While she identified with women's organizations, she refused to be described in feminized terms, maintaining her identity as a rational, scientific practitioner and dedicated experimenter. Some of her ideas reflected a combination of science and feminism characteristic of women's reform in the Progressive Era. For example, she applied theories of evolution to suffrage and used women's health issues to call for improved labor conditions. In other ways, her allegiance to science went far beyond that of most women activists; she was unique among them for doing the actual work of science in the laboratory and the clinic. Her own particular identity and politics had evolved out of an extraordinary life that merged a powerful constellation of issues and influences that signaled changes to come in the twentieth century.

Epilogue

A GAUZE VEIL

Jacobi's defense of vivisection in 1900 was one of her final public battles on behalf of both medical science and medical women. After that, she devoted most of her energy to her private battle with a brain tumor, a condition that finally took her life six years later. She stepped back from her clinical work and political activities and reduced her public appearances. She spent her final years living between her new residence, the home of her daughter at 19 East 47th Street, and the Jacobi cabin at Lake George. Abraham took little part in her health care. Instead, in March 1903, she began to receive treatment from Dr. Helen Baldwin, a New York Infirmary physician.[1] She also enjoyed the arrival of her grandchildren, although her illness barred her from providing any medical assistance with their births. She stayed in touch with her favorite causes, attending the Minneapolis meeting of the National American Woman Suffrage Association and the Alumnae Breakfast at the Twelfth Street School in 1902, where she spoke in public, possibly for the last time.[2]

Jacobi's physical symptoms began to overwhelm her, limiting her mobility and compromising her mental clarity. She tried to remain active, taking short walks with the help of an attendant hired by her husband.[3] Her tremors showed themselves in her handwriting, which fell into an unsteady scrawl.[4] In a note to her younger sister Amy, she explained, "It is strange how little strength I have for writing, and I can only write the first thing in the morning. Later, I get too tired. Oh, illness is a horrid thing, especially if it lasts a year or two or longer."[5] By 1905, her pain had grown unbearable. She asked, "Why cannot *I* die by this time? It is fully time, and there is not use in waiting."[6]

Though she stepped back from medical work after 1900, Mary Putnam Jacobi spent the last years of her life analyzing one final case: her own. In

1903, she began a clinical narrative of her disease and documented anatomical changes, her drug regimen, and the progression of her symptoms.[7] Since the timing of her narrative, simply titled "Case," coincided with the initiation of her care with Helen Baldwin, Jacobi may have wrote it to acquaint Baldwin with her condition and to have a hand in her own treatment. She also shared it with Dr. Charles L. Dana, possibly hoping for his feedback on the case.[8] She clearly needed an outlet for her frustration and fear as a physician who was forecasting her own physical decline and death from a disease she understood all too well.

Jacobi's narrative began with a recollection of her first symptoms, experienced in 1896, while on holiday in Greece. It was then that she first felt an unusual pain in the back of her head. This unfamiliar discomfort lasted only three to five minutes but it returned the next morning in the same area, for the same duration. Over the next four years, the pain continued, worsened, and returned more often, accompanied by nausea and vomiting. On another outing, this time to Yellowstone Park, her pain was "violent," the nausea more extreme, and her mobility limited. She began to have attacks that forced her to remain in bed. "Most frequently upon rising after sitting a long time," she recalled, "perhaps especially in the evening, I would fall to the floor, and experience considerable difficulty in getting up again." She felt no paralysis or cramps but experienced a "slight tremor" in her right hand.[9] As her illness progressed, she described a feeling of heaviness and stiffness in her arm, and documented the "very sharp pain running transversely just below the occiput" (the rear lobe of the brain). It continued to return in the same place, at the same time of day, for a number of years. In a detailed, exacting manner, she traced the changing configuration of the nausea and tremors that accompanied the headaches. She also noted taking phenalgine and nitroglycerine to ease her symptoms.

Although the physical symptoms were painful and debilitating, it was the mental changes that disturbed her most: "I began to lose the initiative which had formerly been so active with me. . . . It seemed as if a gauze veil were thrown over all the objects in which I had formerly been so intensely interested." This feeling was confusing and distressing, she wrote, because of "its sharp contrast with the vivacity and strength of volition which had been a leading characteristic with me all my life."[10] As Jacobi plotted the pattern of her symptoms, she soon realized that she had a brain tumor.

Jacobi had studied brain tumors in detail in the 1880s, writing a medical paper on the subject in her *Essays on Hysteria*.[11] Although she did not offer a detailed etiology of the disease at that time, she agreed with Rudolf Virchow that tumors were a matter of cellular pathology. She believed that invasive cancer cells emerged from normal cells and formed a histological structure that caused local physiological dysfunction in the body.[12] Given her interest in cellular pathology and failed nutrition, a paper on tumors was a logical addition to her neurological volume.

In the 1880s, Jacobi joined other physicians who tried to differentiate signs of tumor from symptoms of nervous disease. She described how brain tumors took many forms, caused a variety of symptoms, and were situated in different locations of the brain. She reported that symptoms included headache, vertigo, vomiting, epileptic convulsions, apoplectiform attacks (strokes), tremors and localized spasms, and impaired vision. Other, nonphysical symptoms included irritability, "maniacal excitement," melancholic depression, and dementia. Jacobi explained that physical pain and discomfort resulted from the "irritation or destruction of the portions of the nerve-tissue in which [tumors] are embedded, or near to which they lie," and from "pressure exercised upon the entire contents of the cranium — nerve tissue, blood-vessels, and lymphatics."[13] While some signs of brain tumor resembled hysterical symptoms, she concluded, tumors were different from other neurological disorders as localized manifestations that damaged the brain.

Foreshadowing her own experience, Jacobi described the typical progression of symptoms of a brain tumor in a middle-aged patient:

> For weeks, or months, the patient will suffer from persistent or periodic headache, usually localized at one spot. . . . After a time there will be attacks of vomiting . . . [which are] dependent upon changes in the position of the body. . . . After the symptoms which have just been enumerated have lasted for a variable length of time, the patient's gait becomes uncertain; he reels or staggers, or shows a tendency to fall forward or backward. This tendency sometimes increases until complete loss of equilibration renders the patient unable to stand, . . . [usually leading to forms of paralysis]."[14]

In 1883, Jacobi felt that treatment options were minimal, with the possible exception of new experimental surgeries. Most tumors "are invariably fatal" but varied in how quickly they killed a patient. "The patient sometimes dies as early as ten or even eight weeks from the appearance of the first symptoms," she explained. "In other cases, these have been prolonged for ten years."[15] She could not have foreseen that she would suffer from a tumor herself for ten years before she died.

Part memoir, part clinical report, Jacobi's "Case" had the characteristics of both a technical, physician narrative and a personal illness narrative. It was professional in its anatomical details and its description of drug regimens yet intimate in its recounting of her travels, her pain, and her growing physical and mental disabilities. Her disturbance with the change in her mental condition is most striking. She prided herself on being healthy for most of her life. In its destruction of her brain capacity and mobility, the tumor took away her solid foundation of good health. This was difficult for a woman who spent her career promoting female fortitude and active womanhood. And though she defined good medicine as rational, positivist, and derived from data, she was unable to filter out her own emotion in her report. With her report, she tried to leave her mark on her own case, and in some ways, tried to manage it by controlling the narrative. Ultimately, she would have the final word on her illness, and could explain how such a robust and accomplished woman had slipped away.

Abraham Jacobi watched Mary's health slowly deteriorate and prepared himself to lose his third wife. The year 1906 was already a difficult one; Carl Schurz passed away on 14 May, and with that, Mary said, "the heaviest blow has fallen."[16] Less than a month later, she succumbed to her illness, dying in her daughter's Manhattan home on 10 June 1906, the anniversary of her son's death, more than twenty years earlier.[17] She was laid to rest in the Jacobi plot at Green-Wood Cemetery, surrounded by Ernst, "The Babies," and Abraham's first and second wives. Her husband mourned in silence, choosing not to eulogize her in public. Instead, women from the New York medical community organized her memorial.

In January of 1907 at the New York Academy of Medicine, the Women's Medical Association of New York City drew together physicians, editors, and women's rights activists to honor her life and work and to attract donors for a fellowship in her name.[18] Both men and women from the medical community paid tribute to her pathbreaking career. Dr. Elizabeth Cushier spoke of her insightful teaching and leadership in the women's community; Dr. Charles L. Dana testified to working side by side with Jacobi; the eminent Dr. William Osler spoke of her many skills and accomplishments that contributed to "the emancipation of women in [the] profession."[19] Osler said he was waiting for "a woman in the profession with an intellect so commanding that she [would] take rank with the Harveys, the Hunters, the Pasteurs, the Virchows, and the

Listers." This woman "will be of the type of mind and training of Mary Putnam Jacobi."[20] At the memorial, Florence Kelley hailed her work in the Consumers' League, and Richard Watson Gilder, editor of *The Century*, praised her writing talents and lauded her fiction, medical articles, and political commentaries.

Also in 1907, the Alumnae Association of the Woman's Medical College of Pennsylvania paid tribute to Jacobi by erecting a memorial tablet in her honor.[21] At the unveiling of the tablet in Philadelphia, her fellow alumnae spoke about her strength and bravery; Charlotte Perkins Gilman expressed her personal thanks to the doctor, whose care revitalized her life and whose intellectual energy served as a model for other women. Friends, family, colleagues, and writers memorialized Mary Putnam Jacobi in a way that reflected her many intersecting medical and political interests.

Nearly twenty years after her death, Mary Putnam Jacobi was memorialized again by women in medicine. In 1925, the Women's Medical Association of New York City resurrected her writings with a published collection of her medical articles.[22] Continuing attention to Jacobi demonstrated her lasting significance for a new generation of women physicians. By publishing some of her most significant work, the Women's Medical Association used Jacobi as a symbol of women's achievements in a medical world that was, by the 1920s, solidly dedicated to the principles of laboratory science, and gradually putting up new gender barriers. Women physicians in 1925 looked to Jacobi as both a medical foremother and a success story, as they faced an uphill professional battle in the early twentieth century.

In the post–World War II era, Mary Putnam Jacobi reappeared when her story was told on the radio, in print, and in film. In 1950, "Within Our Gates," a Philadelphia radio program, "dedicated to decency and human rights," dramatized her life on the air as part of the Community Chest Campaign in support of the Hospital of the Woman's Medical College of Pennsylvania. The program told the story of a spunky girl who refused to act like a "lady" and grew up to be a pioneering woman physician.[23] In 1952, Rhoda Truax published *The Doctor's Jacobi*, a book about a young woman's struggle over adversity and "a perfect partnership and marriage." Written in consultation with her descendants, it was a heroic depiction in a novelistic style, complete with fictional dialogue. Finally, Jacobi was represented in the film *Girl in White* (1952), starring June Allyson as Emily Dunning Barringer, a physician who Jacobi mentored and author of the memoir *Bowery to Bellevue: The Story of New York's First Woman Ambulance Surgeon*.[24] Jacobi's persona can be seen in the film in the character of Dr. Marie Yeomans, an elder doctor who offers guidance and encouragement to women entering the profession. Part of Hollywood's genre of biopics, fueled by the popularity of *Madame Curie* (1943), the film depicts Barringer as a brave young woman who forges her way in a masculine world; she is torn between marriage and her medical career but ultimately finds a way to have both.[25] In the early 1950s, as real women in medicine struggled for recognition, women physicians of the past, like Jacobi and Barringer, were celebrated for their individual victories. They were seen as trailblazers, capturing the optimism and triumphant atmosphere of the postwar period. They were women who challenged the status quo but did so safely in the past.

Since the 1970s, with the surge of scholarship in women's and gender history, and a growing population of women physicians in the United States, Jacobi has reemerged as a significant feminist figure. Other women doctors of the past have drawn great attention, particularly Elizabeth Blackwell, for her historic achievement as the first woman to receive a medical degree. The feminist critique of modern medicine and masculine science in the late twentieth century made Blackwell a popular historical figure, for she was a sympathetic, nurturing physician who believed women could bring special qualities to medicine. More recently, scholars have drawn greater attention to women outside the "sympathetic" model, such as Mary Dixon Jones, Marie Zakrzewska, and Mary Putnam Jacobi. These complex figures are compelling in our own complicated era of gender politics. In what some call a "post-feminist" age, our culture still questions whether female and male doctors are all that different, and how the gender of a physician impacts medical practice, the quality of care, and doctor-patient relationships.[26] In medicine, as in national politics, we continue to debate whether and how gender might affect one's performance.

As we have seen, Jacobi's story enhances our historical understanding of gender, politics, and medical knowledge. Her story adds balance and symmetry to a narrative that once focused on the biases of medical men, showing how women, too, use science for political ends. Medical actors on all sides of the woman question produced scientific knowledge from within a particular social network and cultural milieu; their positions were not so much "biased" as embedded in presumptions about gender. Positivists, like Jacobi, believed that science done right could reveal the truth, and Jacobi in particular believed that truth would lead to greater social harmony and gender equality.

Jacobi's work also complicates broad notions about the masculine nature of scientific knowledge. She worked to promote scientific medicine and gender equality simultaneously, advocating for her sex while denying the importance of sex in practice. And as she challenged the gendering of medicine and ex-perimentalism, she offered a new model of womanhood, one based on science and rationality rather than domesticity and sentimentality. She rallied and inspired, disagreed and disregarded other feminists of her time. She backed the methodologies of some medical men while denying the validity of oth-ers. Her story reveals the multiple meanings of gender and feminism, and the various interpretations of "good science" that coexisted in the late nineteenth century.

Jacobi's research on women's health had a long-term impact, especially her Boylston Prize study, which prompted other women to follow in her footsteps and study menstruation. For example, in the first decade of the twentieth cen-tury, physician Clelia Duel Mosher and psychologist Leta Stetter Hollingworth both continued her efforts to depathologize menstruation and prove women's intellectual capacity with empirical data and scientific arguments.[27] Their work is evidence of the continuing legacy of Edward Clarke. Almost fifty years after *The Question of Rest* was published, women doctors still found it necessary to write against a medical doctrine that characterized menstruation as a biological problem, a sentiment alive and well in the early twentieth century.

Jacobi's rejection of gender dichotomies in the late nineteenth century is truly notable. She made radical assertions in a culture committed to punctu-ating male/female differences. Her arguments built a foundation for other women to use the biological sciences to argue for sex similarities. By 1900, much new work was under way in the social science community to study and demonstrate female intellectual equality, as many women researchers used new methods in psychology and sociology to argue against difference. With New Women as their subjects, these researchers tried to demonstrate women's intellectual capabilities. For example, women like Helen Bradford Thompson Woolley devised tests to measure and compare men's and women's motor skills, sensory abilities, and, ultimately, intelligence. A new generation of women researchers integrated methods in experimental psychology and new genetic information on sex chromosomes to challenge prevailing notions of sex difference.[28]

Jacobi's 1876 rebuttal to Edward Clarke began a string of controversies over biological sex differences at Harvard University that lasted over a century, and reappeared in our own time. In January of 2005, Harvard president Lawrence Summers spoke to the National Bureau of Economic Research Conference on Diversifying the Science and Engineering Workforce and now famously said that women were less successful in the fields of science and engineering because of a "variability of aptitude." He conceded that some social factors contributed to this differential but suggested that new genetic research also supplied some answers. Summers's comments implied that biological differences between men and women explained why men dominated science faculties.[29]

Feminists and many women scientists expressed immediate and impassioned outrage. They also felt a strong sense of déjà vu. Had they traveled back in time to the nineteenth century when many believed that biology was destiny?[30] Some women criticized Summers for downplaying and disregarding discrimination. Nancy Hopkins, an MIT professor of biology, walked out of his lecture in disbelief, particularly since her recent study illustrated how social factors contributed to the secondary status of women at her institution.[31] Other feminists fired back at Summers with new data; a National Academy of Sciences panel, led by Donna E. Shalala, former Secretary of Health and Human Services, said that "outmoded institutional structures" hampered women scientists and that any cognitive differences in men and women were inconsequential.[32] As these responses showed, the Summers controversy was not just about women's abilities but whether genetics or society contributed to the uneven gender representation in the sciences, in effect, sustaining what feels like an endless nature vs. nurture debate. The Summers speech revived a long-standing, historical argument about the nature of gender, and the role of biology in determining sex characteristics. It also resumed an old debate among feminists scholars and strategists: should women seek empowerment by arguing they have unique needs and attributes, or by asserting they are similar and absolutely equal to men in every respect?

Over one hundred years apart, both the Clarke and Summers controversies show that the debates about sex differences remain a central point of contention in American culture. As in the nineteenth century, there is still a strong desire to discover predetermined biological characteristics and provide "hard facts" about both sex similarities and dissimilarities. "Biological determinism" is back in style after years of disregard, and theorists across academic disciplines again use science to show how sex characteristics are "natural" and therefore, inescapable.[33] In the 1990s, a whole new generation of literature, both popular and academic, emerged to argue there are essential cognitive and intellectual differences in men and women.[34] This literature still grows today. For example, Louann Brizendine's *The Female Brain* (2006) argues that there is a neurological basis for why women have more complex emotions, longer memories, and are more empathic than men. The publisher claims that, after reading this book, men will look at women with "brain envy."[35] Or, will they? Does the science of sexual difference help or hinder the cause of gender equality?

Mary Putnam Jacobi believed sexual science was, indeed, the key to gender equality. But she supported a particular sexual science, one based on positivist philosophy, experimental methods, and statistics to prove sex similarities. Though she likely would have bristled at the words of Summers, and disliked today's new science of sex, Jacobi produced knowledge in response to the specific conditions of the Victorian age, in a culture that defined men and women in opposition, and described females as inferior. She grasped the tools available to her and used them to reveal a different truth, that men and women had more in common than not. In contestations over sex differences, science and gender politics go hand in hand today, as they did in the past, but they are also specific to the concerns and conflicts of a particular context and time.

Historically, Mary Putnam Jacobi remains an important figure for her extraordinary life and major accomplishments as both a physician and a leader in the women's rights movement. Her story is not only extremely significant; it is also telling as a portrait of the nineteenth century as a period of transition to modernity. Her experiences followed critical cultural shifts as more Americans began to place their faith in medicine and look to scientific institutions and experts to solve the most intimate and pressing problems. She represented both a new femininity and a new feminism, focusing less on spirituality, self-sacrifice, and domesticity, and more on materiality, self-assertion, and public participation, paving the way for New Women. Her political ideas combined nineteenth-century ideals of socialism, democracy, and republicanism, as well as expertise and reformism, which led to fundamental changes in the Progressive Era. She also reinforced evolutionary explanations for social divisions, ideas that unfortunately plagued medicine for years to come. Jacobi led the charge for a scientific medicine based on the laboratory that, for better or for worse, formed the basis for medical practice in the twentieth century. In 1906, she left the world at a time when women physicians had made great professional strides, but she did not live to see the new frustrations and barriers they faced in the coming decades. Even as she succumbed to a brain tumor, she was still among the faithful, believing in the transformative power of science. Despite the remaining inequalities of her time, she died confident that science would one day lead to social emancipation, not knowing, of course, what problems lay ahead.

Notes

ABBREVIATIONS

Columbia
Columbia University, Rare Book
and Manuscript Library,
New York, N.Y.

Countway
Harvard Medical Library in the Francis A.
Countway Library of Medicine,
Harvard Medical School, Boston, Mass.

Drexel
Archives and Special Collections on Women
in Medicine and Homeopathy, Drexel
University College of
Medicine, Philadelphia, Pa.

HPP
Herbert Putnam Papers,
Manuscript Division, Library of
Congress, Washington, D.C.

HL
Houghton Library, Harvard
University, Cambridge, Mass.

LOC
Library of Congress,
Washington, D.C.

MPJ Papers
Mary Putnam Jacobi Papers, A-26

NYAM
New York Academy of Medicine Library,
Historical Collections, New York, N.Y.

NYCMA
New York City Municipal
Archives, New York, N.Y.

NYPL
New York Public Library, Manuscripts
and Archives Division, Astor, Lenox, and
Tilden Foundations, New York, N.Y.

Pathfinder
Mary Putnam Jacobi, *Mary Putnam
Jacobi, M.D.: A Pathfinder in Medicine,
with Selections from Her Writings and
a Complete Bibliography*, ed. Women's
Medical Association of New York City
(New York: G. P. Putnam's Sons, 1925)

SL
Schlesinger Library on the History
of Women in America, Radcliffe
Institute for Advanced Study, Harvard
University, Cambridge, Mass.

INTRODUCTION

1 Clarke, *Sex in Education*. On Clarke's reception in England, see Burstyn, "Education and Sex," 81.

2 Mary Putnam Jacobi, *Question of Rest*.

3 I use the name "Jacobi" to refer to Mary Putnam Jacobi to be consistent with indexing and also for better readability; I use "Putnam" before her marriage in 1873.

4 For example, see Ehrenreich and English, *For Her Own Good*; Russett, *Sexual Science*; Showalter, *Female Malady*; and Smith-Rosenberg and Rosenberg, "Female Animal," 12–27.

5 I use the term "feminism" to refer broadly to the many forms of activism aimed at advancing the place of women in the nineteenth century. I will also describe and distinguish Jacobi's understanding of feminism in relation to that of other women activists.

6 On analyzing the discourse of women physicians, see Theriot, "Women's Voices," 1–31. To analyze the views of both men and women as political actors, I am also influenced by concepts at the foundation of science studies, such as David Bloor's notion of "symmetry" in the "strong programme." See Bloor, *Knowledge and Social Imagery*.

7 Key published sources on the early life of Mary Putnam Jacobi include Ruth Putnam, *Life and Letters*, and *Pathfinder*. For a novel-like treatment of Mary Putnam Jacobi and Abraham Jacobi, see Truax, *Doctors Jacobi*.

8 Mary C. Putnam, "Theorae ad lienis officium," Medical thesis, Female Medical College of Pennsylvania, 1864, Drexel; Mary C. Putnam, "De la graisse neutre et des acides gras."

9 Morantz-Sanchez, *Sympathy and Science*, 184–202.

10 For other treatments of Jacobi, see Bonner, *To the Ends of the Earth*, 48–54; Gartner, "Fussell's Folly," 470–77; Joy Harvey, "Clanging Eagles," 185–95; Joy Harvey, "'Faithful to Its Old Traditions'?," 323–28; Joy Harvey, "La Visite," 350–71; Joy Harvey, "Medicine and Politics," 107–17; Sicherman, "Paradox of Prudence," 890–912; John Harley Warner, *Against the Spirit of System*, 322–27; and Wells, *Out of the Dead House*, 146–92.

11 Ruth Putnam, *Life and Letters*, 6. On the Putnams of Salem, see Boyer and Nissenbaum, *Salem Possessed*, 110–32. On Israel Putnam and the American Revolution, see Niven, *Connecticut Hero*.

12 The majority of the Putnam family remained in the New York area until the end of the nineteenth century, living on and off in Manhattan and its environs. Following the death of George Palmer Putnam in 1872, the firm became G. P. Putnam's Sons. Putnam Publishing has survived into the twenty-first century as part of the Penguin Group. For the status of Putnam Publishing today, see <http://us.penguingroup.com/static/html/aboutus/history.html>.

13 Mary Putnam Jacobi, "Autobiography," 1902, fragments, p. 5, Folder 3, MPJ Papers, SL.

14 On women, religion, and empowerment, see Brumberg, *Mission for Life*; Cott, "Young Women in the Second Great Awakening," 15–29; and Whitney Cross, *Burned-Over District*. On the widespread influence of women and religion in Victorian society, see Douglas, *Feminization of American Culture*.

15 Tomes, *Gospel of Germs*; Brandt, *No Magic Bullet*; Rosenberg, *No Other Gods*. On scientific motherhood, see Apple, *Perfect Motherhood*.

16 On opposition to women physicians, see Morantz-Sanchez, *Sympathy and Science*, 54, 71–72; and Mary Roth Walsh, *"Doctors Wanted."*

17 Morantz-Sanchez, *Sympathy and Science*, 232.

18 On the state of medical education in the nineteenth century, see Bonner, *Becoming a Physician*, 203–79; Ludmerer, *Learning to Heal*; Morantz-Sanchez, *Sympathy and Science*, 68–70; and Rothstein, *American Medical Schools*, 89–116.

19 On the history of scientific medicine, see Coleman and Holmes, eds., *Investigative Enterprise*; Cunningham and Williams, eds., *Laboratory Revolution in Medicine*; and Romano, *Making Medicine Scientific*. On the debates over science in medicine, see Geison, "Divided We Stand," 67–90; John Harley Warner, "Fall and Rise of Professional Mystery," 110–41; John Harley Warner, "Ideals of Science," 454–78; and John Harley Warner, *Against the Spirit of System.*

20 For more on women physicians in this period of transition, see Morantz-Sanchez, "Feminist Theory and Historical Practice," 51–69; and Tuchman, *Science Has No Sex*, 15.

21 On the school of physiological therapeutics, see John Harley Warner, "Ideals of Science," 456.

22 On the history of nutritional science, see Kamminga and Cunningham, "Science and Culture of Nutrition," 1–14; and McCollum, *History of Nutrition*.

23 Mary Putnam Jacobi, *Physiological Notes*; "Treatment of Incipient Insanity," *Journal of Social Science* 15 (1882): 77–96.

24 Key works by and about Abraham Jacobi include Abraham Jacobi, *Dr. Jacobi's Works* (also known as *Collectanea Jacobi*), and Abraham Jacobi, *Aufsätze, Vorträge, und Reden*. On Abraham Jacobi, see Viner, "Abraham Jacobi and German Medical Radicalism," 434–63; Viner, "Abraham Jacobi and the Origins of Scientific Pediatrics in America," 23–46; and Viner, "Healthy Children." On Jacobi's early years in Germany, see Herzig, *Abraham Jacobi: Die Entwicklung.*

25 Female Child of Abraham and Mary P. Jacobi, b. March 16, 1874, d. March 17, 1874, Buried at Green-Wood Cemetery, March 18, 1874, signed by A. Jacobi, medical attendant, Record of Death #171909, Register of Deaths, Manhattan, NYCMA.

26 For Abraham Jacobi's use of "Grete" for Marjorie, see dedication in Abraham Jacobi, *Aufsätze, Vorträge, und Reden.*

27 Ernst Jacobi, died age seven years, 10 months, and 7 days, d. June 10, 1883, due to "diphtheria," Buried at Green-Wood Cemetery, June 11, 1883, signed by A. Jacobi, medical attendant, Record of Death #460499, Register of Deaths, Manhattan, NYCMA.

28 Mary Putnam Jacobi, *Question of Rest*; Mary Putnam Jacobi, *Essays on Hysteria.*

29 Mary Putnam Jacobi, *"Common Sense."*

30 On issues of public and private in biographical studies, see Alpern, ed., *Challenge of Feminist Biography.*

31 The largest collection of her unpublished correspondence is held in the Mary Putnam Jacobi Papers, A-26, SL. I have found small amounts of material scattered in archives across the United States and in Europe (see bibliography).

32 Marjorie McAneny to Rhoda Truax, 23 February 1952, Rhoda Truax Papers, Drexel.

33 Barringer, *Bowery to Bellevue*, 45.

34 See comments in ibid.; Anna M. Galbraith, "The Life and Genius of Dr. Mary Putnam-

Jacobi, in "Addresses at the Unveiling of a Memorial Tablet," 59–64; and Elizabeth Cushier in Women's Medical Association of New York City, ed., *In Memory of Mary Putnam Jacobi*, 14.

35 For comments on her presence, see Barringer, *Bowery to Bellevue*, 44; and Kate Campbell Hurd Mead, "Forty Years of Medical Progress," in *Seventy-Fifth Anniversary Volume*, Records of the Woman's Medical College of Pennsylvania, 172, Drexel.

36 Elizabeth Cushier, in Women's Medical Association of New York City, ed., *In Memory of Mary Putnam Jacobi*, 12–13; Emily Blackwell, in ibid., 64.

37 Charles L. Dana, in ibid., 38.

38 Charles K. Mills address in "Addresses at the Unveiling of a Memorial Tablet," 67–71, quote on 70.

39 She was talkative by her own description. See Mary Putnam Jacobi to George McAneny, 16 May 1899, Folder 16A, MPJ Papers, SL; and Mary C. Putnam to Edith Putnam, 17 March 1867, Ruth Putnam, *Life and Letters*, 116. M. Carey Thomas said she was "such a talker." See M. Carey Thomas to Mary Garrett, 16 March 1890, Reel 16, no. 45–49, M. Carey Thomas Papers, Bryn Mawr College Library, Special Collections, Bryn Mawr, Pa.

40 Charles L. Dana, in Women's Medical Association of New York City, ed., *In Memory of Mary Putnam Jacobi*, 35; Barringer, *Bowery to Bellevue*, 44.

41 On women who identified with scientific models of medicine, see Morantz-Sanchez, *Sympathy and Science*; Tuchman, *Science Has No Sex*.

42 Morantz-Sanchez, *Sympathy and Science*; More, *Restoring the Balance*.

43 Physician Marie Zakrzewska also argued for genderless science; see Tuchman, *Science Has No Sex*.

44 Margadant, ed., *New Biography*. On gender performance, see Butler, *Gender Trouble*. For another discussion of Jacobi's gender performance, see Wells, *Out of the Dead House*. Wells argues that Jacobi alternated between masculine and feminine discourses and styles of writing.

45 On expertise, credibility, and the politics of knowledge, see Bloor, *Knowledge and Social Imagery*; Collins and Evans, *Rethinking Expertise*; Cozzens and Woodhouse, "Science, Government, and the Politics of Knowledge," 540–48; Shapin, *Social History of Truth*; and Shapin, "Cordelia's Love," 255–75.

46 Scholar Thomas Gieryn ("Boundaries of Science," 405) describes boundary work as "the attribution of selected characteristics to the institution of science (i.e., to its practitioners, methods, stock of knowledge, values, and work organization) for purposes of constructing a social boundary that distinguishes some intellectual activity as non-science." See also Gieryn, "Boundary Work," 781–95.

47 On multiple, historical notions of objectivity, see Daston, "Objectivity and the Escape from Perspective," 110–23; and Daston and Galison, *Objectivity*, 27–53, 115–73.

48 Methodologically, this book has also been influenced by scholarship in science and technology studies that describes the inseparability of science and society, medicine and politics. On scientific research as a social process, see literature in the sociology of scientific knowledge (SSK): for example, Harry Collins, *Changing Order*. On the production of knowledge out of social networks, see work by Bruno Latour, especially *Science in Action*. On the "co-production" of science and society, see Jasanoff, *States of Knowledge*.

For analyses of feminist science and epistemologies, see Harding, *Science Question in Feminism*; Keller and Longino, eds., *Feminism and Science*; and Kohlstedt and Longino, "Women, Gender, and Science Question."

49 On women's use of medical and scientific discourses, see Theriot, "Women's Voices."

50 Peitzman, "Why Support a Women's Medical College?," 576–99. For a specific example, see Lewis, *Our Girls*.

51 National Library of Medicine Symposium, "Women Physicians, Women's Politics, and Women's Health," March 2005; More, Fee, and Parry, *Women Physicians and the Cultures of Medicine*.

52 Morantz-Sanchez, *Sympathy and Science*; More, *Restoring the Balance*.

53 Tuchman, *Science Has No Sex*; Morantz-Sanchez, *Conduct Unbecoming a Woman*.

54 Keller, *Feeling for the Organism*; Keller, *Secrets of Life*. See also Merchant, *Death of Nature*.

55 On the "situatedness" of gender and science, see Kohlstedt and Longino, "Women, Gender, and Science Question." The volume of *Osiris* in which this essay appears includes an essay by Evelyn Fox Keller ("Developmental Biology as a Feminist Cause?" 16–28) on the biologist Christiane Nüsslein-Volhard, which speaks to these issues. See also Sandra Harding, "Rethinking Standpoint Epistemology," and Haraway, "Situated Knowledges." For a comprehensive professional history of women in science, see Rossiter, *Women Scientists in America: Struggles and Strategies to 1940*.

56 Daston, "Objectivity and the Escape from Perspective"; Daston and Galison, *Objectivity*. See also Harding, "Rethinking Standpoint Epistemology," and Haraway, "Situated Knowledges."

57 Jasanoff, *States of Knowledge*; Peter Dear, "Mysteries of State, Mysteries of Nature: Authority, Knowledge and Expertise in the Seventeenth Century," in ibid., 206–24.

58 On post–Civil War transatlantic exchange, see Daniel Rodgers, *Atlantic Crossings*, and Katz, *From Appomattox to Montmartre*. On medical exchanges, see John Harley Warner, *Against the Spirit of System*.

CHAPTER ONE

1 Mary C. Putnam, "Theorae ad lienis officium" ("Theories (with regard) to the Function of the Spleen"), medical thesis, Female Medical College of Pennsylvania, 1864, Drexel (trans. Andrew J. Cain) (emphasis original).

2 Pickstone, *Ways of Knowing*.

3 On women, religion, and empowerment, see Brumberg, *Mission for Life*; Cott, "Young Women in the Second Great Awakening"; Whitney R. Cross, *Burned-Over District*; and Hardesty, *Women Called to Witness*. On the widespread influence of women and religion in Victorian society, see Douglas, *Feminization of American Culture*.

4 For an example, see Sklar, *Catharine Beecher*, 37–42.

5 See Leach, *True Love and Perfect Union*.

6 Stanton, "Has Christianity Benefited Woman?," 389–99.

7 George Palmer Putnam began as an apprentice in a Boston carpet store owned by his relatives. He moved to New York City at the age of fifteen to begin work in the book trade.

See George Haven Putnam, *George Palmer Putnam*. A comprehensive history of George Palmer Putnam's publishing career can be found in Greenspan, *George Palmer Putnam*. On Putnam's partnership with John Wiley, see Greenspan, *George Palmer Putnam*, chap. 3.

8   On George Putnam's early publishing career, see Greenspan, *George Palmer Putnam*, chaps. 3–5. For George Palmer Putnam's own account of his earliest work in the book trade, see excerpts from "Rough Notes of Thirty Years in the Trade," in George Haven Putnam, *George Palmer Putnam*, 17–25.

9   Greenspan, *George Palmer Putnam*, 212–17.

10 Mary Putnam Jacobi, "Autobiography," 1902, Folder 3, MPJ Papers, SL. Knowing the reading public was hungry for a distinct nationalistic literature, George Putnam carved out a specific niche in the market for American writings to overshadow publishers who often relied on reprinting works from Europe. See Greenspan, *George Palmer Putnam*, 285–321.

11 Greenspan, *George Palmer Putnam*, 368–73.

12 Stampp, *America in 1857*, chap. 8.

13 Greenspan, *George Palmer Putnam*, 373–74.

14 Mary Putnam Jacobi, "Autobiography," 1902, Folder 3, MPJ Papers, SL.

15 Ruth Putnam, *Life and Letters*, 44–45. The family was forced to relocate from their most recent home in Yonkers to Morrisania in the Bronx, and they traveled to Manhattan via the Harlem trains.

16 Long, *Revival of 1857–58*, 72.

17 George Palmer Putnam quoted in Nott, *Memoir of Abner Kingman Nott*, 266; George Haven Putnam, *Memories of My Youth*, 76–79.

18 George Palmer Putnam quoted in Nott, *Abner Kingman Nott*, 266. This reference is to Mary, since her sister Edith would have been about twelve years old that year and a little young to be baptized into the church.

19 George Haven Putnam, *Memories of My Youth*, 78.

20 Mary C. Putnam, "Minnie's List of Virtues and Vices," 1853, in Victorine Haven Putnam Ledger Book, Container 1, HPP.

21 George Haven Putnam, *Memories of My Youth*, 23–24.

22 Mary C. Putnam to Catherine Palmer Putnam, October 1854, Folder 5, MPJ Papers, SL (emphasis added).

23 Mary C. Putnam to George Haven Putnam, 1857, Folder 6, MPJ Papers, SL.

24 George Haven Putnam, *Memories of My Youth*, 78–79.

25 Abner Kingman Nott quoted in Nott, *Abner Kingman Nott*, 210.

26 Reverend Abner Kingman Nott, "Jesus and the Resurrection," in Nott, *Abner Kingman Nott*, 273–90.

27 Mary C. Putnam to Mary Swift, c. 1859, Ruth Putnam, *Life and Letters*, 55–56.

28 George Palmer Putnam, "Eulogy to Kingman Nott," in Nott, *Abner Kingman Nott*, 267. In a letter to his family, Nott referred to a Fourth of July celebration in Melrose, spent cruising in a rowboat in the Harlem River and under High Bridge. He was probably in the company of the Putnams. See Nott, *Abner Kingman Nott*, 218.

29 George Palmer Putnam quoted in Nott, *Abner Kingman Nott*, 266 (emphasis original).

30 Ruth Putnam, *Life and Letters*, 56–57.

31 Nott, *Abner Kingman Nott*, 252–55.

32 Mary C. Putnam to Mary Swift, c. 1859, Ruth Putnam, *Life and Letters*, 55.

33 George Haven Putnam, *Memories of My Youth*, 78.

34 Mary C. Putnam to Mary Swift, c. 1859, Ruth Putnam, *Life and Letters*, 54.

35 On nineteenth-century "literary domestics," see Kelley, *Private Woman, Public Stage*.

36 Brumberg, *Body Project*, xx–xxi; Jane H. Hunter, *How Young Ladies Became Girls*, 38–90.

37 Thirty-sixth Annual Report of the New York Infirmary, 1889, in Daniel, "'Cautious Experiment,'" *Medical Woman's Journal* 49 (November 1942): 343. The Woman's Medical College of the New York Infirmary received the memorial fund of Lydia F. Wadleigh, facilitated in part by Mary Putnam Jacobi, who was on the memorial committee.

38 Mary Putnam enrolled in the school in 1857. See Ruth Putnam, *Life and Letters*, 45–46. On the institution's goals and reference to the domestic "prison-house," see Hon. S. S. Randall, "Introductory Address," as well as Mary C. Putnam, "Woman's Right to Labor," in *Graduates' Reunion*, 1–3, 62–71, also in Folder 27, MPJ Papers, SL.

39 Hunter, *How Young Ladies Became Girls*, 5, 169.

40 For the best accounts of the Putnam home life, see Anna B. Warner, *Susan Warner*. See also letters between George Palmer Putnam and Victorine Haven (Putnam), HPP.

41 On Putnam family life on Staten Island, see Anna B. Warner, *Susan Warner*, 286–350 passim.

42 On Sedgwick, see Greenspan, *George Palmer Putnam*, 228–31.

43 On literary guests to the Putnam home on Staten Island, see George Haven Putnam, *Memories of My Youth*, 25–26. On Putnam's dealings with Bremer, see Greenspan, *George Palmer Putnam*, 259–60. Fredrika Bremer would later support the entrance of women into medicine, saying, "That women have a natural feeling and talent for the vocation of physicians is proved by innumerable instances . . . and it is a shame and a pity that men have not hitherto permitted these to be developed by science." Quoted in Morantz-Sanchez, *Sympathy and Science*, 47. On Susan Warner, see Grace Overmyer, "Susan Warner," in *Notable American Women*, 3:543–45.

44 Quotation from Anna B. Warner, *Susan Warner*, 283.

45 Kelley, *Private Woman, Public Stage*, 18–19, 150–51.

46 Mary Putnam Jacobi, "An Appreciation," Ruth Putnam, *Life and Letters*, 359.

47 Susan Warner, *Wide, Wide World*.

48 Anna B. Warner, *Susan Warner*, 294.

49 Susan Warner to Anna B. Warner, 28 September 1850, Staten Island, quoted in Anna B. Warner, *Susan Warner*, 295, 296, 305. Mary also spent time at the Warner home on Constitution Island near West Point. See Ruth Putnam, *Life and Letters*, 24.

50 On Fredrika Bremer and the Putnams, see Greenspan, *George Palmer Putnam*, 259–61.

51 Anna B. Warner, *Susan Warner*, 373, quoted in Ruth Putnam, *Life and Letters*, 32.

52 For an account of the founding of *Putnam's Monthly*, see Greenspan, *George Palmer Putnam*, chap. 9. See also *Putnam's* magazine, first issues in 1853. George William Curtis wrote the lead article, "The Potiphar Papers," which was a satire of New York's fashionable elite. Unlike *Harper's Monthly*, *Knickerbocker*, and *Godey's*, *Putnam's* did not include reprints of foreign articles but contained exclusively American compositions. Financial concerns forced Putnam to abandon it in 1854 until after the Civil War.

53 Greenspan, *George Palmer Putnam*, 293.

54 George Haven Putnam, *Memories of My Youth*, 46, 54.

55 Ibid., 54.

56 Ibid., 51–52. Originals of the "local paper" do not survive.

57 Mary C. Putnam, "The Three Paths of Life," 1851, Folder 23, MPJ Papers, SL; see also Mary C. Putnam, "Life: What Is It?," 1852, Folder 23, MPJ Papers, SL.

58 Mary C. Putnam, "Life in the Country," "Queen Marie Antoinette," "Napoleon Bonaparte," and "Revolutions." For other examples, see "Aims and Ends," "An Adventure in California," and "The Philosopher's Stone," all unpublished, c. 1857–59, Folders 24–25, MPJ Papers, SL.

59 Mary C. Putnam, "A Fragment at the Thought of Her Twelfth Birthday," 2 August 1854, Folder 5, MPJ Papers, SL.

60 Mary C. Putnam, "Aims and Ends," c. 1857–59, Folder 25, MPJ Papers, SL (emphasis original).

61 Mary C. Putnam, "Truth," c. 1857–59, Folder 25, MPJ Papers, SL.

62 Susan Wells (*Out of the Dead House*, 147, 155) discusses how Putnam disguised her gender and performed gender in her writings.

63 Mary C. Putnam, "Hair Chains," 50–96. Also published in the *Atlantic Monthly*, November 1861, 534–49.

64 Mary C. Putnam, "Hair Chains," 90.

65 Mary C. Putnam, "Effeminacy," c. 1857–59, Folder 25, MPJ Papers, SL.

66 Mary C. Putnam, "The Nineteenth Century," c. 1857–59, Folder 25, MPJ Papers, SL.

67 Mary C. Putnam, "The Moral Significance of William the Conqueror," c. 1857–59, Folder 24, MPJ Papers, SL (emphasis added).

68 Ruth Putnam, *Life and Letters*, 47, 61. According to Ruth Putnam, the school was run by a woman named Miss Gibson and Putnam received her private lessons in Greek from a Polish immigrant and political exile named Dr. Kreitzer.

69 On the feminization of teaching, see Jo Anne Preston, "Domestic Ideology," 531–51.

70 Putnam reflected back on teaching in her 1865 essay/address "Woman's Right to Labor," 66–67.

71 Ruth Putnam, *Life and Letters*, 47; Mary C. Putnam, "Found and Lost," 1–49; also published in *Atlantic Monthly*, April 1860, 391–407.

72 See Jane Tompkins, afterword, in Susan Warner, *Wide, Wide World*, 585.

73 Mary C. Putnam, "Conversations with Dr. Anderson," June 1862, Folder 26, MPJ Papers, SL. On women and conversion narratives, see Brumberg, *Mission for Life*, 34–35, 107–44. On the First Baptist Church, see Hansell, *Reminiscences of Baptist Churches*.

74 When she started her sessions with Anderson, she retained her belief in the doctrines of grace but refused to accept the idea of "absolute faith."

75 Mary C. Putnam, "Conversations with Dr. Anderson," June 1862, Folder 26, MPJ Papers, SL. He told her: "You are in the midst of a great trial and temptation, out of which I trust that God in his own good time will deliver you, and bring you back to a firmer standing and brighter vision than you had before."

76 Mary C. Putnam to Rev. Dr. Anderson, 19 April 1863, Ruth Putnam, *Life and Letters*, 58.

77 Ibid.

78 Ibid., 58–59. She wrote, "If one cannot believe in the mystery of God without the Trinity, in the mercy of God and the vicariousness of pure love without Atonement, in the hatefulness of sin without eternal punishment, why then I suppose it is best that men should believe these partial symbols of the vast ideas which would else escape them. But there is a point where doctrines shrivel."

79 Mary C. Putnam, "Conversations with Dr. Anderson," June 1862, Folder 26, MPJ Papers, SL.

80 Ibid.

81 Ibid. Rejecting the idea of future punishment, Putnam believed that it did not prevent the human transgression of divine law: "Why should not these dreams of goodness and truth that haunt our footsteps, be anticipations glimmering in the future, as well as reminiscences drifted from the past[?]"

82 A few years later, Putnam cited her training with Blackwell and Percy as evidence of instruction prior to arriving at the Female Medical College of Pennsylvania. See "Minute Book of the Faculty of the Female Medical College of Pennsylvania," 10 and 12 March 1864, 172, 176–77, Drexel. On the New York Medical College (not the New York Medical College for Women), see Spiegal, "New York Medical College," 293–315.

83 Elizabeth Blackwell to Barbara Smith Bodichon, 25 April 1860, Elizabeth Blackwell Papers, Columbia. See also Sahli, *Elizabeth Blackwell*, 147.

84 Elizabeth Blackwell, "Medical Education," *Annual Report of the New York Infirmary*, 1860, quoted in Daniel, "A Cautious Experiment," *Medical Woman's Journal* 47 (February 1940): 40.

85 New York College of Pharmacy Lecture Leaflet, 1861–62, in Wimmer, *College of Pharmacy*, 55.

86 On cell theory, see Ackerknecht, *Rudolf Virchow*, 57–58; Roderick E. McGrew, *Encyclopedia of Medical History* (New York: McGraw-Hill, 1985), 52–54; and W. F. Bynum and Roy Porter, *Companion Encyclopedia of the History of Medicine* (New York: Routledge, 1994), 1:105–9. See also Virchow, *Cellular Pathology*.

87 Wimmer, *College of Pharmacy*, 51. For more on the college, see Ballard, *History of the College of Pharmacy*, and Rusby, *College of Pharmacy*.

88 Kremers, *Kremers and Urdang's History of Pharmacy*. On pharmacy education, see ibid., chap. 14.

89 George Palmer Putnam to Mary C. Putnam, 13 February 1861, Ruth Putnam, *Life and Letters*, 60 (emphasis original).

90 See Commencement Program, College of Pharmacy, 1863, in Wimmer, *College of Pharmacy*, 56. While Putnam's thesis does not survive, we can assume it reflected her chemistry training and described the chemical filtering process of dialysis. See also "College of Pharmacy Commencement," 8.

91 "College of Pharmacy Commencement," 8.

92 Wimmer, *College of Pharmacy*, 57. Although the New York College of Pharmacy had a troubled beginning, it experienced greater stability after 1870 with the expansion of formal pharmaceutical education nationally. In 1904, after graduating more than three thousand pharmacists, the college merged with Columbia University and continued to train students in pharmaceutical sciences. For a history of the merger, see ibid.

93 At the end of the nineteenth century, the slow process of professionalization allowed for a number of women to study and practice in the field of pharmacy. See Gallagher, "From Family Helpmeet to Independent Professional," 60; and Ward, "Hygeia's Sisters," 1–54.

94 Mary Putnam may have worked in soldiers' hospitals during the war, but evidence is limited. See George Haven Putnam (studying in Germany) to Mary C. Putnam, 1862, fragment quoted in Ruth Putnam, *Life and Letters*, 63. He said, "Mother makes me quite anxious in telling me of your work in the soldiers' hospitals. It is worrying to think of your being exposed to a danger which I can neither prevent nor share. Do take care of yourself and remember how valuable you are to all of us."

95 Greenspan, *George Palmer Putnam*, 400–405. See also George Palmer Putnam, "Before and After the Battle," 231–50.

96 Upon arriving in Louisiana, she presented letters to the adjutant general and the quartermaster's department to explain her visit. Mary had previously met the quartermaster general, Colonel Holabird, socially in New York. His wife was a cousin to Mary Swift, Mary Putnam's former teacher and friend from the Twelfth Street School. Letters from the Swifts in New York provided the introduction she needed to acquire housing at the quartermaster general's home as she searched for her brother. See Ruth Putnam, *Life and Letters*, 64.

97 Haven learned of the ensuing war while studying abroad in Germany. He returned to New York to volunteer for the Union army and enrolled in the 176th Division of New York Volunteers. See George Haven Putnam, *Memories of My Youth*, 231–32, 241.

98 Ibid., 264.

99 Ibid., 265, 266.

100 Ibid., 266.

101 Ibid.

102 Ibid.

103 Ibid.

104 Ibid., 266–67.

105 Ibid., 285. Haven wrote that she returned to New York in early 1864, but it was more likely to be late 1863.

106 Ruth Putnam, *Life and Letters*, 66.

107 Ibid., 65–66; George Haven Putnam, *Memories of My Youth*, 266.

108 Ruth Putnam, *Life and Letters*, 83–84. See clippings of *New Orleans Times* articles in Folder 28, MPJ Papers, SL.

109 George Haven Putnam, *Prisoner of War*.

110 Alex McDonald, U.S. Sanitary Commission, to Mary C. Putnam, 29 December 1864, George Palmer Putnam Collection, MS 117, Rauner Special Collections, Dartmouth College Library, Hanover, N.H.

111 On women teaching the freedmen, see Hoffman, *Woman's "True" Profession*.

112 Certificate of Commission, National Freedmen's Relief Association, issued to Mary C. Putnam, "Teacher," 22 December 1864, George Palmer Putnam Collection, MS 117, Rauner Special Collections, Dartmouth College Library, Hanover, N.H.

113 Rules and Regulations, National Freedmen's Relief Association, George Palmer Putnam

Collection, MS 117, Rauner Special Collections, Dartmouth College Library, Hanover, N.H.

114 Attie, "Warwork and the Crisis of Domesticity in the North," 247–59; Faust, *Mothers of Invention*; Schultz, *Women at the Front*.

115 Mary C. Putnam, "Theorae ad lienis officium," Medical thesis, Female Medical College of Pennsylvania, 1864, Drexel.

116 Ibid.

117 Ibid.

118 On medical theses at the Female/Woman's Medical College of Pennsylvania, see Wells, *Out of the Dead House*, 80–121.

119 Today, we understand the spleen as

> a large unpaired organ situated in the left upper part of the abdominal cavity be-
> tween the stomach and the left kidney, behind the left lower ribs and underneath the
> left hemidiaphram. . . . It has a fibrous structure occupied by blood and lymphoid
> tissue. The spleen has several functions: in fetal life and in the newborn it is a site
> of red blood cell formation, a function to which it can revert in later life under
> certain conditions; it acts as a reservoir of blood; it sequesters and destroys aging or
> imperfect blood cells; it is part of the immunological system, producing antibodies,
> plasma cells and lymphocytes; it is also part of the reticulo-endthelial system. None
> of these functions, however, is vital or unique, and surgical removal of the spleen
> (occasionally necessary after abdominal trauma) does not usually produce obvious
> ill-effects in adults. Removal is also needed in some blood diseases. (*Oxford Medical
> Companion*, 919)

120 For history of knowledge on the spleen, see Crosby, "Historical Sketch of Splenic Function and Splenectomy," 52–55; and McClusky et al., "Tribute to a Triad," pt. 1, 311–25, and
pt. 2, 514–26.

121 *Oxford Medical Companion*.

122 McClusky et al., "Tribute to a Triad," pt. 1, 320–24.

123 For some of their work on the spleen, see Gray, *On the Structure and Use of the Spleen*;
Thomson, *Practical Treatise on the Diseases of the Liver*; and Kölliker, *Manual of Human
Microscopical Anatomy*.

124 Mary C. Putnam, "Theorae ad lienis officium," Medical thesis, Female Medical College of
Pennsylvania, 1864, Drexel. She quotes Twining's description of leukemia in her thesis as
it was understood in the nineteenth century: "The symptoms of this malady are complete
fatigue, paleness and the poor circulation of blood in the capillaries. One's extremities
become chilly because of the lack of blood getting to them, and the skin is dry and cor-
rugated. The abdomen swells up, breathing becomes more rapid, and a stinking smell is
emitted from the body. There is emotional despair, clouding both body and mind, and
also muscular debility."

125 On the intersection of women's medical education and the efforts to raise standards, see
Morantz-Sanchez, *Sympathy and Science*, 68–72.

126 *The Female Medical College of Pennsylvania, Annual Announcement*, 1863, 14–15; Wells, *Out
of the Dead House*, 80–121.

127 Morantz-Sanchez, *Sympathy and Science*, 28–63.

128 Drachman, *Hospital with a Heart*; Morantz-Sanchez, *Sympathy and Science*, 81–84; Tuchman, *Science Has No Sex*; Tuchman, "Situating Gender," 34–57; Tuchman, "'Only in a Republic,'" 121–42.

129 The college changed its name in 1867, becoming the Woman's Medical College of Pennsylvania.

130 For a history of the college, see Peitzman, *New and Untried Course*. See also Clara Marshall, *Woman's Medical College of Pennsylvania*.

131 Minute Book, Faculty, Female Medical College of Pennsylvania, 3 February 1864, 163, 165, Drexel.

132 Ibid., 26 February 1864, 168–69.

133 Ibid., 169.

134 Ibid., 12 March 1864, 172.

135 Ibid., 176–77.

136 For another treatment of this controversy, see Gartner, "Fussell's Folly," 470–77.

137 Edwin Fussell joined the faculty in 1853 and a few years later became dean. His uncle, Dr. Bartholomew Fussell, was one of the college founders. Edwin Fussell was a staunch supporter of temperance and a strong abolitionist who, while living in Indiana, was attacked by a mob for his antislavery activism. See Ellwood Harvey, "Report of the Delaware County Medical Society," 318–19.

138 Minute Book, Faculty, Female Medical College of Pennsylvania, 10 March 1864, 174, Drexel (emphasis original).

139 Ibid., 12 March 1864, 175.

140 Edwin Fussell to the faculty of the Female Medical College of Pennsylvania, 27 February 1864, 195–96, in the Minute Book, Faculty, Female Medical College of Pennsylvania, Drexel.

141 Minute Book, Faculty, Female Medical College of Pennsylvania, 27 March 1864, 198–99, Drexel.

142 Fussell, "Introductory Address," 10 (emphasis original). Fussell's return was short-lived; he resigned from the college again in October 1865 for reasons unknown. Ellwood Harvey reported that Fussell served as chair of the Principles and Practice of Medicine until 1868. See Ellwood Harvey, "Report of the Delaware County Medical Society," 318. However, the Faculty Minutes report his resignation in 1865. I thank Steve Peitzman for pointing out this discrepancy.

143 Mary Putnam Jacobi, "Women in Medicine," 161–62. 144. See *Reports and Transactions of the Annual Meetings*, 1888–1900.

144 *Reports and Transactions of Annual Meetings*, 1888–1900.

145 Cleveland studied at the Maternité Hospital in Paris. See Mary Putnam Jacobi, "Woman in Medicine," 158.

146 Ibid., 166.

147 Tuchman, *Science Has No Sex*, 177–98.

148 Morantz-Sanchez, *Sympathy and Science*, 167.

149 Bonner, *To the Ends of the Earth*, 27.

150 For a portrait of Mayer, see Wimmer, *College of Pharmacy*, 53.

151 Victorine Haven Putnam to Mary Caroline [cousin], 5 April 1865, Ruth Putnam, *Life and Letters*, 75–76; Truax, *Doctors Jacobi*, 44–49.

152 Mary C. Putnam to George Palmer Putnam, August 1865, Ruth Putnam, *Life and Letters*, 80–81.

153 Wimmer, *College of Pharmacy*, 57; "Eighteenth Annual Meeting of the American Pharmaceutical Association." Notes from the meeting state that Mayer "is supposed to be dead, as the most diligent inquiry of his friends in New York have not availed to find his whereabouts."

154 George Palmer Putnam to Mary C. Putnam, c. fall 1863, quoted in Ruth Putnam, *Life and Letters*, 67.

155 Ibid., 67–68.

156 Ibid., 67 (emphasis original).

CHAPTER TWO

1 Mary C. Putnam to George Palmer Putnam, 12 November 1868, Ruth Putnam, *Life and Letters*, 202. Putnam was quoting a line from Robert Browning's poem "Bishop Blougram's Apology" (1855). The line reads: "Our interest's on the dangerous edge of things."

2 On August Comte, see Pickering, *August Comte*.

3 On positivism in the Second Empire, see Charlton, *Positivist Thought in France*. See also Simon, *European Positivism*.

4 On transnational history, see Rodgers, *Atlantic Crossings*. On American responses to French political conflicts in the 1860s, see Katz, *From Appomattox to Montmartre*.

5 For other treatments of Putnam in Paris, see Bonner, *To the Ends of the Earth*, 48–54; Joy Harvey, "'Faithful to Its Old Traditions'?," 323–28; Joy Harvey, "La Visite," 350–71; Joy Harvey, "Medicine and Politics," 107–17; and John Harley Warner, *Against the Spirit of System*, 322–27. Joy Harvey also connects Putnam's medicine and politics.

6 As John Harley Warner (*Against the Spirit of System*, chaps. 1 and 2) argues, the city's popularity was not a measure of how "advanced" medical knowledge really was in the French academy but a reflection of the needs and aspirations of American medical students, who desired clinical experience and the prestige that came with a Paris education.

7 Ibid., 24–31, 5.

8 Ibid., 165.

9 Ibid., chaps. 9–10.

10 Bernard, *Introduction to the Study of Experimental Medicine*. On Bernard, see also Holmes, *Claude Bernard and Animal Chemistry*; Lesch, *Science and Medicine in France*, 197–224; and Normandin, "Claude Bernard," 495–528.

11 Bidelman, *Pariahs Stand Up!*, 3–32; Moses, *French Feminism*, 1–15.

12 Henri Montanier, "La femme médecin," *Gazette des Hôpitaux* 34 (1868): 1–2, as quoted in Bonner, *To the Ends of the Earth*, 52 n. 87.

13 McMillan, *France and Women*, 101–3.

14 Moses, *French Feminism*, 127–72.

15 The determination to maintain traditional gender roles in French society was most strongly articulated through the writings of historian Jules Michelet. Historians believe

Michelet represented the backlash against feminist activism during the 1848 revolutions, and a larger cultural backlash against more liberal interpretations of female roles in the 1860s. In his work *Le Femme*, Michelet used new medical knowledge about the physical inferiority of women in his moral campaign against the expansion of women's rights. See Moses, *French Feminism*, 158–61.

16 Mary C. Putnam to Victorine Haven Putnam, 16 April 1867, Ruth Putnam, *Life and Letters*, 121.

17 Ibid., 120–21.

18 Mary C. Putnam to George Palmer Putnam, 12 November 1867, Ruth Putnam, *Life and Letters*, 153.

19 Mary C. Putnam to Victorine Haven Putnam, 13 November 1866, Ruth Putnam, *Life and Letters*, 103.

20 Ibid., 22 April 1867, 124–25.

21 Mary C. Putnam to Edith Putnam, 30 September 1866, Ruth Putnam, *Life and Letters*, 97.

22 On Elizabeth Blackwell's own medical education in Paris at the Maternité, see Elizabeth Blackwell, *Pioneer Work*, 90–128.

23 John Harley Warner, *Against the Spirit of System*, 318–22.

24 Elizabeth Blackwell, *Pioneer Work*, 100.

25 Mary C. Putnam to Victorine Haven Putnam, 3 December 1866, Ruth Putnam, *Life and Letters*, 104.

26 Ibid., 13 November 1866, 100–101.

27 Dr. Benjamin Ball was a colleague of Jean-Martin Charcot, who worked with him on studies of old age and senility. See Charcot, *Leçons Cliniques*.

28 Mary C. Putnam to Victorine Haven Putnam, 13 November 1866, Ruth Putnam, *Life and Letters*, 102.

29 Mary C. Putnam, "Letters to the *Medical Record*," in *Pathfinder*, 3–4, 12–13, 50–51.

30 On Charcot at the Salpêtrière, see Goldstein, *Console and Classify*, 326–38. For another view of Charcot, see Showalter, *Female Malady*, 147–54.

31 Mary C. Putnam to Victorine Haven Putnam, 13 November 1866, Ruth Putnam, *Life and Letters*, 102.

32 Mary C. Putnam, "Letters to the *Medical Record*," *Pathfinder*, 8–9. Putnam told readers of the *Medical Record* about Moreau's belief that genius was a form of neuroses.

33 Moreau, *Hashish and Mental Illness*. Moreau's book was originally published in 1845.

34 Mary C. Putnam to Victorine Haven Putnam, 16 April 1867, Ruth Putnam, *Life and Letters*, 122. On Putnam and Paris clinics, see works by Joy Harvey.

35 Ibid., 123.

36 Ibid., 22 April 1867, 128.

37 Ibid., 16 April 1867, 122.

38 "Jean-François Jarjavay," in *Dictionnaire de Biographie Française*, 478; Ruth Putnam, *Life and Letters*, 130.

39 Mary C. Putnam to Edith Putnam, 5 May 1867, Ruth Putnam, *Life and Letters*, 129.

40 Mary C. Putnam to George Palmer Putnam, 1 February 1867, and Mary C. Putnam to Victorine Haven Putnam, 14 February 1867, Ruth Putnam, *Life and Letters*, 111.

41 Mary C. Putnam to Victorine Haven Putnam, 29 May 1867, Ruth Putnam, *Life and Letters*, 139.

42 On the rise of laboratory science in Paris medicine, see John Harley Warner, *Against the Spirit of System*, 294, 334–35.

43 Cornil and Ranvier, *Manual of Pathological Histology*, v.

44 See Mary C. Putnam, "De la graisse neutre et des acides gras."

45 Mary C. Putnam, "Letters to the Medical Record," *Pathfinder*, 1–170.

46 "George Frederick Shrady," in *Dictionary of American Medical Biography*, 680–81; James J. Walsh, *History of Medicine in New York*, 2:350.

47 Putnam's letters in the *New York Evening Post* were unsigned. Although difficult to verify as Putnam's, several entries cover topics of interest to her. See, for example, *New York Evening Post*, 7 January, 8 January, 21 January, 4 February 1867; and Mary C. Putnam to Edith Putnam, 21 February 1867, Ruth Putnam, *Life and Letters*, 112–13. On the challenges of writing for the *Post*, see Ruth Putnam, *Life and Letters*, 151, 153, 157.

48 Several articles from Paris were published later in Mary Putnam Jacobi, *Stories and Sketches*. In *Putnam's Monthly*, see "Imagination and Language," "Study of Still-Life, Paris," "Sermon at Notre-Dame," "Martyr to Science," and "Concerning Charlotte." She also contributed "Some of the French Leaders" to *Scribner's Monthly*.

49 Mary C. Putnam, "Martyr to Science," 212–61, quotes on 233.

50 For another discussion of her letters to the *Medical Record*, see Joy Harvey, "'Faithful to Its Old Traditions'?," 323–28.

51 For example, see P. C. M., "Letters to the *Medical Record*," *Pathfinder*, 4, 12, 17, 51.

52 Ibid., 81.

53 Ibid., 82.

54 Ibid., 143–70. Albuminuria refers to the presence of albumin in urine, sometimes a sign of kidney disease.

55 Mary C. Putnam to Victorine Haven Putnam, 29 May 1867, Ruth Putnam, *Life and Letters*, 139–40.

56 Mary C. Putnam to George Palmer Putnam, 12 November 1867, Ruth Putnam, *Life and Letters*, 152.

57 Ibid.

58 Ibid.

59 Ibid., 152–53.

60 Procés-Verbal de L'Assemblée de Professeurs, Faculté de Médecine de Paris, 23 November 1867, AJ16-6255, Archives Nationales, Paris. For Putnam's account, see Ruth Putnam, *Life and Letters*, 155–57.

61 Procés-Verbal de L'Assemblée de Professeurs, Faculté de Médecine de Paris, 23 November 1867, AJ16-6255, Archives Nationales, Paris.

62 On the popularity of Robin's histology courses among American students, see John Harley Warner, *Against the Spirit of System*, 294; and Ruth Putnam, *Life and Letters*, 158.

63 Mary C. Putnam to Victorine Haven Putnam, 25 January 1868, Ruth Putnam, *Life and Letters*, 167 (emphasis original).

64 For a later example of a woman physician referencing the petticoat, see Van Hoosen, *Petticoat Surgeon*.

65 Mary C. Putnam to Victorine Haven Putnam, 25 January 1868, Ruth Putnam, *Life and Letters*, 168.

66 "Joseph-Arsène Danton," *Dictionnaire de Biographie Française*, ed. Roman D'Amat et al. (Paris: Librairie Letouzey et Ané, 1965), 142.

67 Mary C. Putnam to Victorine Haven Putnam and George Palmer Putnam, 24 June 1868, Ruth Putnam, *Life and Letters*, 179. Putnam decided to "boldly" approach Danton. Although he had expected a visit from Putnam, Danton pretended to be naïve about her case, and tested her by requesting that she explain herself and prove her readiness. He finally agreed to put the authorization into motion, and told Putnam to wait for a letter of approval from the rector.

68 The letter was from the vice-rector of the academy to the dean of faculty (Vice-Recteur, Université de France, to Adolphe Wurtz, Dean, Faculté de Médecine de Paris, 4 June 1868, AJ16-6823, Archives Nationales, Paris).

69 Matriculation Record of Mary C. Putnam, Faculté de Médecine de Paris, AJ16-6823, Archives Nationales, Paris.

70 Mary C. Putnam to Victorine Haven Putnam and George Palmer Putnam, 24 June 1868, Ruth Putnam, *Life and Letters*, 178–84, quote on 180.

71 Joy Harvey shows how Putnam used her social network to facilitate her admission to the Paris school of medicine. See Harvey, "La Visite," 351; and John Harley Warner, *Against the Spirit of System*, 326.

72 Horvath-Peterson, *Victor Duruy*, 47; Moses, *French Feminism*, 173–75.

73 Horvath-Peterson, *Victor Duruy*, 154–55.

74 Schultze, "La femme-médecin au XIXe siècle," 15–17.

75 Bonner, *To the Ends of the Earth*, 53–54.

76 Duruy, *Notes et souvenirs*, 196.

77 Ibid., 196–98.

78 Empress Eugenie to Victory Duruy, 1870, ibid., 198.

79 On the Reclus see Dunbar, *Élisée Reclus*; Fleming, *Anarchist Way to Socialism*; Fleming, *Geography of Freedom*; and Ishill, *Elisée and Elie Reclus*.

80 Fleming, *Anarchist Way to Socialism*, 244.

81 Mary C. Putnam to Edith Grace Putnam, 24 March 1868, Ruth Putnam, *Life and Letters*, 172.

82 Mary C. Putnam to Victorine Haven Putnam, 29 October 1868, Ruth Putnam, *Life and Letters*, 197. On the Reclus and Putnam at Vascoeuil, see also Dunbar, *Élisée Reclus*, 53–55.

83 Mary C. Putnam to Victorine Haven Putnam, 2 April 1868, Ruth Putnam, *Life and Letters*, 174.

84 Noémi Reclus to George Palmer Putnam and Victorine Haven Putnam, c. June 1871, Ruth Putnam, *Life and Letters*, 282.

85 Mary C. Putnam to George Palmer Putnam, 15 August 1871, Ruth Putnam, *Life and Letters*, 293.

86 Reclus, *La Commune de Paris*.

87 Fleming, *Anarchist Way to Socialism*, 67–70.

88 Ibid., 71–72.

89 According to Dunbar (*Élisée Reclus*, 11), Paul Vidal de la Blache (1845–1918), a Sorbonne professor, gave him this title. On Reclus and American slavery, see Fleming, *Anarchist Way to Socialism*, 48.

90 Fleming, *Anarchist Way to Socialism*, 145. Human geography is defined as the study of the relationship between people and their environments.

91 Ibid., 149.

92 Ibid., 144–62; Fleming, *Geography of Freedom*, 112–39.

93 Mary C. Putnam to Victorine Haven Putnam, 9 December 1866, Ruth Putnam, *Life and Letters*, 105.

94 On Comte's use and criticism of certain sciences and their methods, see Pickering, *August Comte*, 561–624.

95 On Fourier, see Moses, *French Feminism*, 90–98.

96 Mary C. Putnam to Victorine Haven Putnam, 22 September 1868, Ruth Putnam, *Life and Letters*, 191.

97 Mary Putnam Jacobi to Edmund C. Stedman, 24 January 1876, Columbia; Mary Putnam Jacobi to Elizabeth Blackwell, 25 December 1888, Manuscript Division, Blackwell Family Papers, 0320T, LOC; Mary Putnam Jacobi, "Reply to Professor Munsterberg," unpublished essay, c. 1880, Folder 30, MPJ Papers, SL; Mary Putnam Jacobi, *Value of Life*, 87.

98 Mary C. Putnam to Victorine Haven Putnam, 11 March 1869, Ruth Putnam, *Life and Letters*, 208 (emphasis original).

99 Ibid., 29 October 1868, 194.

100 Ibid., 195, 194.

101 Reclus Wedding Statement, Élisée Reclus Papers, NAF 22909: 10–14, Manuscript Collections, Bibliothèque Nationale de France, Paris.

102 Mary C. Putnam to Victorine Haven Putnam, 5 January 1868, Ruth Putnam, *Life and Letters*, 162.

103 Mary C. Putnam to Élisée Reclus, 28 June 1870, Élisée Reclus Papers, NAF 22914: 346–47, Manuscript Collections, Bibliothèque Nationale de France, Paris.

104 Mary Putnam Jacobi, "Sermon at Notre Dame," 166–211.

105 Ibid., 172, 179, 187–88, 195, 209, 210, 211.

106 Mary C. Putnam to George Palmer Putnam, 12 November 1868, Ruth Putnam, *Life and Letters*, 201.

107 Ibid., 201 (emphasis original). Putnam added, "I had not much to do with the borderland here, since I merely described a state of things peculiar to one country, and which would by no means be true of England or America" (Ruth Putnam, *Life and Letters*, 202).

108 Mary C. Putnam to Victorine Haven Putnam, 25 January 1868, Ruth Putnam, *Life and Letters*, 170–71.

109 Ibid., 11 November 1869, 222.

110 Ibid., 14 August 1870, 255.

111 Mary C. Putnam to George Palmer Putnam, 4 September 1870, Ruth Putnam, *Life and Letters*, 256, 267.

112 Mary C. Putnam to Victorine Haven Putnam, 15 September 1870, Ruth Putnam, *Life and Letters*, 271.

113 Mary C. Putnam to George Palmer Putnam, 2 February 1871, Ruth Putnam, *Life and Letters*, 277.

114 Mary C. Putnam to George Palmer Putnam, Paris, c. 28 September 1870, Container 10, Folder 3, HPP (emphasis added).

115 Mary C. Putnam to George Palmer Putnam, 2 February 1871, Ruth Putnam, *Life and Letters*, 275; Mary C. Putnam to Family, c. February 1871, fragment, HPP.

116 Mary C. Putnam to George Palmer Putnam, 2 February 1871, Ruth Putnam, *Life and Letters*, 276.

117 Ibid., 26 December 1870, 272.

118 This is similarly noted by Katz, *From Appomattox to Montmarte*, who discusses how Americans viewed the Paris Commune with their own nationalist lens.

119 The leadership included moderate republicans Jules Favre, Jules Simon, Jules Ferry, and Ernest Picard; the radicals Léon Gambetta and Henri Rochefort; and the conservative Jules Trochu. The new government tried to expand the National Guard, win the war against Prussia, and defend the new republic.

120 Eichner, *Surmounting the Barricades*; Gullickson, *Unruly Women of Paris*.

121 On the declaration of the republic and the history of the Commune, see Tombs, *Paris Commune*, and Shafer, *Paris Commune*.

122 Mary Putnam Jacobi, "Some of the French Leaders," 390–443. Her frustration can also be seen in "Clubs of Paris," 105–9.

123 Mary Putnam Jacobi, "Some of the French Leaders," 390.

124 Ibid., 442.

125 On American impressions of French politics, see Katz, *From Appomattox to Montmarte*, chap. 3.

126 "The Magazines for August," *The Nation*, 3 August 1871, as quoted in Ruth Putnam, *Life and Letters*, 294.

127 R. W. Gilder to George Haven Putnam, 4 August 1871, Ruth Putnam, *Life and Letters*, 296. Mary Putnam was outraged by the accusation and asked her father to write to *The Nation* in her defense. Instead, her brother, Haven, replied to the publishing company. The incident sheds light on the reception of information about French politics in America. It is possible that *The Nation* did not believe a woman was capable of writing a knowledgeable piece about a complex ideological conflict, and assumed that a young American woman in Paris would know only the language, but not the politics. But it is also likely that the accusation emerged from the competitive publishing market in the early 1870s. *The Nation*, a weekly paper, and *Scribner's Monthly* both published articles on French politics and vied for New York readers. Putnam's informed critique of the conflict may have seemed "foreign" to readers who expected a distanced perspective from a young American woman living in Paris.

128 Mary C. Putnam to George Haven Putnam, 7 May 1871, Ruth Putnam, *Life and Letters*, 277–79.

129 Ibid., 278.

130 Fleming, *Anarchist Way to Socialism*, 95–100.

131 Élisée Reclus to Fanny L'Herminez, 29 July 1871, Élisée Reclus Papers, NAF 22913: 68–69, Manuscript Collections, Bibliothèque Nationale de France, Paris.

132 Noémi Reclus to George Palmer Putnam, c. 1871, Ruth Putnam, *Life and Letters*, 282.

133 Mary C. Putnam to Victorine Haven Putnam, 29 July 1871, Ruth Putnam, *Life and Letters*, 286 (emphasis original).

134 Mary C. Putnam, "De la graisse neutre et des acides gras." Putnam received "*tres satisfait*"

on four of her exams and *"bien"* on one of them. On her thesis exam, she received *"extreme-ment satisfait,"* the highest possible grade. See list of "Examens," Commission Scolaire, Faculté de Médecine de Paris, AJ16-6255, Archives Nationales, Paris.

135 Mary C. Putnam, "De la graisse neutre et des acides gras."

136 On Bernard and the chemical/physiological debate, see Holmes, *Claude Bernard and Animal Chemistry*, 1–33. In his *Cours de Philosophie Positive, III* (1838), August Comte also addressed physiology and chemistry as systems of analysis. The extent of Comte's influence on Claude Bernard and other scientists during the Second Empire has been debated by historians. On the relationship between Bernard and Comte, see Holmes, *Claude Bernard and Animal Chemistry*, 403–6, 454–55; and Charlton, *Positivist Thought in France*, 72–85.

137 Claude Bernard quoted in Weber, *Nineteenth-Century Science*, 315–16.

138 Mary C. Putnam to Victorine Haven Putnam, 29 July 1871, Ruth Putnam, *Life and Letters*, 287.

139 *Archives de Médecine*, July 1871, quoted in Ruth Putnam, *Life and Letters*, 291.

140 Mary C. Putnam to Victorine Haven Putnam, 13 January 1870, Ruth Putnam, *Life and Letters*, 233.

141 "Miss Putnam," *Le Figaro*, 1871, Ruth Putnam, *Life and Letters*, 288–89.

142 *Archives de Médecine*, July 1871, Ruth Putnam, *Life and Letters*, 290–91.

143 She also thanked other mentors, including Doctors Hérard, Ball, Chereau, Moreau (de Tours), Raige-Delorme, Cornil, Martin-Damourette, Fort, and Sappey. See Mary C. Putnam, "Dédicace," in "De la graisse neutre et des acides gras."

144 Mary C. Putnam to Victorine Haven Putnam, 28 August 1871, Paris, Ruth Putnam, *Life and Letters*, 298.

CHAPTER THREE

1 Mary C. Putnam to Victorine Haven Putnam, 13 January 1870, Ruth Putnam, *Life and Letters*, 235.

2 Reported by her sister, Ruth Putnam, *Life and Letters*, 309–10. George Palmer Putnam died of a heart attack at the age of fifty-eight on 20 December 1872. See obituary, "George Palmer Putnam, Publisher," *New York Times*, 21 December 1872. For another account, see Greenspan, *George Palmer Putnam*, 476.

3 Mary C. Putnam to Victorine Haven Putnam, 13 January 1870, Ruth Putnam, *Life and Letters*, 233. Mary Putnam Jacobi taught at the Woman's Medical College from 1871 to 1889, serving as a lecturer on materia medica from 1871 to 1872, professor of materia medica from 1872 to 1873, and professor of materia medica and therapeutics from 1873 to 1889. See *Pathfinder*, xvii; and Woman's Medical College of the New York Infirmary, *Annual Catalogue and Announcement*, 1871–89.

4 For example, see Mary Putnam, "Some Details in the Pathogeny of Pyemia and Septice-mia," 171–200.

5 For a record of her admission to the Medical Society of the County of New York, see Minutes of the Comitia Minora, 27 November 1871, Records of the Medical Society of the County of New York, NYAM; Mary Corinna Putnam, "Particulars for Permanent

Record of Members," 10 January 1872, Records of the Medical Society of the County of New York, NYAM.

6 See Abraham Jacobi and Mary C. Putnam, Certificate of Marriage, 22 July 1873, NYCMA.

7 Mary Putnam Jacobi to Elizabeth Blackwell, 25 December 1888, Blackwell Family Papers, 0320T, LOC.

8 James J. Walsh, *History of Medicine in New York*.

9 Wallace and Burrows, *Gotham*; Bender, *New York Intellect*.

10 For more on the New York Positivist Society, see Harp, *Positivist Republic*, chap. 2.

11 David, *Positivist Primer*, 6.

12 Ibid., 7.

13 See Harp, *Positivist Republic*, 40. See Harp's appendix for a list of the writers, educators, and professionals who attended meetings of the New York Positivist Society.

14 On the "spiritual crisis," see Paul A. Carter, *Spiritual Crisis of the Gilded Age*.

15 "A Positivist Celebration," *Springfield Daily Republican*, 8 April 1872, 6.

16 On Jacobi's participation in the New York Positivist Society, see "From New York," *Springfield Daily Republican*, 31 January 1872, 5.

17 Leach, *True Love and Perfect Union*, 153–57.

18 Mary C. Putnam, "Christianity Not for Reformers, but for Come-Outers," c. 1873, Folder 25, MPJ Papers, SL. Although this unpublished essay is filed in her papers under writings for 1857–59, it most likely was composed after 1873. Several factors point to this, including the fact that she would have been only about seventeen in 1859. Also, Ruth Putnam's bibliography claims this essay was one of several contributions to "The Fraternity — a social literary club," dated 1873. See Ruth Putnam, *Life and Letters*, 353–54. Finally, the tone and language match those in other writings from this later period of her life.

19 Mary C. Putnam, "Christianity Not for Reformers, but for Come-Outers," c. 1873, Folder 25, MPJ Papers, SL.

20 Mallock, *Is Life Worth Living?*; on Mallock, see Mallock, *Memoirs of Life and Literature*, and editor's preface to Mallock, *New Paul and Virginia*.

21 Mary Putnam Jacobi, *Value of Life*.

22 Ibid., 89–90.

23 Ibid., 61.

24 Charlton, *Positivist Thought in France*, 9.

25 Mary Putnam Jacobi, *Value of Life*, 222.

26 Ibid., 89.

27 On the history of nutrition, see Kamminga and Cunningham, "Science and Culture of Nutrition," 1–14. See also several nineteenth-century medical textbooks and dictionaries; for example, Quain, ed., *Dictionary of Medicine*, 1050; and Dalton, *Treatise on Physiology*. On Bernard and nutrition, see Holmes, "Claude Bernard," 8–9.

28 Mary Putnam Jacobi, *Value of Life*, 92.

29 Ibid., 85–87.

30 Ibid., 85.

31 Ibid., 95–96.

32 On evolutionary socialism, see Pittenger, *American Socialists*, 19–22.

33 See Mary Putnam Jacobi, *Value of Life*, 87. On Saint-Simon and Fourier, see Moses, *French Feminism*, chaps. 3 and 4; and Taylor, *Political Ideas of the Utopian Socialists*, 21–24, 39–68, 100–131. On Fourier, see also Guarneri, *Utopian Alternative*. Fourier quoted in Taylor, *Political Ideas of the Utopian Socialists*, 113.

34 Mary Putnam Jacobi, "Reply to Professor Munsterberg," unpublished essay, c. 1880, Folder 30, MPJ Papers, SL.

35 Harp, *Positivist Republic*, 17–20; Leach, *True Love and Perfect Union*, 153–57; Newman, *White Women's Rights*.

36 Mary Putnam Jacobi, *Value of Life*, 253.

37 Stepan and Gilman, "Appropriating the Idioms of Science," 72–103.

38 Anderson, "Black Responses to Darwinism," 247–66.

39 Swetlitz, "American Jewish Responses," 209–45.

40 Mary Putnam Jacobi, "Social Aspects," 168. Her by-line is incorrect, printed as "Mary E. Putnam Jacobi" rather than "Mary C."

41 Mary Putnam Jacobi, "Women in Medicine," 197.

42 Mary Putnam Jacobi, "Social Aspects," 173.

43 Mary Putnam Jacobi, "Shall Women Practice Medicine?," *Pathfinder*, 389.

44 Mary Putnam Jacobi, "Married Women's Right to Compensation," 66.

45 Mary Putnam Jacobi, "Social Aspects," 171.

46 Mary Putnam Jacobi, *Essays on Hysteria*, 66.

47 Mary Putnam Jacobi, "Social Aspects," 173.

48 Ibid., 174 (emphasis original).

49 Ibid., 174.

50 Ibid., 173.

51 On scientific motherhood, see Apple, *Mothers and Medicine*. On the application of science to domestic work, see Stage and Vincenti, eds., *Rethinking Home Economics*.

52 Mary Putnam Jacobi, "Inaugural Address," *Pathfinder*, 356.

53 Mary Putnam Jacobi, "School of Medicine for Women" (courtesy of NYAM).

54 Ibid., 25.

55 Ibid., 25.

56 Ibid., 15–16.

57 Mary Putnam Jacobi, "Inaugural Address," *Pathfinder*, 334.

58 On the sympathetic model, see Morantz-Sanchez, *Sympathy and Science*. On the construction of physician empathy, see More and Milligan, eds., *Empathic Practitioner*.

59 Mary Putnam Jacobi, "Inaugural Address," *Pathfinder*, 335.

60 Ibid., 347–48.

61 Mary Putnam Jacobi, "Shall Women Practice Medicine?," *Pathfinder*, 373.

62 Mary Putnam Jacobi to Elizabeth Blackwell, 25 December 1888, Blackwell Family Papers, 0320T, LOC.

63 Ibid.

64 Mary C. Putnam, "Woman's Right to Labor," in *Graduates' Reunion*, 64. Other examples of her rebuttal against the "unsexed" accusation can be found in an early article, under the name "Mary Israel," "Sketches of Character: No. XVI," *New Orleans Times*, MPJ Papers, SL. See also Mary Putnam Jacobi, "Reply to Professor Munsterberg," unpublished essay,

c. 1880, Folder 30, MPJ Papers, SL; and Mary Putnam Jacobi, "Shall Women Practice Medicine?," *Pathfinder*, 372.

65 On her roles as a physician, see *Pathfinder*, xv–xvi. Several of her medical articles draw from patients treated at the infirmary. On her role in management, see Minutes, Medical Board of the New York Infirmary, 1892–99, Records of the New York Infirmary, New York Downtown Hospital. On the children's ward, see Daniel, "'A Cautious Experiment,'" *Medical Woman's Journal* 48 (July 1941): 199.

66 For example, she called for an honors program, requiring more clinical experience from students via out-practice (home visits) and adding a bedside exam to students' final examinations, as was done in France and Germany. See Excerpts, College Faculty Minutes, 2 November 1888, in Daniel, "'A Cautious Experiment,'" *Medical Woman's Journal* 48 (September 1941): 273–74.

67 See, for example, Association for the Advancement of the Medical Education of Women, *Report of the Association for the Advancement of the Medical Education of Women*. On her donations, see M. P. Jacobi, "Memorial to Trustees of the Infirmary," in Daniel, "'A Cautious Experiment,'" *Medical Woman's Journal* 48 (October 1941): 305. On her proposals and resignation, see Excerpts, College Faculty Minutes, 2 November 1888, 4 January 1889, 12 January 1889, 25 January 1889, in Daniel, "'A Cautious Experiment,'" *Medical Woman's Journal* 48 (September 1941): 272–76.

68 Elizabeth Blackwell to Mary C. Putnam, 31 December 1871, in Ruth Putnam, *Life and Letters*, 306. Excerpts, College Faculty Minutes, 8 December 1871, in Daniel, "'A Cautious Experiment,'" *Medical Woman's Journal* 48 (January 1941): 11.

69 Elizabeth Blackwell to Mary C. Putnam, 31 December 1871, Ruth Putnam, *Life and Letters*, 307.

70 Morantz-Sanchez, *Sympathy and Science*, 72–76.

71 On Blackwell's views of science, see Morantz-Sanchez, "Feminist Theory and Historical Practice," 51–69.

72 Elizabeth Blackwell, "Erroneous Method in Medical Education," 38–39. Also cited in Morantz-Sanchez, "Feminist Theory and Historical Practice." See also Elizabeth Blackwell, *Address Delivered at the Opening of the Woman's Medical College*.

73 For observations on the Eleventh Ward, see Daniel, "'A Cautious Experiment,'" *Medical Woman's Journal* 46 (May 1939): 127–28. See also Sahli, *Elizabeth Blackwell*, 129–30. On the history of disease and immigration in New York in the nineteenth century, see Kraut, *Silent Travelers*; Charles E. Rosenberg, *Cholera Years*.

74 Woman's Medical College of the New York Infirmary, *Annual Catalogue and Announcement*, 1869–70, 4.

75 *Brief History of the Woman's Medical College*, 1897; *Annual Report of the New York Infirmary for Women and Children*, 1890, 7–9. See also Abram, *"Send Us a Lady Physician,"* 84–88; Daniel, "'A Cautious Experiment,'" *Medical Woman's Journal* 47 (January 1940): 10–12, 263; Tuchman, *Science Has No Sex*, 80–88; *The New York Infirmary: A Century of Devoted Service, 1854–1954* (New York: New York Infirmary, 1954). On Blackwell and the Infirmary, see also Sahli, *Elizabeth Blackwell*; Frances Farley, "New York Infirmary for Women and Children."

76 Woman's Medical College of the New York Infirmary, *Annual Catalogue and Announcement*, 1870–71, 3–6.

77 Morantz-Sanchez, *Sympathy and Science*, 72–78.

78 Woman's Medical College of the New York Infirmary, *Annual Catalogue and Announcement*, 1870–71, 4.

79 Morantz-Sanchez, *Sympathy and Science*, 74–76.

80 Mary Putnam Jacobi suggested that many of the city's male physicians, with roots in radical politics, helped open doors for women. See her "Women in Medicine," 190–91.

81 Historians have described the poor state of American medical education at midcentury. See Morantz-Sanchez, *Sympathy and Science*, 68–70. See also Kaufman, *American Medical Education*.

82 Morantz-Sanchez, *Sympathy and Science*, 69.

83 Mary Putnam Jacobi, "On Atropine," *Pathfinder*, 205.

84 Elizabeth Blackwell to Mary C. Putnam, 31 December 1871, Ruth Putnam, *Life and Letters*, 307.

85 Ibid. (emphasis original).

86 Mary Putnam Jacobi, "On Atropine," *Pathfinder*, 204–5.

87 Mary Putnam Jacobi, "Progress in Medical Education," 584.

88 Ibid.

89 Mary Putnam Jacobi, "School of Medicine for Women," 12.

90 Jacobi's final examination questions reveal the range of knowledge expected from students upon completion of her course. See Woman's Medical College of the New York Infirmary, *Annual Catalogue and Announcement*, 1884, 27–31.

91 Ibid., 6–11.

92 Ibid., 7.

93 Wells, *Out of the Dead House*, 193–226.

94 Woman's Medical College of the New York Infirmary, *Annual Catalogue and Announcement*, 1884, 8.

95 On the history of the study of anatomy, see Sappol, *Traffic of Dead Bodies*; Wells, *Out of the Dead House*.

96 Sappol, *Traffic of Dead Bodies*, 88.

97 Woman's Medical College of the New York Infirmary, *Annual Catalogue and Announcement*, 1884, 8.

98 Mary Putnam Jacobi, "School of Medicine for Women," 12.

99 Elizabeth Blackwell, "Erroneous Method in Medical Education," 43. See also Morantz-Sanchez, *Sympathy and Science*, 191.

100 Elizabeth Blackwell, "Scientific Method in Biology," 111–12, 117. Also quoted in Abraham Jacobi, "Abraham Jacobi Address," 77–78.

101 Elizabeth Blackwell to Emily Blackwell, 18 January 1875, Blackwell Family Papers, MC-411, Box 3, Folder 47, SL.

102 Elizabeth Blackwell, "Erroneous Method in Medical Education," 35.

103 Ibid., 37, 41.

104 Ibid., 45.

105 Ibid., 43 (emphasis added).

106 Woman's Medical College of the New York Infirmary, *Annual Catalogue and Announcement*, 1884, 8, 10; ibid., 1885, 8.

107 Ibid., 1884, 7 (emphasis original).

108 On Jacobi and Blackwell's disagreement about vivisection, see Mary Putnam Jacobi to Elizabeth Blackwell, 25 December 1888, Blackwell Family Papers, 0320T, LOC. See also Morantz-Sanchez, "Feminist Theory and Historical Practice."

109 Mary Putnam Jacobi to Elizabeth Blackwell, 25 December 1888, Blackwell Family Papers, 0320T, LOC.

110 Emily Blackwell, "Woman's Medical College Justified."

111 Mary Putnam Jacobi, "Shall Women Practice Medicine?," *Pathfinder*, 372 (emphasis added).

112 Ibid.

113 Rossiter, *Women Scientists in America*. On the association of science and masculinity in western culture, see Keller, *Reflections on Gender and Science*; Harding, *Science Question in Feminism*; Noble, *World Without Women*; and Schiebinger, *Mind Has No Sex?*. On the history of human experimentation, see Susan Lederer, *Subjected to Science*.

114 Warner, *Therapeutic Perspective*; Morantz-Sanchez, "Feminist Theory and Historical Practice," 57.

115 Mary Putnam Jacobi, "On Atropine," *Pathfinder*, 222, fn. 3.

116 Mary Putnam Jacobi, "Remarks Upon the Action of Nitrate of Silver," *Pathfinder*, 291–94.

117 Mary C. Putnam, "Phenomena Attending Section of the Right Restiform Body," 17–18. In this study, (Putnam) Jacobi also examined the relationship between nervous dysfunction and nutritional failure.

118 For Abraham Jacobi's short contribution to this discussion, see ibid., 18.

119 Mary Putnam Jacobi, "Practical Study of Biology," *Pathfinder*, 462.

120 Mary Putnam Jacobi, "On Atropine," *Pathfinder*, 204–39. Atropine is understood today to smooth muscle spasms or to dilate the pupil of the eye.

121 Ibid., 209.

122 Ibid., 222–23. See fn. 3 for a reference to experiments on rabbits. See p. 223 for a second therapeutic application on a patient with vertigo at the Dispensary for Nervous Diseases.

123 On the lack of regulation, see Lederer, *Subjected to Science*, 1–26.

124 For example, see Mary Putnam Jacobi, *Question of Rest*.

125 Mary Putnam Jacobi, "Acute Fatty Degeneration of the New-Born," *Pathfinder*, 313, 316, 322, 325. Originally published in *The American Journal of Obstetrics*, 1878.

126 Ibid., 313.

127 Ibid., 316, 322, 325.

128 On the sphygmograph, see Frank, "Telltale Heart," 211–90.

129 Mary Putnam Jacobi, "Sphygmographic Experiments," *Pathfinder*, 299–310; Mary Putnam Jacobi, "Provisional Report on the Effect of Quinine," 33–43.

130 Mary Putnam Jacobi, "Practical Study of Biology," *Pathfinder*, 461.

131 For example, see "Mary Putnam Jacobi's Letter of Protest," 110–14.

132 Mary Putnam Jacobi, "Practical Study of Biology," *Pathfinder*, 459.

133 Ibid., 461.

134 Ibid., 459. On the British antivivisection movement and the 1876 legislation limiting the practice, see Richard D. French, *Antivivisection and Medical Science*, 112–76.

135 Mary Putnam Jacobi, "Practical Study of Biology," *Pathfinder*, 459.

136 Mary Putnam Jacobi, "Women in Medicine," 191; Mary Putnam Jacobi, "Opening Lecture on Diseases of Children," *Pathfinder*, 403–18.

CHAPTER FOUR

1 Mary Putnam Jacobi, "Reply to Professor Munsterberg," unpublished essay, c. 1880, 10, Folder 30, MPJ Papers, SL. Hugo Munsterberg (1863–1916) was a German American psychologist.

2 On defining science, see Thomas F. Gieryn on "boundary-work," in Gieryn, "Boundaries of Science," 405; and Gieryn, "Boundary-Work and the Demarcation of Science," 781–95.

3 Here, I apply the science studies literature on expertise and the politics of knowledge. For example, see Collins and Evans, *Rethinking Expertise*; Cozzens and Woodhouse, "Science, Government, and the Politics of Knowledge," 540–48; Shapin, *Social History of Truth*; and Shapin, "Cordelia's Love," 255–75.

4 Daston and Galison, *Objectivity*, 27–50.

5 For more on women physicians and the politics of knowledge, see Theriot, "Women's Voices," 1–31. For more on situated knowledge and examples of scientific contestations over race (instead of gender), see Stepan and Gilman, "Appropriating the Idioms of Science."

6 Mary Putnam Jacobi, "Modern Female Invalidism," *Pathfinder*, 482. Elizabeth Cady Stanton made a similar statement in a lecture called "Our Girls." She said, "I would have girls regard themselves not as adjectives but as nouns" (quoted in Brumberg, *Body Project*, xxxii).

7 Mary Putnam Jacobi, "Modern Female Invalidism," *Pathfinder*, 478–82.

8 Mary Putnam Jacobi, *Question of Rest*, 109.

9 On the history of menstruation, see Brumberg, *Body Project*; Smith-Rosenberg and Rosenberg, "Female Animal," 12–27; Bullough and Voght, "Women, Menstruation, and Nineteenth-Century Medicine," 28–37; and Vostral, *Under Wraps*. For Vostral's discussion of Jacobi, see 35–42.

10 Mary Putnam Jacobi, *Question of Rest*, 171, 182, 115.

11 Mitchell, *Lectures on Diseases of the Nervous System*, 95–96.

12 Hewitt, *Pathology, Diagnosis, and Treatment of the Diseases of Women*, 159. On the physiological approach to neurology and mental disease, see Blustein, *Preserve Your Love for Science*.

13 Mary Putnam Jacobi to Elizabeth Blackwell, 25 December 1888, New York, Blackwell Family Papers, 0320T, LOC.

14 Elizabeth Blackwell, "Human Element in Sex," 3, 19, 32. For another interpretation, see Krug, "Women Ovulate," 51–72.

15 Frances Emily White, "Woman's Place in Nature," 297, 300; Edward T. Morman, "Frances Emily White," in *American National Biography*, eds. John A. Garraty and Mark C. Carnes (New York: Oxford University Press, 1999), 23:203–4.

16 See Tuchman, *Science Has No Sex*, 75–79.

17 Ibid.; Tuchman, "'Only in a Republic,'" 121–42; "Situating Gender," 34–57.

18 Morantz-Sanchez, *Conduct Unbecoming a Woman*, 114–37.

19 Mary Putnam Jacobi, *Question of Rest*, 62, 224, 226.

20 Horowitz, *Power and Passion*, 86–89, 250–52.

21 M. Carey Thomas to Mary Garrett, 8 April 1892, Outgoing Correspondence, Reel 16, no. 902-14, M. Carey Thomas Papers, Bryn Mawr College Library, Special Collections, Bryn Mawr, Pa.

22 Mary Putnam Jacobi to Elizabeth Blackwell, 25 December 1888, Blackwell Family Papers, 0320T, LOC.

23 On these techniques of measuring nutrition, see Holmes, *Claude Bernard*; Romano, *Making Medicine Scientific*. New technologies for measuring hemoglobin, the hemocytometer and hemoglobinometer, emerged in the 1880s. They monitored the number of red blood corpuscles in patients and measured the amount of hemoglobin. See Wailoo, *Drawing Blood*, 24.

24 Clarke, *Sex in Education*, 126; Zschoche, "Dr. Clarke Revisited," 545–69.

25 Clarke, *Sex in Education*, 13.

26 Ibid., 19.

27 Mary Putnam Jacobi, "Mental Action and Physical Health," 257–306.

28 Ibid., 259, 263.

29 Ibid., 258.

30 Ibid., 281, 263, 261, 258.

31 For a history of mind/body dualism, see Curti, *Human Nature in American Thought*, 187–93; Russett, *Sexual Science*, 112–66. On reflex theory, see Shorter, *From Paralysis to Fatigue*, 40–68; and Morantz-Sanchez, *Conduct Unbecoming a Woman*, 116–17.

32 Mary Putnam Jacobi, "Mental Action and Physical Health," 272.

33 Ibid., 284. See also 271–72, 274–75.

34 Ibid., 274. Here, Jacobi is probably quoting from Jules Michelet's *La Femme*, to which she refers on pages 261, 273.

35 Mary Putnam Jacobi, "Mental Action and Physical Health," 279–82.

36 Ibid., 293.

37 On education and the hygiene of both teachers and pupils, see Mary Putnam Jacobi, "Educational Needs," 299–304, and Mary Putnam Jacobi, "Modern Female Invalidism," *Pathfinder*, 481.

38 Mary Putnam Jacobi, "Mental Action and Physical Health," 303.

39 Ibid., 301–2.

40 Dr. Morrill Wyman quoted in letter, C. Alice Baker to Mary Putnam Jacobi, 7 November 1874, Folder 10, MPJ Papers, SL. On C. Alice Baker, see "Charlotte Alice Baker (1833–1909)," in *American Women Historians, 1700s–1990s: A Biographical Dictionary*, ed. Jennifer Scanlon and Shaaron Cosner (Westport, Conn.: Greenwood Press, 1996), 10; and "Charlotte Alice Baker," in *The Biographical Cyclopaedia of American Women*, ed. Mabel Ward Cameron (New York: Halvord Publishing Co., 1924), 1:345–47.

41 Minutes of the Boylston Prize Committee, 5 June 1876, DE-10, Boylston Prize Committee Records, Countway.

42 C. Alice Baker to Mary Putnam Jacobi, 7 November 1874, Folder 10, MPJ Papers, SL.

43 Mary F. Eastman offered Baker help in procuring statistics for Jacobi. See Mary F. Eastman to "Miss Baker," Mary F. Eastman Letter, E-13, SL.

44 Mary Putnam Jacobi, "Mental Action and Physical Health," 258.

45 Mary Roth Walsh, *"Doctors Wanted,"* 26–32, 165–75. Harriot Hunt applied to Harvard in both 1847 and 1850, unsuccessfully.

46 John Harley Warner, *Against the Spirit of System*, 336; Tuchman, *Science Has No Sex*, 173–74.

47 On the changing discourses of gynecology, see Morantz-Sanchez, "Female Patient Agency," 69–88.

48 Mary Putnam Jacobi to Richard M. Hodges, 6 June c. 1876, Boylston Prize Committee Records, DE-10, Countway.

49 Mary Putnam Jacobi, *Question of Rest*.

50 Ibid.; Richard M. Hodges to Mary Putnam Jacobi, 6 June 1877, Boylston Prize Committee Records, DE-10, Countway.

51 Mary Putnam Jacobi to Richard M. Hodges, 8 June 1877, Boylston Prize Committee Records, DE-10, Countway. Jacobi told Hodges that she would try to correct the error, and suggested inserting the prize questions and rules in future printings. The "Boylston Medical Prize Questions" did appear in some versions of her *Question of Rest*.

52 Mary Putnam Jacobi, *Question of Rest*, 27, 31. Jacobi distributed 1,000 questionnaires but received only 268 answers. Her use of statistics reflected the movement toward a "trust in numbers." On the history of statistics, see Theodore M. Porter, *Rise of Statistical Thinking* and *Trust in Numbers*.

53 Mary Putnam Jacobi, *Question of Rest*, 62.

54 Ibid., 62–63.

55 Ibid., 227.

56 Ibid., 109.

57 Jacobi later expanded on her menstruation theory when she studied the etiology of endometritis. See Mary Putnam Jacobi, "Studies in Endometritis" (1885), 596–606.

58 Mary Putnam Jacobi, *Question of Rest*, 115.

59 On the sphygmograph, see Frank, "Telltale Heart," 211–90. See also Romano, *Making Medicine Scientific*, 79–86.

60 See Jacobi's sphygmographic tracings, inserts in *Question of Rest*. See also her laboratory studies on urea in ibid., 140–41.

61 Ibid., 146–48.

62 Ibid., 202.

63 Ibid., 165.

64 Ibid., 14–15.

65 Emmet, *Principles and Practice of Gynaecology*, 147–52. For a discussion of ovulation and another interpretation of *Question of Rest*, see Laqueur, *Making Sex*, 220–25.

66 Mary Putnam Jacobi, *Question of Rest*, 13.

67 On the plethoric explanation, see ibid., 8, 12–13.

68 Marsh and Ronner, *Empty Cradle*, 84–85; Laqueur, *Making Sex*, 214.

69 Jacobi said clearly, "Reproduction is essentially a process of nutrition." Here she quotes Claude Bernard. See Mary Putnam Jacobi, *Question of Rest*, 82, 100.

70 Ibid., 167–68.

71 "The Question of Rest for Women during Menstruation" (book review), *Medical Record* 13 (1878): 14.

72 "Reviews and Book Notices," 511.

73 Bowditch, "Question of Rest." See W. P. Garrison to Henry Pickering Bowditch, 3 August 1877, Countway.

74 See discussion by Mundé, "Report on the Progress of Gynecology," 127–73.

75 Goodman, "The Cyclical Theory of Menstruation," 673–94.

76 Engelmann, "American Girl of To-day," 15.

77 Stephenson, "On the Menstrual Wave," 287–94, Other proponents of the wave idea are noted in Novak, *Menstruation and Its Disorders*, 85.

78 Mary Putnam Jacobi, "Stephenson Wave," 92.

79 For example, see Mary Putnam Jacobi, "Studies in Endometritis," 18 (1885): 36–50, 113–28, 262–83, 376–86, 519–31, 596–606, 802–46, 915–32; and 19 (1886): 352–86. See also "Some Considerations on Endometritis," 468–70. These articles are also discussed in Wells, *Out of the Dead House*, 186–87.

80 Mary Putnam Jacobi, "Studies in Endometritis" (1885), 386, 519, 520.

81 Ibid. (1885), 602; (1886), 385–86.

82 Alexander Agassiz to Mary Putnam Jacobi, 16 May 1878, Folder 12, MPJ Papers, SL; letter from Mary Putnam Jacobi and nine others to the president and overseers of Harvard University, *Annual Reports of the President and Treasurer of Harvard College, 1881–1882* (Cambridge, Mass.: University Press, John Wilson and Son, 1882), Appendix I, 133–34 (Sequence 749–50); Mary Roth Walsh, *"Doctors Wanted,"* 173–75, 233.

83 "Hysteria," *Oxford English Dictionary*, 1991, 585–86.

84 On the history of hysteria, see Smith-Rosenberg, "The Hysterical Woman: Sex Roles and Role Conflict in Nineteenth-Century America," in *Disorderly Conduct*, 197–216; Showalter, *Female Malady*; Maines, *Technology of Orgasm*; and Shorter, *From Paralysis to Fatigue*. On anorexia nervosa as a form of hysteria, see Brumberg, *Fasting Girls*.

85 For other women physicians who interpreted hysteria, see Theriot, "Women's Voices," 11–15.

86 On nervousness and neurasthenia, see Lutz, *American Nervousness*; Schuster, "Personalizing Illness and Modernity," 695–722; and Sicherman, "Uses of a Diagnosis," 33–54.

87 Mitchell, *Fat and Blood*; Mitchell, *Wear and Tear*.

88 On motor hysteria, see Shorter, *From Paralysis to Fatigue*, 95–112, 201.

89 Mitchell, *Lectures on Diseases of the Nervous System*, 14, 217, 220.

90 Ibid., 227.

91 Cervetti, "S. Weir Mitchell Representing 'a hell of pain,'" 69–96.

92 Mitchell, *Lectures on Diseases of the Nervous System*, 222, 228, 222, 230.

93 On Weir Mitchell as misogynist, see Wood, "'Fashionable Diseases,'" 25–52. For an opposing view, see Morantz, "Perils of Feminist History," 649–60. For more on Weir Mitchell in cultural and literary context, see Cervetti, "S. Weir Mitchell and His Snakes," 119–33; Cervetti, "S. Weir Mitchell Representing 'a hell of pain,'" 69–96; Denise D. Knight, "'All the Facts of the Case,'" 259–77; Schuster, "Personalizing Illness and Modernity," 695–722; and Tuttle, "Letters from Elizabeth Stuart Phelps," 83–94.

94 Schuster, "Personalizing Illness and Modernity."

95 Mary Putnam Jacobi, "Some Considerations on Hysteria," 7.

96 Ibid., 2, 7, and 70.

97 Ibid., 7.

98 On the shifting models of hysteria and psychosomatic illness, see Shorter, *From Paralysis to Fatigue*, 201, 208, 220, 233.

99 Mary Putnam Jacobi, "Modern Female Invalidism," *Pathfinder*, 480.

100 Mary Putnam Jacobi, "Some Considerations on Hysteria," 67–80. For her later interest in psychological issues, see, for example, Mary Putnam Jacobi, "Suggestion in Regard to Suggestive Therapeutics," *Pathfinder*, 483–93.

101 Mary Putnam Jacobi, *Essays on Hysteria*.

102 Russett, *Sexual Science*, 109, 113.

103 Mary Putnam Jacobi, "Some Considerations on Hysteria," 2.

104 Ibid., 2, 4–5.

105 Albert Eulenberg quoted in Mary Putnam Jacobi, *Essays on Hysteria*, 65–66.

106 Mary Putnam Jacobi, "Some Considerations on Hysteria," 70–73. On the Butler Health Lift, see Todd, *Physical Culture*.

107 Mary Putnam Jacobi, "Some Considerations on Hysteria," 74; see figs. 8 and 9 for examples of how she illustrated increased circulation and nutrition.

108 See Todd, *Physical Culture*; Verbrugge, *Able-Bodied Womanhood*; and Whorton, *Crusaders for Fitness*.

109 Mary Putnam Jacobi, "Use of Electricity," 60–73. See also Longo, "Electrotherapy in Gynecology," 343–66; and Rosner, "Professional Context," 64–82.

110 Maines, *Technology of Orgasm*.

111 Mary Putnam Jacobi, "Case of Uterine Fibroid," 807.

112 Longo, "Electrotherapy in Gynecology," 344; Engelmann, "Use of Electricity in Gynecological Practice," 207–355. Despite the interest in using electricity, many gynecologists remained committed to surgery.

113 Mary Putnam Jacobi, "Some Considerations on Hysteria," 70, 68.

114 On the history of gynecological surgery, see Morantz-Sanchez, *Conduct Unbecoming a Woman*, and McGregor, *From Midwives to Medicine*.

115 Mary Putnam Jacobi, "Cystic Ovaries," 705. She presented this case to the New York Pathological Society on 28 May 1884.

116 Mary Putnam Jacobi, "Some Considerations on Hysteria," 79–80.

117 Ibid., 80. On the return or increase of symptoms after surgery, see comments by Mary Putnam Jacobi, "The President," in *Reports and Transactions of the Annual Meetings*, 1890, 80–82.

118 See Morantz-Sanchez, *Conduct Unbecoming a Woman*, 174–76.

119 On the history of chlorosis and anemia, see Brumberg, "Chlorotic Girls," 1468–77; and Wailoo, *Drawing Blood*, 17–45.

120 Jacobi and White, *On the Use of the Cold Pack*, 3–4.

121 Ibid., 48–49 (emphasis mine).

122 Mary Putnam Jacobi to S. Weir Mitchell, c. 1891, S. Weir Mitchell Papers, Box 10, Series 4.4, Folder 15, College of Physicians of Philadelphia, Historical Library, Philadelphia. Also published as "Mary Putnam Jacobi's Letter of Protest," 110–14.

123 See Records of the Section on Neurology and Psychiatry, vol. 1, Records of the New York

Academy of Medicine, NYAM; Minutes of the New York Neurological Society, NYAM. Mary Putnam Jacobi was admitted to the New York Neurological Society on 20 April 1877 and made Corresponding Secretary on 6 April 1880.

124 Blustein, *Preserve Your Love for Science*, 162–80.

125 S. Weir Mitchell to Mary Putnam Jacobi, c. 1902, Folder 17, MPJ Papers, SL.

126 Mitchell, *Characteristics*.

127 "Mary Putnam Jacobi's Letter of Protest," 112.

128 See Lane, *To Herland and Beyond*; Rudd and Gough, eds., *Charlotte Perkins Gilman*.

129 Wegener, "'What a Comfort a Woman Doctor Is!,'" 45–73.

130 Knight, ed., *Abridged Diaries of Charlotte Perkins Gilman*, 213.

131 Charlotte Perkins Gilman address in "Addresses at the Unveiling of a Memorial Tablet," 66.

132 On Gilman, see Lane, *To Herland and Beyond*, and Ganobcsik-Williams, "Intellectualism of Charlotte Perkins Gilman," 16–41. For another take on Gilman's racial ideology, with references to Jacobi, see Newman, *White Women's Rights*, especially chap. 6.

133 Knight, ed., *Abridged Diaries*, 213.

134 Gilman, *Living*, 291.

135 Edmund B. Wilson, *Cell in Development and Inheritance*.

136 See Gilman, *Human Work*. On *Human Work*, see Lane, *To Herland and Beyond*, chap. 10.

137 Mary Putnam Jacobi, *Physiological Notes*, 3, 1–2, 4, 2, 1 (emphasis added).

138 Tomlinson, "From Rousseau to Evolutionism," 246–54.

139 Newman, *White Women's Rights*, 132–37.

140 On feminism and evolutionary biology, see Hamlin, "Beyond Adam's Rib"; Kohlstedt and Jorgensen, "'Irrepressible Woman Question,'" 267–93; and Paxton, *George Eliot and Herbert Spencer*.

141 Charlotte Perkins Gilman address in "Addresses at the Unveiling of a Memorial Tablet," 66.

142 Ibid., 66.

143 Mary Putnam Jacobi, "Case of Absent Uterus," 511. Her colleague was Dr. Willy Meyer, a consulting physician at the New York Infirmary and professor of clinical surgery at the Woman's Medical College of the New York Infirmary; he was also a nephew to Abraham Jacobi and his first wife, Fanny Meyer Jacobi. See Boas and Meyer, *Alma Farm*, 88–90.

144 According to Alice Dreger (*Hermaphrodites*, 11, 29), the nineteenth-century definition of sex relied on the gonads; the presence of ovaries or testes was the most important determinant of sex. Therefore, missing or mixed (male and female) gonads placed an individual in hermaphroditic categories.

145 Ibid., 25–27; Fee, "Nineteenth-Century Craniology," 415–33; Russett, *Sexual Science*.

146 On the two-sex model, see Laqueur, *Making Sex*. On hermaphrodism, see Dreger, *Hermaphrodites*; Reis, "Impossible Hermaphrodites," 411–41; and Fausto-Sterling, *Sexing the Body*.

147 Mary Putnam Jacobi, "Case of Absent Uterus," 538.

148 Ibid., 510.

149 Ibid., 512–15; Dreger, *Hermaphrodites*, 68–75; Laqueur, *Making Sex*, 10, 169, 171.

150 Mary Putnam Jacobi, "Case of Absent Uterus," 513, 530.

151 Ibid., 537–38.

152 Ibid., 512. "Case of absent uterus with persistence of urogenital sinus (ug), which combines the urethra and vagina," from *Dictionnaire Encyclopédie Sciences Médical*, 1888, vol. 13, art. "Hermaphrodites."

153 Mary Putnam Jacobi, "Case of Absent Uterus," 513, 518.

154 Ibid., 521–22.

155 Mary Putnam Jacobi, "Case of Absent Uterus," 523. For more on this case, see Barbin, *Herculine Barbin*, and Dreger, *Hermaphrodites*, 51–52.

156 Mary Putnam Jacobi, "Case of Absent Uterus," 544.

157 Ibid., 534–35; Dreger, *Hermaphrodites*, 68–70.

158 Paul Le Gendre in Bouchard, *Traité de Pathologie Générale*, vol. 1, 283. Le Gendre translated in Mary Putnam Jacobi, "Case of Absent Uterus," 534–35.

159 Geddes and Thomson, *Evolution of Sex*; Mary Putnam Jacobi, "Case of Absent Uterus," 531–33.

160 Mary Putnam Jacobi, "Case of Absent Uterus," 533.

161 Ibid., 535 (emphasis original).

162 Ibid., 541.

163 Ibid., 539.

164 Ibid., 541.

165 See Schiebinger, *Mind Has No Sex?*, and Harth, *Cartesian Women*.

166 Mary Putnam Jacobi, "Shall Women Practice Medicine?" *Pathfinder*, 390.

167 Mary Putnam Jacobi, "Case of Absent Uterus," 539–40.

168 Ibid., 530, 542.

CHAPTER FIVE

1 Mary Putnam Jacobi, "Women in Medicine," 184. She was accepted to the medical society on 22 November 1871 and officially approved/elected on 27 November 1871. See Medical Society of the County of New York, Minutes of the Comitia Minora, November 1871, NYAM; Ruth Putnam, *Life and Letters*, 301–3.

2 Mary C. Putnam to Victorine Putnam, Summer 1872, Ruth Putnam, *Life and Letters*, 311 (emphasis original).

3 Abraham Jacobi and Mary C. Putnam, Marriage Certificate, 22 July 1873, NYCMA; Abraham Jacobi, *Infant Diet* (1874); Truax, *Doctors Jacobi*, 169–70.

4 For another historical discussion of their relationship, see Joy Harvey, "Clanging Eagles," 185–95.

5 On Abraham Jacobi's youth in Germany, see Herzig, *Entwicklung*, 14–20; Viner, "Healthy Children," 26–28. Several different spellings of his father's name appear in different sources: "Eleasar" in Herzig, "Eleaser" in Viner, and "Eleazar" on the Abraham Jacobi and Mary C. Putnam marriage certificate.

6 Cole, *Franz Boas*, 8–9, 13–14.

7 Viner, "Healthy Children," 27–28; Cole, *Franz Boas*, 14–16. On the politics and social conflict of the *Vormärz*, see Sperber, *Rhineland Radicals*, chaps. 2 and 3.

8 Viner, "Healthy Children," 28–31, 34.

9 Ibid., 59. See letters from Abraham Jacobi to Fanny Meyer, 1850–51, in Herzig, *Entwicklung*, 81–106.

10 Quotation is from Herzig (ibid., 10): "Für Jacobi bedeutete Demokratie die totale Gegnerschaft zum Absolutismus."

11 Ibid., 10–11.

12 Viner, "Healthy Children," 61–62; Herzig, *Entwicklung*, 26–29.

13 Virchow quoted in Ackerknecht, *Rudolf Virchow*, 46.

14 Ibid., 45–46.

15 Ibid., 137–45; quotation on 40.

16 Ibid., 45, 137–45, 164; Viner, "Healthy Children," 68–71. On science in medicine in the German context, see Tuchman, *Science, Medicine*.

17 On Jacobi's trial and imprisonment, see Viner, "Healthy Children," 36–42; and Herzig, *Entwicklung*, 47–51. According to Rhoda Truax, a tale circulated in the family that Jacobi escaped because there was a rumor he would be released only to be captured and charged again. A friendly jailer supposedly let him go early so that he could escape and quickly visit his family and Fanny Meyer, now his fiancée, before fleeing to England. See Truax, *Doctors Jacobi*, 155–56; and Viner, "Abraham Jacobi and German Medical Radicalism," 437.

18 *Karl Marx, Frederick Engels*, 355, 352–53.

19 Ibid., 353. Also quoted in Viner, "Abraham Jacobi and German Medical Radicalism," 437–38.

20 Ibid.

21 Ibid., 358.

22 Nadel, *Little Germany*, 1.

23 On the motivations for German immigration, see ibid., 15–21. On divisions of labor in Little Germany, see ibid., 62–90.

24 Viner, "Abraham Jacobi and German Medical Radicalism," 441–42.

25 Viner, "Healthy Children," 113–16; Viner, "Abraham Jacobi and German Medical Radicalism," 442–48. On other German radicals in American medicine, see Tuchman, *Science Has No Sex*.

26 Abraham Jacobi, "Address at the Twenty-Fifth Jubilee," 62–63.

27 Zelizer, *Pricing the Priceless Child*. See also Gary Cross, *Cute and the Cool*.

28 Viner, "Abraham Jacobi and the Origins of Scientific Pediatrics in America," 24–31.

29 "Abraham Jacobi," in *Dictionary of American Medical Biography*, 389–90.

30 Mary Putnam Jacobi to George McAneny, 16 May 1899, Folder 16A, MPJ Papers, SL.

31 Mary C. Putnam to Victorine Haven Putnam, 29 May 1867, Ruth Putnam, *Life and Letters*, 141.

32 Mary C. Putnam to Edith Putnam, 17 March 1867, Ruth Putnam, *Life and Letters*, 116.

33 Mary C. Putnam to Victorine Haven Putnam, 29 May 1867, Ruth Putnam, *Life and Letters*, 141.

34 Leach, *True Love and Perfect Union*, 3–4, 167–79. Joy Harvey, "Clanging Eagles."

35 In 1865, after her first engagement ended, Mary told her father that she needed a husband who was her superior. See Mary C. Putnam to George Palmer Putnam, August 1865, Ruth Putnam, *Life and Letters*, 81; and Mary Putnam Jacobi, "Shall Women Practice Medicine?," *Pathfinder*, 389–90.

36 Morantz-Sanchez, *Sympathy and Science*, 135–40; More, *Restoring the Balance*, 23–25.

37 Mary Putnam Jacobi, "Shall Women Practice Medicine?" *Pathfinder*, 385, 382, 389.

38 Abraham Jacobi Household (misspelled "Jacoby"), 110 West 34th Street, New York City, New York, U.S. Census Bureau, *Tenth Census of the United States, 1880*, and U.S. Census Bureau, *Twelfth Census of the United States, 1900*.

39 Mary Putnam Jacobi, "Inaugural Address," *Pathfinder*, 353.

40 Addresses are from the Jacobi Burial Records: Julius Jacobi, d. 12 August 1855, Late Residence at Forsythe 30, New York; Fanny Jacobi, d. 16 September 1856, Late Residence at 89 Christie St., New York, Jacobi Family Burial Records, Archives of Green-Wood Cemetery, Brooklyn, N.Y.

41 Ibid.; see Fanny Jacobi, b. Germany, d. age 23, 17 September 1856, Phlebitis, Death Record, NYCMA. There is a discrepancy between the death record and burial record. The death record says she lived twenty-three years and died on 17 September, while the burial record says she died on 16 September, at age twenty-five.

42 See Cole, *Franz Boas*, 16. See Franz Boas correspondence with Abraham Jacobi, c. 1880–1917, Franz Boas Collection, B B61, American Philosophical Society, Philadelphia.

43 Marriage of Abraham Jacobi and [Kate] Rosalie Dessafo, 2 June 1862, NYCMA. Records of her origins are contradictory. Truax states her last name was "Rabbe." See Truax, *Doctors Jacobi*, 160. Their marriage record says she was born in Georgia, her death certificate says Augusta, Georgia, but the 1870 census (U.S. Census Bureau, *Ninth Census of the United States*) states her place of birth as Florida.

44 Amity Street is now W. 3rd in Greenwich Village. Address noted on Death Record, Kate Rosalie Jacobi, d. 27 April 1871, Record #86049, NYCMA.

45 According to the 1870 census, her main occupation was "Keeping H" (keeping house). See the entry for "Kate Jacoby [*sic*]": A. Jacobi Household (misspelled "Jacoby"), New York City, Ward 20, District 19, p. 39, U.S. Census Bureau, *Ninth Census of the United States, 1870*.

46 Mary Putnam Jacobi to George McAneny, c. 27 October 1898, Folder 16A, MPJ Papers, SL; see also Truax, *Doctors Jacobi*, 160.

47 A Female Child of Dr. Jacobi, d. 26 January 1863, Stillborn; A Child of Dr. Jacobi, d. 26 September 1863, Stillborn, Jacobi Family Burial Records, Archives of Green-Wood Cemetery, Brooklyn, N.Y.

48 Death Record, Mary Jacobi, d. 14 September 1865, NYCMA; A Female Child of Dr. Jacobi, d. 14 September 1865, Stillborn, Jacobi Family Burial Records, Archives of Green-Wood Cemetery, Brooklyn, N.Y.

49 Death Record, A Male Infant of Dr. A. Jacobi [and Kate], c. 18 March 1868, Record #5082, NYCMA.

50 Death Record, Kate Rosalie Jacobi, d. 27 April 1871, Record #86049, NYCMA. "Nephritis" is a kidney disease caused by inflammation or infection.

51 See Mary Putnam Jacobi, *Question of Rest*, 62, 224, 226; M. Carey Thomas to Mary Garrett, 8 April 1892, Reel 16: Outgoing Correspondence to Mary Garrett, Jan. 1890–Aug. 1892, #902–914, M. Carey Thomas Papers, Bryn Mawr College Library, Special Collections, Bryn Mawr, Pa.

52 Death Record, "A Female Child of Abraham and Mary P. Jacobi," d. 17 March 1874, Record #171909, NYCMA.

53 On atelectasis pulmonum, see nineteenth-century texts on diseases of children, such as Meigs and Pepper, *Practical Treatise*, 134–43.

54 Mary Putnam Jacobi to John Bishop Putnam, 23 August 1875, Ruth Putnam, *Life and Letters*, 318.

55 Mary Putnam Jacobi to Victorine Haven Putnam, 29 May 1875, Container 13, Folder 3, HPP (emphasis original).

56 Ibid., 4 July 1875 (emphasis original).

57 Hiawatha Island Deed, 17 September 1867, Courtesy of the McAneny Family Collection.

58 For background on the history of Lake George, and Jacobi's history there, see O'Brien, *Great and the Gracious*, 121–44; and Boas and Meyer, *Alma Farm*, 48–65.

59 Boas and Meyer, *Alma Farm*, 21–47.

60 Truax, *Doctors Jacobi*, 183–84. The story was also recalled in Marjorie McAneny to Shirley Putnam O'Hara, n.d., Container 4, HPP.

61 Mary Putnam Jacobi to Victorine Haven Putnam, 14 August 1875, Hiawatha Island, Container 13, Folder 3, HPP.

62 Mary Putnam Jacobi to Victorine Haven Putnam, 25 June 1876, Between Scilly Islands and Land's End, Container 13, Folder 4, HPP.

63 Mary Putnam Jacobi to Victorine Haven Putnam, 14 August 1875, Hiawatha Island, Container 13, Folder 3, HPP.

64 Ibid.

65 Victorine Haven Putnam to Amy Putnam, 21 January 1877, Container 5, HPP. "Mary" is most likely a reference to a Mary Louise, a family visitor, who stayed with Mary Putnam Jacobi, according to ibid., c. 25 February 1877.

66 Victorine Haven Putnam to Amy Putnam, 4 February 1877, Container 5, HPP.

67 Ibid., 12 February 1877.

68 Mary Putnam Jacobi to Victorine Haven Putnam, 14 August 1875, Container 13, Folder 3, HPP.

69 Victorine Haven Putnam to Amy Putnam, 21 January 1877, Container 5, HPP.

70 Megan Marshall, *Peabody Sisters*.

71 Mary Putnam Jacobi to Mary Tyler Peabody Mann, 28 January 188[?], Reel 38, Horace Mann Collection, microfilm edition, Massachusetts Historical Society, Boston.

72 On the Jacobi-Schurz bond, see comments by George McAneny and others, Dedication of the Abraham Jacobi–Carl Schurz Memorial Park, Bolton Landing, Lake George, 13 June 1936, courtesy Mount Sinai School of Medicine Archives, Levy Library, New York, N.Y.

73 Mary Putnam Jacobi to Victorine Haven Putnam, 14 August 1875, Hiawatha Island, Container 13, Folder 3, HPP.

74 For their collaboration, see Jacobi and White, *On the Use of the Cold Pack*.

75 Abraham Jacobi to Mary Putnam Jacobi, 21 March c. 1883, Folder 21, MPJ Papers, SL (emphasis original).

76 Ibid.

77 Ernst Jacobi, Death Record, d. 10 June 1883, Record #460499, NYCMA.

78 Mary Putnam Jacobi to Toni and Sophie Boas, 27 February 1884, Lakewood, NYAM.

79 Ibid.

80 Mary Putnam Jacobi to "Mrs. Curtis," 4 September 1883, Rye, N.Y., Folder 13, MPJ Papers, SL.

81 Ibid.

82 Boas and Meyer, *Alma Farm*, 54–55; O'Brien, *Great and the Gracious*, 130–32.

83 See Calling Card, Mary Putnam Jacobi to Fanny Garrison Villard, June 1890, Fanny Garrison Villard Papers, Ms Am 1321, HL. On Fanny Garrison Villard, see *Notable American Women*, 3: 520–22.

84 Mary Putnam Jacobi to George McAneny, 19 December 1898, Folder 16A, MPJ Papers, SL.

85 Interview with Ernest McAneny (grandson of Abraham Jacobi) by David Nicholson, 29 October 1998, p. 20, Riverdale Country School, Riverdale, New York.

86 As Russell Viner has said, "Like the majority of his fellow socialists, [Jacobi] discarded revolution as a form of social change unnecessary in a democratic republic. . . . It was at social and economic inequality that the Forty-Eighters [in America] aimed their reforms." See Viner, "Healthy Children," 112.

87 Abraham Jacobi, "Inaugural Address, Including Paper on Infant Asylums," 155.

88 Ibid., 152–53.

89 Abraham Jacobi, "Physical Cost of Women's Work," 8.

90 Abraham Jacobi, "Inaugural Address, Including Paper on Infant Asylums," 127–32, quote on 132.

91 Abraham Jacobi, "Women Physicians in America," 307, 314, 307.

92 Abraham Jacobi, "Inaugural Address, Including Paper on Infant Asylums," 138–39; Abraham Jacobi, "Women Physicians in America," 312.

93 Abraham Jacobi, "Inaugural Address, Including Paper on Infant Asylums," 137–38.

94 Mary Putnam Jacobi, "Women in Medicine," 184.

95 Ibid.

96 Records of the New York Obstetrical Society, 19 March to 21 May 1878, Minute Book, Box 3, 1874–82, NYAM.

97 Abraham Jacobi, "Women Physicians in America," 314.

98 Ibid., 311.

99 Abraham Jacobi, "Physical Cost of Women's Work," 6.

100 Ibid., 4.

101 Abraham Jacobi, "Remarks," 375; Mary Putnam Jacobi, "Education of Girls."

102 Abraham Jacobi, "Inaugural Address, Including Paper on Infant Asylums," 155, 152–53.

103 See Zelizer, *Pricing the Priceless Child*; Cross, *Cute and the Cool*.

104 Stern and Markel, *Formative Years*, 4.

105 Abraham Jacobi, "History of Pediatrics," 92.

106 Abraham Jacobi, "Treatment of Infant Diarrhea," 185; King, *Children's Health in America*, 74–76.

107 For a history of infant feeding, see Apple, *Mothers and Medicine*.

108 Abraham Jacobi, *Infant Diet* (1873). The Jacobi treatise was published long before Luther Emmett Holt's classic manual, *The Care and the Feeding of Children* (1894).

109 Abraham Jacobi, *Infant Diet* (1873), 38–39.

110 Ibid., 36. Abraham Jacobi claimed anyone could follow his instructions because they required "little money and as little brain as a human being raising infants ought to be permitted to have."

111 *Infant Diet* (1873), 28.

112 Abraham Jacobi, *Infant Diet* (1874). Both editions were published by the Putnam family publishing house.

113 Ibid., iii, iv, v.

114 Ibid., viii.

115 Ibid., 14–20.

116 Ibid., 20–34.

117 Ibid., 43.

118 Ibid., 43–45.

119 Ibid., vii, 50, 60.

120 Ibid., 55.

121 Ibid., 116. To lower the child's temperature, they suggested administering cold baths, giving infants water to drink rather than breast milk, and supplementing milk with small doses of brandy or whiskey to work as a stimulant.

122 Mary Putnam Jacobi later edited the Uffelmann manual for an audience of "educated women" interested in the "technical" details and science of infant care. See "Editor's Preface" in Uffelmann, *Manual of the Domestic Hygiene of the Child*, v–vi.

123 Bridgewater M. Arnold to Rhoda Truax, 15 April 1952, Rhoda Truax Papers, Drexel. Arnold's grandfather was Dr. Alexander S. Hunter, "twice president of the New York County Medical Society elected in 1890 and apparently knew the Jacobis quite well."

124 For a history of Mount Sinai, see Hirsh and Doherty, *First Hundred Years*, and Aufses and Niss, *This House of Noble Deeds*.

125 See "Opponents of the Old Code" and *Report of the Association for Preventing the Re-Enactment in the State of New York of the Present Code of Ethics*. For a summary of the controversy over the AMA Code, see John Harley Warner, "Ideals of Science," and Rosenkrantz, "Search for Professional Order," 219–32.

126 Viner, "Abraham Jacobi and the Origins of Scientific Pediatrics in America," 26–31.

127 John Harley Warner, *Against the Spirit of System*, 334–35.

128 Ibid., 348–49; Tuchman, *Science Has No Sex*, 236–38.

129 Abraham Jacobi, "Some Remarks," 343; "General Therapeutics," 32; "Phases in the Development of Therapy," 25. In numerous addresses and essays, especially in his essays on therapeutics, Abraham Jacobi warned against dependence on the external laboratory; see *Dr. Jacobi's Works*, 4:23–26, 78–79, 176; "Some of the Benefits," 385–406. On his support of vivisection, see "Address at the Dedication," 315–42; and "Oration at the Semi-Centennial," 353–72.

130 Mary Putnam Jacobi, "Indication for Quinine in Pneumonia," *Pathfinder*, 419–45, quote on 444 (emphasis original).

131 Ibid., 432.

132 Ibid., 434.

133 Ibid., 439.

134 Ibid., 444.

135 Ibid., 419–45.

136 Morantz-Sanchez, *Sympathy and Science*, 190, 200; Tuchman, *Science Has No Sex*, 236–38.

137 "Discussion on Diphtheria," 84–93; also quoted in Hammonds, *Childhood's Deadly Scourge*, 51, 238 n. 14. On her knowledge of bacteriology, see Mary Putnam Jacobi, "Discoveries of Pasteur, Koch, and Others," 954–57.

138 On the history of diphtheria, and another discussion of the Jacobis, see Hammonds, *Childhood's Deadly Scourge*, 17–18.

139 Abraham Jacobi, *Treatise on Diphtheria*.

140 Ibid., 132–33.

141 Hammonds, *Childhood's Deadly Scourge*, 27–28.

142 Abraham Jacobi, *Treatise on Diphtheria*, 231–34; Hammonds, *Childhood's Deadly Scourge*, 25.

143 Hammonds, *Childhood's Deadly Scourge*, 52.

144 Abraham Jacobi, *Treatise On Diphtheria*, 50.

145 Abraham Jacobi, "Diphtheria and Diphtheritic Affections," 351–70.

146 Hammonds, *Childhood's Deadly Scourge*, 22–24; Abraham Jacobi, *Treatise on Diphtheria*, 49–50.

147 Abraham Jacobi, *Treatise on Diphtheria*, iv.

148 Abraham Jacobi praises Virchow for his "conservatism" on bacteriology. See Abraham Jacobi, "Inaugural Address," 149–69, reference on 162–63.

149 Hammonds, *Childhood's Deadly Scourge*, 52; K. Codell Carter, "Koch's Postulates," 369–72.

150 Hammonds, *Childhood's Deadly Scourge*, 30–36.

151 Abraham Jacobi, "Inaugural Address," 163, 167.

152 Ibid., 165–66.

153 Ibid., 167.

154 Abraham Jacobi, "Diphtheria Spread by Adults," 446, 447–48 (emphasis original).

155 Ibid., 444.

156 Truax, *Doctors Jacobi*, 198; Abraham Jacobi Household (misspelled "Jacoby"), 110 West 34th Street, New York City, U.S. Census Bureau, *Tenth Census of the United States, 1880*.

157 Abraham Jacobi, "Diphtheria Spread by Adults," 447. Also quoted in Hammonds, *Childhood's Deadly Scourge*, 33.

158 Abraham Jacobi, "Local Treatment of Diphtheria," 325–32.

159 Mary Putnam Jacobi, "Croup and Diphtheria," 125; Mary Putnam Jacobi, "Cerebro-Spinal Meningitis," 237.

160 Mary Putnam Jacobi to Mrs. Curtis, 4 September 1883, Folder 13, MPJ Papers, SL. On Dr. Edward Curtis, see Hammonds, *Childhood's Deadly Scourge*, 48.

161 Mary Putnam Jacobi quoted in "Discussion on Diphtheria," 87.

162 Mary Putnam Jacobi, *Physiological Notes*, 29, 24. For more on this study, see Chapter 4.

163 Marjorie's complaint was reported by Ruth Putnam, *Life and Letters*, 322. Truax (*Doctors Jacobi*, 207–8) also suggests that Marjorie was a research subject for her mother's "Experiment in Primary Education"; Truax consulted Marjorie while writing *The Doctors Jacobi*.

164 Marjorie McAneny to Rhoda Truax, 23 February 1952, Rhoda Truax Papers, Drexel.
165 Mary Putnam Jacobi to Marjorie Jacobi, 3 July 1889, Folder 14, MPJ Papers, SL.
166 "Meeting of Trustees and Associate Members, Barnard College," 11 November 1891; Barnard Yearbook, 1898; Report of the Dean, Barnard College, 1895, all Barnard College Archives, New York.
167 Record of Marjorie Jacobi, "Records, Registration, Fees, Time Schemes and Other Academic Data of the First Ten Years of Barnard College, 1889 through 1899"; Barnard Yearbook, 1898; Marjorie Jacobi, "Employer's Liability," Thesis, Class of 1899, all Barnard College Archives, New York.
168 According to Rhoda Truax, Abraham preferred the name Margarethe over Marjorie, wanting to name his daughter after the late Mrs. Carl Schurz, who had died in childbirth years before at the age of forty-four. See Truax, *Doctors Jacobi*, 189–90. See also Abraham Jacobi, *Aufsätze, Vorträge, und Reden*.
169 Abraham Jacobi, *Aufsätze, Vorträge, und Reden*, dedication and xxvi.
170 George McAneny, "Reminiscences of George McAneny," Oral History, Columbia. On McAneny's philosophy on the city and political reform, see his lectures, such as "The Use of City Government." On his relationship with Schurz, see his Scrapbook, Clippings, Death of Carl Schurz, all in the George McAneny Collection, Columbia. On McAneny's roll in subway expansion and city politics, see also Derrick, *Tunneling the Future*, and Hood, *722 Miles*.
171 Mary Putnam Jacobi to George McAneny, 7 October 1898, Folder 16A, MPJ Papers, SL; Marjorie McAneny to Shirley Putnam O'Hara, 3 February 1941, Container 4, HPP.
172 On her Barnard Alumnae Questionnaire, Marjorie McAneny said she "never worked." See Marjorie Jacobi McAneny, Barnard Alumnae Questionnaire, c. 1956, Class of 1899, Barnard College Archives, New York.
173 George McAneny to Green-Wood Cemetery Staff, 11 July 1919, Archives of Green-Wood Cemetery, Brooklyn, N.Y. (emphasis added).

CHAPTER SIX

1 "Education of Girls," 18.
2 Hamlin, "Beyond Adam's Rib"; Kohlstedt and Jorgensen, "'Irrepressible Woman Question,'" 267–93; Newman, *White Women's Rights*; Paxton, *George Eliot and Herbert Spencer*; Pittenger, *American Socialists*.
3 Jacobi was on the Executive Committee of the National Association for Sanitary and Rural Improvement; see "Methods of Sanitarians," 8. Jacobi was invited to speak at the Congress of Women for Improved Dress; see "Fair by Women for Charity," 8. Her anticorruption activities took place in the League for Political Education and the Woman's Municipal League; see "Women Are at Work," 5; "Woman's Political Work," 21; and "Women Against the Tiger," 5.
4 DuBois, "Working Women," 34–58. See also DuBois, *Harriot Stanton Blatch*; Graham, "Suffrage Renaissance," 157–78; and McDonald, "Organizing Womanhood."
5 Mary Putnam Jacobi to Agatha Schurz, c. 1894, Folder 15, MPJ Papers, SL.
6 Mary Putnam Jacobi to Richard W. Gilder, c. 26 January 1890, Richard Watson Gilder Papers, Century Collection, NYPL.

7   On nineteenth-century views of animals, see Turner, *Reckoning with the Beast*. See also Jones, *Valuing Animals*.

8   Lederer, *Subjected to Science*, 28.

9   For discussions on the history of pain, see Pernick, *Calculus of Suffering*, and Turner, *Reckoning with the Beast*. On views about pain in antebellum America, see Halttunen, "Humanitarianism," 303–34.

10 For more on Leffingwell, see Woolsey and Burke, "Playwright," 235–58; Leffingwell, "Does Vivisection Pay?," 391–99; and Leffingwell, "On Vivisection in America," 133–68.

11 Leffingwell, "Does Vivisection Pay?," 395, 391, 392 (emphasis original).

12 On Bigelow's opposition, see Lederer, *Subjected to Science*, 54; *Anti-Vivisection* 2 (March 1895): 13; and *Vivisection: Hearing*, 57. On Matthew C. Woods, see *Anti-Vivisection* 2 (March 1895): 13; and *Vivisection: Hearing*, 12–16. On Lawson Tait, see Berdoe, "Does Vivisection Help?," 956–58; and Risdon, *Robert Lawson Tait*. See the journal *Anti-Vivisection*, 1893–97, produced by the Illinois Anti-Vivisection Society, Aurora, Ill. Some issues and other pamphlets are housed in the Blackwell Family Papers, MC-411, Box 15, Folders 214–16, SL.

13 Rev. John C. Kimball, *Anti-Vivisection* 5 (June 1897): 63–64. For more men opposed to vivisection, see Peabody and Ingersoll, *Personal Experiences*, and Salt, *Animals' Rights*.

14 On the gendering of the anti-vivisection movement, see Lederer, "Moral Sensibility," 59–73.

15 Buettinger, "Women and Antivivisection," 857–72; Lederer, *Subjected to Science*, 27, 29, 36, 39. It was common for WCTU women to unite temperance with other strands of social reform. See Bordin, *Woman and Temperance*, 98, 109. For the WCTU's work in Wyoming against the juvenile death penalty and in favor of woman suffrage, see Brumberg, *Kansas Charley*, 166–71.

16 On British activism, see Ferguson, *Animal Advocacy*; and Elston, "Women and Anti-Vivisection," 259–94. Elston describes how vivisection also produced conflict within British feminist organizations that were torn between supporting women doctors and opposing animal experimentation (pp. 281–86).

17 *Anti-Vivisection* 2 (December 1894).

18 *Anti-Vivisection* 2 (August/September 1894): frontispiece; *Anti-Vivisection* 2 (December 1894): frontispiece.

19 *Anti-Vivisection* 2 (December 1894): 10.

20 Alice Stone Blackwell, "Abominable Practice," 340.

21 Kimball, "Woman's Medical College and Vivisection," 153.

22 Mary Putnam Jacobi, "Does Vivisection Help?," 157–58.

23 On the controversy over gynecological surgery, see Morantz-Sanchez, *Conduct Unbecoming a Woman*.

24 On Jacobi's testimony, see *Vivisection: Hearing*. On the Senate hearing, see Woolsey and Burke, "Playwright," and Gossel, "William Henry Welch," 397–419.

25 Gossel, "William Henry Welch," 418.

26 For more on the defense of vivisection, see "'Vivisection.'"

27 *Vivisection: Hearing*, 58–61, quotes on 60, 58.

28 Ibid., 60.

29 Woolsey and Burke, "Playwright," 247.

30 William Welch quoted in Lederer, *Subjected to Science*, 58.

31 "Additional Statement of Matthew Woods, of Philadelphia," *Vivisection: Hearing*, 169. Woods, president of the Pennsylvania Society for the Prevention of Cruelty to Animals, quotes Shakespeare on vivisection, claiming he "was among the first of moderns who condemned it, because of its effect in 'hardening human hearts.'" For background on Woods, see Woolsey and Burke, "Playwright," 243.

32 *Vivisection: Hearing*, 217.

33 Ibid.

34 Ibid.

35 Ibid., 60.

36 Robinson, "Malice and Vindictiveness," cited in Buettinger, "Women and Antivivisection," 867–68.

37 See Guerrini, *Experimenting with Humans and Animals*, and Lederer, *Subjected to Science*.

38 *Vivisection: Hearing*, 60.

39 Mary Putnam Jacobi, "Letter from Dr. Mary Putnam Jacobi," 44.

40 Mary Putnam Jacobi to Agatha Schurz, c. 1894, Folder 15, MPJ Papers, SL (emphasis added).

41 Mary Putnam Jacobi, "Letter from Dr. Mary Putnam Jacobi," 44.

42 Mary Putnam Jacobi, "Two Representative Women," 410.

43 Jacobi, "Letter from Dr. Mary Putnam Jacobi," 44 (emphasis original).

44 See the Jacobi/Stone Blackwell exchange in the following articles: "A.S.B." [Alice Stone Blackwell], "Women and Prohibition," 157; Mary Putnam Jacobi, "Dr. Mary Putnam-Jacobi on Prohibition," 160; Mary Putnam Jacobi, "Rights of Majorities," 194.

45 "Concerning Women," 401. Jacobi held meetings at her home in early February, early March, and late April of 1894. See column by Blake, "Our New York Letter." See also Josephine Shaw Lowell to Annie (Rice?), 29 April 1894, quoted in Stewart, *Philanthropic Work*, 136.

46 DuBois, "Working Women," 39.

47 Suffragists had long viewed the constitutional convention as an opportunity to argue on behalf of woman suffrage. On the 1867 suffrage campaign at the New York State Constitutional Convention, see DuBois, *Feminism and Suffrage*, 66–67, 87.

48 On the 1894 campaign, see DuBois, "Working Women," 36–37. On the political history of New York, see McCormick, *From Realignment to Reform*.

49 Stanton, *Eighty Years and More*, 451; New York State Woman Suffrage Association, *1894, Constitutional-Amendment Campaign Year*.

50 Mary Putnam Jacobi, "Report of the 'Volunteer Committee' in New York City," in New York State Woman Suffrage Association, *1894, Constitutional-Amendment Campaign Year*, 217–20.

51 Blake, "Our New York Letter," 10 March 1894, 77.

52 *Woman's Journal*, 7 April 1894, 109.

53 Stanton, *Eighty Years and More*, 451.

54 Hunter Graham, "Suffrage Renaissance," 161–65.

55 Mary Putnam Jacobi, "Woman Suffrage Question"; Mary Putnam Jacobi et al. "Shall Women Vote?," pamphlet, n.d., in *History of Women* (microfilm), Reel 951, no. 9224 (New Haven: Research Publications, Inc., 1977).

56 Mary Putnam Jacobi, "Two Representative Women," 406, 410.

57 Mary Putnam Jacobi, "Dr. Putnam Jacobi on the 'Antis,'" 198. Jacobi was especially frus- trated with a group of women commissioners to the Woman's Board at the World's Fair who rejected suffrage despite their public representation of women's interests. See also, "No Compromise with 'Antis,'" 8.

58 "Suffragists on the Warpath," 9.

59 Susan B. Anthony to Clara Colby, 3 February 1894, Rochester, cc3(8), Clara Colby Pa- pers, Huntington Library, San Marino, Calif. (emphasis original). Anthony reported to Colby that she was going to hear Jacobi's speech at the Albany Convention. See Susan B. Anthony to Clara Colby, 30 May 1894, Rochester, cc3(24), ibid.

60 See *1894, Constitutional-Amendment Campaign Year*, 8–9; and Mary Putnam Jacobi, "Ad- dress on Behalf of the Women of the City of New York Before the Committee on Suffrage of the State Constitutional Convention," 31 May 1894, reprinted in Mary Putnam Jacobi, *"Common Sense,"* 199–236. For reports on Jacobi and the suffrage hearings in Albany, see "Women Pleading at Albany," 2; and "On the Ballot for Women," 8.

61 *1894, Constitutional-Amendment Campaign Year*, 9.

62 Mary Putnam Jacobi, "Address on Behalf of the Women of the City of New York," in *"Common Sense,"* 200.

63 Ibid., 220–21.

64 Ibid., 209, 203–4, 206.

65 Ibid., 227.

66 Ibid., 210–11.

67 Ibid., 211.

68 Mary Putnam Jacobi, "Woman Suffrage Question," 820; see also Jacobi's argument in "Address on Behalf of the Women of the City of New York," in *"Common Sense,"* 212.

69 *1894, Constitutional-Amendment Campaign Year*, 16.

70 Mary Putnam Jacobi to Carl Schurz, 2 August 1894, Ruth Putnam, *Life and Letters*, 331.

71 Francis M. Scott quoted in *1894, Constitutional-Amendment Campaign Year*, 11.

72 Mary Putnam Jacobi, *"Common Sense."*

73 Paine, *Common Sense.*

74 Mary Putnam Jacobi, *"Common Sense,"* 16. On progress, women, and evolution, see Gra- ham, "Suffrage Renaissance," 167–68; and Newman, *White Women's Rights.*

75 Mary Putnam Jacobi, *"Common Sense,"* 16–25.

76 Ibid., 67.

77 Ibid., 74–75.

78 On the suffragist's use of evolutionary and racial discourses, see Newman, *White Women's Rights.* For Newman's take on Jacobi and racialized rhetoric, see ibid., 64–65, 151, 155.

79 Mary Putnam Jacobi, *"Common Sense,"* 137–38.

80 Ibid., 138.

81 The New York *Home Journal* quoted in "Dr. Jacobi's New Book," 262. For another sup- portive review of Jacobi's *"Common Sense,"* see *Popular Science Monthly* 47 (1895): 272.

82 Mary Putnam Jacobi, *"Common Sense"* (1915 edition).

83 "Literature," 151–52.

84 "Two Views of Woman Suffrage," 8.

85 Mary Putnam Jacobi, "Status and Future of the Woman Suffrage Movement," c. 1902, Folder 34, MPJ Papers, SL.

86 Jean Brooks Greenleaf, "Dr. Mary Putnam-Jacobi's Study Courses," in *1894, Constitutional-Amendment Campaign Year*, 239. Jacobi created the syllabi for these courses, which included a reading list of civic manuals, history books, women's rights texts, and suffrage newspapers and pamphlets. *Civil Government in the United States*, written by John Fiske, a historian and follower of Herbert Spencer, served as the primary textbook for the club.

87 Unfortunately, it was often responsible for promoting "educated suffrage," a stance bent on the exclusion of the illiterate and uneducated voters at the polls. The League for Political Education publicly supported pro-suffrage assembly and senatorial candidates and continued petition drives.

88 "Civil Service Outlook," 13.

89 "Women Against the Tiger," 5. See also "Women Are at Work," 5, and "Woman's Political Work," 21.

90 On the failed Massachusetts referendum, see Graham, "Suffrage Renaissance," 159–61.

91 Mary Putnam Jacobi, "From Massachusetts to Turkey," 6–8. On Charlotte Perkins Gilman's references to "the harem" as commentary on gender roles in the East, see Newman, *White Women's Rights*, 142.

92 Mary Putnam Jacobi, "From Massachusetts to Turkey," 3.

93 Mary Putnam Jacobi, *Question of Rest*, 232.

94 For Jacobi's leadership positions, see Nathan, *Story of an Epoch-Making Movement*, Appendix D and Appendix E, 132–33; and Consumers' League of the City of New York, *Annual Report*, 1896 and 1897.

95 On Jacobi's role in the Women's Conference of the Society for Ethical Culture, see "For Relief of the Hungry," 5.

96 Mary Putnam Jacobi, *"Common Sense,"* 190.

97 Gilman, *Women and Economics*.

98 Extracts from the Report of Alice Woodbridge, read at the Meeting of the Working Women's Society, 1890, Appendix A, in Nathan, *Story of an Epoch-Making Movement*, 129–30. On the history of labor and department stores, see Benson, *Counter Cultures*.

99 On Lowell, see Waugh, *Unsentimental Reformer*, and Stewart, *Philanthropic Work*.

100 Nathan, *Story of an Epoch-Making Movement*, 18–19; Ruth Putnam on the Consumers' League in Ruth Putnam, *Life and Letters*, Appendix E, 380–81.

101 The *New York Times* quoted in Nathan, *Story of an Epoch-Making Movement*, 21.

102 Ibid., 21–23.

103 Ibid., 25–27.

104 Lowell quoted in Stewart, *Philanthropic Work*, 346.

105 On "girl advocacy" and moral reform, see Peiss, *Cheap Amusements*; Odem, *Delinquent Daughters*; and Kunzel, *Fallen Women*.

106 Mary Putnam Jacobi to Agatha Schurz, Bolton Landing, c. 1894, Folder 15, MPJ Papers, SL.

107 Lowell quoted in Stewart, *Philanthropic Work*, 344.

108 Lowell quoted in ibid., 338.

109 Mary Putnam Jacobi, "The Property Rights of Employees," published in ibid., 350–56.

Jacobi tried to discern between "good" labor rendered for personal services with fair compensation and labor expended solely for the accumulation of fortunes. Greater rewards were received by those who worked for the "personal welfare" of others, she said.

110 Ibid., 352, 355–56.

111 Ibid., 354.

112 Ibid., 50. See also Waugh, *Unsentimental Reformer*, 199–200.

113 On Kelley and the Consumers' League, see Sklar, *Florence Kelley*, 309–11.

114 Florence Kelley's address, in Women's Medical Association of New York City, ed., *In Memory of Mary Putnam Jacobi*, 25–30, quote on 28.

115 Alice Hamilton carried on this work in the early twentieth century. See Sicherman, *Alice Hamilton*.

116 Florence Kelley's address, in Women's Medical Association of New York City, ed., *In Memory of Mary Putnam Jacobi*, 30 (emphasis original).

117 Mary Putnam Jacobi, "Address Before the Women's Medical Association about 1900," in *Pathfinder*, 494.

118 Ibid., 498.

119 Mary Putnam Jacobi "Women in Medicine"; Morantz-Sanchez, *Sympathy and Science*, 144–83, 232–65. On women's medical societies, see Marrett, "On the Evolution of Women's Medical Societies," 434–48.

120 In 1885, the Association for the Advancement of the Medical Education of Women changed its name to the Women's Medical Association. See *Pathfinder*, xxv.

121 Mary Putnam Jacobi, "Address at the Semi-Centennial of the Woman's Medical College of Pennsylvania, 1900," typescript, 6, Folder 33, MPJ Papers, SL.

122 On the founding of the Alumnae Association of the Woman's Medical College of Pennsylvania, see Peitzman, *New and Untried Course*, 61–62.

123 Mary Putnam Jacobi, "Circular Letter to the Alumnae of the Woman's Medical College of Pennsylvania," in *Reports and Transactions of the Annual Meetings*, 1890, 72.

124 Mary Putnam Jacobi quoted in ibid., 1895, 24–25.

125 Mary Putnam-Jacobi, President, "Circular Letter to the Alumnae of the Woman's Medical College of Pennsylvania," in ibid., 1890, 73.

126 For a summary of the Hopkins campaign, see Alan Mason Chesney Archives, *Women's Medical Fund*. See also Morantz-Sanchez, *Sympathy and Science*, 84–87.

127 Paul S. Boyer, "Mary Elizabeth Garrett," in *Notable American Women*, 2:21–22; Horowitz, *Power and Passion*.

128 Alan Mason Chesney Archives, *Women's Medical Fund*, 12.

129 Ibid., 14.

130 Mary Putnam Jacobi to M. Carey Thomas, 24 October [n.d.], Reel 163, no. 510–12, M. Carey Thomas Papers, Bryn Mawr College Library, Special Collections, Bryn Mawr, Pa.

131 M. Carey Thomas to Mary Garrett, 16 March 1890, Reel 16, no. 45–49, ibid.

132 M. Carey Thomas to Mary Garrett, 15 April 1890, Reel 16, no. 65–69, ibid. Thomas here could have been referring to either Miss Alice Lyon or Eliza Sinclair Lyon, both members of the New York branch of the WFC. See Alan Mason Chesney Archives, *Women's Medical Fund*, List of Committees, 5.

133 Mary Putnam Jacobi, "On the Opening of the Johns Hopkins School to Women," 633–34.

134 "Temptation of Johns Hopkins," 550.

135 Mary Putnam Jacobi, "'Temptation of Johns Hopkins,'" 588–89. See also the response of Emily Blackwell, "'The Temptation of Johns Hopkins,'" *Medical Record*, 6 December 1890, 650.

136 See "Preliminary Announcement" reprinted in Alan Mason Chesney Archives, *Women's Medical Fund*, 16–17, which said: "Men and women will be admitted on the same terms."

137 Osler, "On the Opening of the Johns Hopkins Medical School to Women," 635; Morantz-Sanchez, *Sympathy and Science*, 87.

138 Osler, "On the Opening of the Johns Hopkins Medical School to Women," 635. "The past history of the chemical, physiological, and pathological departments of the Johns Hopkins University is a sufficient guarantee for the character of the scientific work of the medical school," he added in defense of the groundbreaking development.

139 See Morantz-Sanchez, *Sympathy and Science*, 232–65.

EPILOGUE

1 Helen Baldwin, M.D., attended Jacobi from March 1903 until her death in 1906, serving as the main witness on the death certificate. See Death Record, Mary Corinna Putnam Jacobi, d. 10 June 1906, "Cerebellar Tumor and Bronchopneumonia," Record #18762, NYCMA.

2 "Address at the Annual Alumnae Breakfast," Wadleigh School (Twelfth Street School), March 1902, in Ruth Putnam, *Life and Letters*, 336–40.

3 Mary Putnam Jacobi to Amy Putnam, c. 15 July 1905, Folder 19, MPJ Papers, SL.

4 See letters Mary Putnam Jacobi to Amy Jacobi, 1903–5, MPJ Papers, SL.

5 Mary Putnam Jacobi to Amy Putnam, c. 15 July 1905, Folder 19, MPJ Papers, SL.

6 Mary Putnam Jacobi to Ruth Putnam, c. 13 June 1905, Folder 19, MPJ Papers, SL (emphasis original).

7 Mary Putnam Jacobi, "Case," 1903, Folder 35, MPJ Papers, SL.

8 Dr. Charles L. Dana in Women's Medical Association of New York City, ed., *In Memory of Mary Putnam Jacobi*, 39.

9 Mary Putnam Jacobi, "Case," 1903, Folder 35, MPJ Papers, SL.

10 Ibid.

11 Mary Putnam Jacobi, "Tumors of the Brain," in *Essays on Hysteria*, 81–139.

12 Ibid., 136; Patterson, *Dread Disease*, 14–16.

13 Mary Putnam Jacobi, *Essays on Hysteria*, 81.

14 Ibid., 122–23.

15 Ibid., 136.

16 Mary Putnam Jacobi quoted in Ruth Putnam, *Life and Letters*, 343.

17 Death Record, Mary Corinna Putnam Jacobi, d. 10 June 1906, "Cerebellar Tumor and Bronchopneumonia," Record #18762, NYCMA. For obituaries, see "Dr. M. P. Jacobi's Death"; Henry Brown Blackwell, "In Memoriam," 95; "Mary Putnam Jacobi," *New York*

Tribune, 12 June 1906; *New York Eve Staats Zeitung*, 15 June 1906; and "A Woman of Greatness," *Brooklyn Eagle*, 12 June 1906. Abraham Jacobi outlived Mary by many years, dying in 1919.

18 Women's Medical Association of New York City, ed., *In Memory of Mary Putnam Jacobi*.

19 Ibid., 8.

20 Ibid., 6.

21 "Addresses at the Unveiling of a Memorial Tablet."

22 Ruth Putnam, *Life and Letters*; *Pathfinder*.

23 Transcript, Mary Putnam Jacobi, "Within Our Gates," recorded 26 October 1950, Drexel. Marie Zakrzewska was also the subject of a radio program in 1942 called "The Cavalcade of America"; see Tuchman, *Science Has No Sex*, 1.

24 Truax, *Doctors Jacobi*; Barringer, *Bowery to Bellevue*.

25 On medicine and American film, see Reagan, Tomes, and Treichler, eds., *Medicine's Moving Pictures*, especially Naomi Rogers, "American Medicine," 199–238.

26 See, for example, Liz Savage and Andrea Widener, "Physician Characteristics Are Associated with Quality of Cancer Care," *Journal of the National Cancer Institute* 100 (2008): 157; and "The Sex of Your Surgeon May Matter," *New York Times*, 29 January 2008.

27 Hollingworth, *Functional Periodicity*; Mosher, "Normal Menstruation," 178–79, and, more importantly, Mosher, *Health and the Woman Movement*.

28 Rosalind Rosenberg, *Beyond Separate Spheres*; Hollingworth, *Functional Periodicity*; Mosher, "Normal Menstruation," 178–79; Mosher, *Health and the Woman Movement*.

29 Lawrence H. Summers, "Remarks at NBER Conference on Diversifying the Science and Engineering Workforce," 14 January 2005, <http://www.president.harvard.edu/speeches/2005/nber.html>. For coverage of the event, see Marcella Bombardieri, "Summers' Remarks on Women Draw Fire," 17 January 2005, <http://www.boston.com/news/education/higher/articles/2005/01/17/summers_remarks_on_women_draw_fire>; and Michael Dobbs, "Harvard Chief's Comments on Women Assailed; Academics Critical of Remarks about the Lack of Gender Equality," 19 January 2005, <http://www.washingtonpost.com/wp-dyn/articles/A19181–2005Jan18.html>.

30 See remarks by Helen Lefkowitz Horowitz, "Clanging Chains, Once Again: Harvard's Long Tradition of Putting Women in their Place," SAQ Online (The Magazine of Alumnae and Friends of Smith College), <http://saqonline.smith.edu/article.epl?issue_id=9&article_id=783>.

31 Hopkins chaired an MIT research committee on gender discrimination. See "A Study on the Status of Women Faculty in Science at MIT," <http://web.mit.edu/fnl/women/women.html>. See also comments of Denice D. Denton, then chancellor designate of UC Santa Cruz, during the conference in Sam Dillon, "Harvard Chief Defends His Talk on Women," *New York Times*, 18 January 2005; "NOW Calls for Resignation of Harvard University's President," 20 January 2005, <http://www.now.org/press/01-05/01-20-Harvard.html>.

32 Cornelia Dean, "Institutions Hinder Female Academics, Panel Says," *New York Times*, 18 September 2006. For a rebuttal, see John Tierney's op-ed, "Academy of P.C. Sciences," *New York Times*, 26 September 2006.

33 On the renewed interest in nature vs. nurture, and scientific practice, see recent comments

by Evelyn Fox Keller in Cornelia Dean, "Theorist Drawn into Debate 'That Will Not Go Away,'" *New York Times*, 12 April 2005.

34 For example, see Blum, *Sex on the Brain*; Kimura, *Sex and Cognition*; Moir and Jessel, *Brain Sex*; Rhoads, *Taking Sex Differences Seriously*; and Sax, *Why Gender Matters*. Claiming to balance biological and social factors is Hines, *Brain Gender*.

35 Brizendine, *Female Brain*.

Bibliography

MANUSCRIPT SOURCES

France

Paris

  Archives Nationales

    Faculté de Médecine de Paris, AJ16

    Victor Duruy Papers, AP114

    Bibliothèque Nationale de France, Manuscript Collections

    Élisée Reclus Papers, NAF 22909–22919

United States

Boston, Mass.

  Harvard Medical Library in the Francis A. Countway Library of Medicine, Harvard
      Medical School

    Boylston Prize Committee Records, DE-10

      Mary Putnam Jacobi Correspondence

  Massachusetts Historical Society

    Horace Mann Collection, microfilm edition, 40 reels (Boston: Massachusetts
      Historical Society, 1989)

Brooklyn, N.Y.

  Archives of Green-Wood Cemetery

    Jacobi Family Burial Records

Bryn Mawr, Pa.

  Bryn Mawr College Library, Special Collections

    M. Carey Thomas Papers

Cambridge, Mass.

  Houghton Library, Harvard University

    Joseph Ishill Papers, MS Am 1614

    Fanny Garrison Villard Papers, MS Am 1321

Henry Villard Papers, MS Am 1322
Schlesinger Library on the History of Women in America, Radcliffe Institute for
    Advanced Study, Harvard University
    Blackwell Family Papers, MC-411
    Mary F. Eastman Letter, E-13
    Mary Putnam Jacobi Papers, A-26
    Corinna Lindon Smith Papers, MC-433
Hanover, N.H.
    Rauner Special Collections, Dartmouth College Library
    George Palmer Putnam Collection, MS 117
New York, N.Y.
    Barnard College Archives, Barnard College
    Barnard College Announcements, 1899–1903
    Barnard Yearbook, 1898
    Marjorie Jacobi, "Employer's Liability," Thesis, Class of 1899
    Marjorie Jacobi McAneny, Barnard Alumnae Questionnaire, c. 1956, Class of 1899
    "Meeting of Trustees and Associate Members, Barnard College," 11 November 1891
    Record of Marjorie Jacobi, "Records, Registration, Fees, Time Schemes and Other
        Academic Data of the First Ten Years of Barnard College, 1889 through 1899"
    Columbia University, Rare Book and Manuscript Library
    Elizabeth Blackwell Papers
    Mary Putnam Jacobi Correspondence with Christine Ladd Franklin, Edmund C.
        Stedman, Seth Low
    George McAneny Papers
    George Haven Putnam Collection
    "Reminiscences of George McAneny," Oral History, 1949
    Cornell University, Weill Medical College, Medical Center Archives
    Records of the Women's Medical Association of New York City
    Mount Sinai School of Medicine, Levy Library
    Mount Sinai Archives
    Miscellaneous Holdings
    New York Academy of Medicine Library, Historical Collections
    Abraham Jacobi Papers
    Letter, Mary Putnam Jacobi to Toni and Sophie Boas, 1884
    Records of the Medical Society of the County of New York
    Records of the New York Academy of Medicine
    Records of the New York Neurological Society
    Records of the New York Obstetrical Society
    New York City Municipal Archives
    County of New York, Manhattan, Register of Births, Deaths, and Marriages
    New York Public Library, Manuscripts and Archives Division, Astor, Lenox, and Tilden
        Foundations
    Richard Rogers Bowker Papers
    Richard Watson Gilder Papers, Century Company Records

New York Downtown Hospital, Archive
  Records of the New York Infirmary
Philadelphia, Pa.
  American Philosophical Society
    Franz Boas Collection, Correspondence with Abraham Jacobi, c. 1880–1917, B B61
  Drexel University College of Medicine, Archives and Special Collections on Women in
      Medicine and Homeopathy
    Mary C. Putnam, "Theorae ad lienis officium [Theories with regard to the function
        of the spleen]," Medical thesis, Female Medical College of Pennsylvania, 1864
        (translated by J. Cain)
      Records of the Female Medical College of Pennsylvania
      Records of the Woman's Medical College of Pennsylvania
      Rhoda Truax Papers
      "Within Our Gates" Transcript
  College of Physicians of Philadelphia, Historical Library
    Records of the Mount Sinai Outdoor Department
Princeton, N.J.
  Princeton University Library, Rare Books and Special Collections
    Abraham Jacobi Papers, C0724
San Marino, Calif.
  Huntington Library
    Clara Colby Papers
Washington, D.C.
  Library of Congress
    Manuscript Division
      Elizabeth Blackwell Papers
      Blackwell Family Papers, 0320T
      George Palmer Putnam Papers, MMC-3588
      Herbert Putnam Papers, 0630X
      Ruth Putnam Papers, MMC-0131
    Prints and Photographs
      Herbert Putnam Papers, LOT 11490
      Portraits of Herbert Putnam's Family and Friends
  National Library of Medicine, History of Medicine Division
    Abraham Jacobi Papers

PUBLISHED PRIMARY SOURCES

*Works by Mary Putnam Jacobi can be found under Jacobi, Mary Putnam; P. C. M.;
and Putnam, Mary C.*

"Addresses at the Unveiling of a Memorial Tablet in Honor of Mary Putnam-Jacobi."
  Woman's Medical College of Pennsylvania Alumnae Association Transactions (1907): 56–71.
Annual Report of the New York Infirmary for Women and Children, 1883, 1884, 1888, 1890, 1891.

Anti-Vivisection, 1893–97 (Aurora, Ill.: Illinois Anti-Vivisection Society).

Association for the Advancement of the Medical Education of Women. *Report of the Association for the Advancement of the Medical Education of Women, with Addresses Delivered at Union League Hall, Tuesday, March 26th, 1878.* New York: G. P. Putnam's Sons, 1878.

Barbin, Herculine. *Herculine Barbin: Being the Recently Discovered Memoirs of a Nineteenth-Century Hermaphrodite.* Introduction by Michel Foucault. Translated by Richard McDougall. New York: Pantheon, 1980.

Barringer, Emily Dunning. *Bowery to Bellevue: The Story of New York's First Woman Ambulance Surgeon.* New York: W. W. Norton & Company, 1950.

Berdoe, Edward. "Does Vivisection Help?" *The Century* 40 (1890): 956–58.

Bernard, Claude. *An Introduction to the Study of Experimental Medicine (1865).* Translated by Henry Copley Greene. New York: Dover Publications, 1957.

Blackwell, Alice Stone. "An Abominable Practice." *The Woman's Journal*, 22 October 1892, 340.

———. "Women and Prohibition." *The Woman's Journal*, 18 May 1889, 157.

Blackwell, Elizabeth. *Address Delivered at the Opening of the Woman's Medical College of the New York Infirmary, November 2, 1868.* New York: Edward O. Jenkins, 1869.

———. "Erroneous Method in Medical Education." In *Essays in Medical Sociology*, 2:35–45.

———. *Essays in Medical Sociology.* 2 vols. New York: Arno Press, 1972.

———. "The Human Element in Sex: Introduction." In *Essays in Medical Sociology*, 1:1–17.

———. "Scientific Method in Biology." In *Essays in Medical Sociology*, 2:87–150.

———. *Pioneer Work for Women.* London: J. M. Dent and Sons, 1914.

Blackwell, Emily. "Woman's Medical College Justified." *The Woman's Journal*, 22 May 1897, 161.

Blackwell, Henry Brown (signed H. B. B.). "In Memoriam: Dr. Mary Putnam Jacobi." *The Woman's Journal*, 16 June 1906, 95.

Blake, Lillie Devereux. "Our New York Letter." *The Woman's Journal*, February–June 1894.

Bouchard, Charles Jacques. *Traité de Pathologie Générale.* 6 vols. Paris: G. Masson, 1895.

Bowditch, Henry Pickering. "The Question of Rest." *The Nation*, 13 September 1877.

Brackett, Anna C. *The Education of American Girls: Considered in a Series of Essays.* New York: G. P. Putnam's Sons, 1874.

"A Brief History of the Women's Medical College of the New York Infirmary for Women and Children," 1897. In Women's Medical College of the New York Infirmary Collection of Publications, National Library of Medicine, Microfilm no. 27010650R.

Charcot, Jean-Martin. *Leçons cliniques sur les maladies des vieillards et les maladies chroniques.* Edited by B. Ball. Paris: Adrien Delahaye, 1867.

"Civil Service Outlook: George McAneny Addresses the League for Political Education on the Prospects of Reform." *New York Times*, 5 December 1897, 13.

Clarke, Edward H. *Sex in Education; or, A Fair Chance for the Girls.* Boston: James R. Osgood and Company, 1873.

"College of Pharmacy Commencement." *New York Times*, 20 March 1863, 8.

"'Common Sense Applied to Woman Suffrage.'" *Popular Science Monthly* 47 (1895): 272.

"Concerning Women." *The Woman's Journal*, 17 December 1881, 401.

Consumers' League of the City of New York. *The Consumers' League of the City of New York, Annual Reports*, 1896, 1897, 1899, 1900.

Cornil, André-Victor, and Louis-Antoine Ranvier. *A Manual of Pathological Histology*. Translated by E. O. Shakespeare and J. Henry C. Simes. Philadelphia: Henry C. Lea, 1880.

Dalton, John C. *A Treatise on Human Physiology*. Philadelphia: H. C. Lea, 1875.

Daniel, Annie Sturges. "'A Cautious Experiment': The History of the New York Infirmary for Women and Children and the Women's [*sic*] Medical College of the New York Infirmary; Also Its Pioneer Founders, 1853–1899." *Medical Woman's Journal* 46 (May 1939): 125–31; (June 1939): 168–74; (July 1939): 196–202; (August 1939): 229–38; (September 1939): 269–77; (October 1939): 295–99, 309; (November 1939): 335–39; (December 1939): 357–60.

———. "'A Cautious Experiment.'" *Medical Woman's Journal* 47 (January 1940): 10–12; (February 1940): 40–45; (March 1940): 67–69; (April 1940): 97–101; (May 1940): 135–39, xi; (June 1940): 167–71; (July 1940): 199–204, 228; (August 1940): 234–39; (September 1940): 263–68, 282; (October 1940): 296–300; (November 1940): 323–29, 345; (December 1940): 357–62, 370.

———. "'Cautious Experiment.'" *Medical Woman's Journal* 48 (January 1941): 10–13; (February 1941): 33–39; (March 1941): 74–79, 91; (April 1941): 102–4, 123; (May 1941): 134–38; (June 1941): 167–73; (July 1941): 197–99, 216; (August 1941): 233–40; (September 1941): 272–78, 288; (October 1941): 301–7; (November 1941): 331–38, 346; (December 1941): 364–71.

———. "'A Cautious Experiment.'" *Medical Woman's Journal* 49 (January 1942): 12–15, 26; (February 1942): 37–40, 59; (March 1942): 71–74; (April 1942): 105–9; (May 1942): 137–38; (June 1942): 165–66, 189; (July 1942): 208–12, 228; (August 1942): 241–43; (September 1942): 274–75; (October 1942): 306–10, 324; (November 1942): 342–44; (December 1942): 373–75, 392.

David, C. G. (aka David G. Croly). *Positivist Primer: Being A Series of Familiar Conversations on the Religion of Humanity*. New York: David Wesley & Co., 1871.

"Discussion on Diphtheria." *Quarterly Bulletin of the Clinical Society of the New York Post-Graduate Medical School and Hospital* 1 (1885): 84–93.

"Dr. Jacobi's New Book." *The Woman's Journal*, 18 August 1894, 262.

"Dr. M. P. Jacobi's Death Ends a Brilliant Career." *New York Times*, 12 June 1906, 9.

Duruy, Victor. *Notes et souveneirs, 1811–1894*. Vol. 2. Paris: Librairie Hachette, 1902.

———. "Une Conquête du féminisme sous le Second Empire: Fondation d'une école pour l'instruction medical des femmes." 1870. *Bulletin enseignement public au Maroc* 41 (1954): 51–61.

E. A. "Woman as a Physician." *The Commercial*, 30 September 1877.

"The Education of Girls: Dr. Mary Putnam Jacobi Discusses Phases of It Before the Mothers' Congress." *New York Times*, 21 November 1897, 18.

"Eighteenth Annual Meeting of the American Pharmaceutical Association, Held at Baltimore." *American Journal of Pharmacy* (November 1870).

Emmet, Thomas Addis. *The Principles and Practice of Gynaecology*. Philadelphia: Henry C. Lea, 1879.

Engelmann, George J. "The American Girl of To-day: The Influence of Modern Education on Functional Development." *Transactions of the American Gynecological Society* 25 (1900): 8–45.

———. "The Use of Electricity in Gynecological Practice." *Transactions of the American Gynecological Society* 11 (1887): 207–355.

"Fair by Women for Charity: To Show Artistic and Healthful Garments." *New York Times*, 17 February 1894, 8.

The Female Medical College of Pennsylvania, Annual Announcements, 1863–65.

"For Relief of the Hungry." *New York Times*, 27 December 1893, 5.

"From New York." *Springfield Republican*, 31 January 1872, 5.

Fussell, Edwin. "Introductory Address." *Announcement of the Sixteenth Annual Session of the Female Medical College of Pennsylvania* (1865), 8–16.

Geddes, Patrick, and J. Arthur Thomson. *The Evolution of Sex*. London: Walter Scott, 1889.

Gilman, Charlotte Perkins. *Human Work*. New York: McClure, Phillips & Co., 1904.

———. *The Living of Charlotte Perkins Gilman: An Autobiography*. New York: Harper & Row, 1975.

———. *Women and Economics: A Study of the Economic Relation Between Men and Women as a Factor in Social Evolution*. Berkeley: University of California Press, 1998.

———. *The Yellow Wallpaper*. New York: The Feminist Press, 1973.

Goodman, John. "The Cyclical Theory of Menstruation." *American Journal of Obstetrics and Diseases of Women and Children* 11 (1878): 673–94.

Graduates' Reunion: Senior Department of School No. 47, Twelfth St., New York. New York: Hurd and Houghton, 1865.

Gray, Henry. *On the Structure and Use of the Spleen*. London: John W. Parker and Son, 1854.

Hansell, George H. *Reminiscences of Baptist Churches and Baptist Leaders in New York City and Vicinity, from 1835–1898*. Philadelphia: American Baptist Publication Society, 1899.

Harvey, Ellwood. "Report of the Delaware County Medical Society, Edwin Fussell, M.D., 1813–1882." *Transactions of the Medical Society of Pennsylvania* 14 (1882): 318–19.

The Health-Lift Company. *The Health-Lift, Reduced to a Science, Cumulative Exercise: A Thorough Gymnastic System in Ten Minutes Once a Day*. New York: The Health-Lift Company, 1876.

Hewitt, Graily. *The Pathology, Diagnosis, and Treatment of the Diseases of Women*. Vol. 2. New York: Bermingham & Co., 1883.

Hollingworth, Leta Stetter. *Functional Periodicity: An Experimental Study of the Mental and Motor Abilities of Women during Menstruation*. New York: Teachers College, Columbia University, 1914.

Holt, Luther Emmett. *The Care and Feeding of Children: A Catechism for the Use of Mothers and Children's Nurses*. New York: D. Appleton and Company, 1894.

Howe, Julia Ward, ed. *Sex and Education: A Reply to Dr. E. H. Clarke's "Sex in Education."* Boston: Roberts Brothers, 1874.

Ishill, Joseph. *Elisée and Elie Reclus: In Memoriam*. Berkeley Heights, N.J.: The Oriole Press, 1927.

Jacobi, Abraham. "Abraham Jacobi Address." In *In Memory of Dr. Elizabeth Blackwell and Emily Blackwell*, edited by Women's Medical Association of New York City, 67–82. New York: New York Academy of Medicine, 1911.

———. "Address at the Dedication of the Bender Laboratory, Albany." *Albany Medical Annals* (1896). Reprinted in *Dr. Jacobi's Works*, 7:315–41.

———. *Address at the Twenty-Fifth Jubilee of the German Dispensary of New York.* Reprinted in *Dr. Jacobi's Works*, 8:59–75.

———. *Aufsätze, Vorträge, und Reden.* 2 vols. New York: Press of Stettiner, Lambert, and Co., 1893.

———. "Biographical Sketch of Ernst Krackowizer, M.D., Address Delivered Before the New York Academy of Medicine" (1875). Reprinted in *Aufsätze, Vorträge, und Reden,* 1:357–93.

———. "Address on the Claims of Paediatric Medicine." *Transactions of the American Medical Association* 31 (1880): 709–14.

———. "Diphtheria Spread by Adults." *New York Medical Journal,* September (1884). Reprinted in *Dr. Jacobi's Works*, 3:439–48.

———. *Dr. Jacobi's Works: Collected Essays, Addresses, Scientific Papers, and Miscellaneous Writings* (aka *Collectanea Jacobi*). Vol. 1–8. Edited by William J. Robinson. New York: The Critic and Guide Company, 1909.

———. "General Therapeutics." In *Therapeutics of Infancy and Childhood, 3rd Edition.* Philadelphia: J. B. Lippincott Co., 1903. Reprinted in *Dr. Jacobi's Works*, 2:9–46.

———. "The History of Pediatrics and Its Relation to Other Sciences and Arts." *American Medicine* 8 (1904). Reprinted in *Dr. Jacobi's Works*, 1:55–93.

———. "Inaugural Address." *Transactions of the New York Academy of Medicine* 5 (1885): 149–69.

———. "Inaugural Address, Including a Paper on Infant Asylums, Medical Society of the County of New York, 4 December 1871." *New York Medical Journal,* January (1872). Reprinted in *Aufsätze, Vorträge, und Reden,* 1:125–86.

———. *Infant Diet: A Paper Read Before the Public Health Association of New York.* New York: G. P. Putnam's Sons, 1873.

———. *Infant Diet: Revised, Enlarged, and Adapted to Popular Use by Mary Putnam Jacobi, M.D.* New York: G. P. Putnam's Sons, 1874.

———. "Local Treatment in Diphtheria." *Therapeutic Gazette* (March 1894). Reprinted in *Dr. Jacobi's Works*, 2:325–32.

———. "Monism in Medicine: Address to the Association of Graduates of Medical Colleges of New York City." *Annals of Gynecology and Pediatry* 18 (1905): 57–67.

———. "On Diphtheria and Diphtheritic Affections." *American Medical Times,* August 1860. Reprinted in *Dr. Jacobi's Works*, 3:351–70.

———. "Oration at the Semi-Centennial of the New York Academy of Medicine." *Medical Record,* March 1897. Reprinted in *Dr. Jacobi's Works*, 7:353–71.

———. "Part of Inauguration Address of the President of the Medical Society of the County of New York, November 7, 1870." *Medical Record,* December 1870. Reprinted in *Aufsätze, Vorträge, und Reden,* 1:117–23.

———. "Phases in the Development of Therapy." *Yale Medical Journal* (July 1905). Reprinted in *Dr. Jacobi's Works*, 4:9–46.

———. "The Physical Cost of Women's Work." Reprinted from *Charities and the Commons,* 2 February 1907, 1–8.

———. "Remarks at the Anniversary of the New York German Medical Society" (1898). Reprinted in *Dr. Jacobi's Works*, 7:373–75.

———. "Report of the Committee Appointed to Co-Operate with the New York Society for the Prevention of Cruelty to Children, 1881." *Transactions of the Medical Society of the State of New York* (1881). Reprinted in *Aufsätze, Vorträge, und Reden*, 1:431–51.

———. "Rudolf Virchow, An Address Introductory to the Course of Lectures of the Term 1881–1882, Delivered in the Lecture Room of the College of Physicians and Surgeons, New York." *Medical Record*, October 1881. Reprinted in *Aufsätze, Vorträge, und Reden*, 1:479–521.

———. "Some of the Benefits Derived from Medical Libraries." *Cleveland Medical Journal* (November 1906). Reprinted in *Dr. Jacobi's Works*, 8:385–406.

———. "Some Remarks on the Practice of Medicine as a Career." *Medical Record*, April 1909. Reprinted in *Dr. Jacobi's Works*, 8:339–48.

———. *A Treatise on Diphtheria*. New York: William Wood & Co., 1880.

———. "Treatment of Infant Diarrhea and Dysentery." *American Journal of Obstetrics and Diseases of Women and Children*, July 1879. Reprinted in *Dr. Jacobi's Works*, 2:185–217.

———. "Women Physicians in America." *Deutsche Medicinische Wochenschrift* 25 (1896). Reprinted in *Dr. Jacobi's Works*, 7:305–14, trans. from the German.

Jacobi, Mary Putnam. "Acute Fatty Degeneration of the New-Born." *American Journal of Obstetrics and Diseases of Women and Children* 2 (1878): 499. Reprinted in *Pathfinder*, 311–25.

———. "Acute Mania after Operations." *Medical Record* 35 (1889): 446–48.

———. "Address before the Women's Medical Association about 1900." Reprinted in *Pathfinder*, 494–500.

———. "An Address Delivered at the Commencement of the Woman's Medical College of the New York Infirmary, May 30, 1883." *Archives of Medicine* 10 (1883): 59. Reprinted in *Pathfinder*, 391–402.

———. "Anomalous Malformation of the Heart." *Medical Record* 7 (1872): 111–12.

———. "Ataxia in a Child." *Medical Record* 51 (1897): 761–65.

———. "The Blood Count in Anaemia and Certain Nervous Affections." *Medical Record* 53 (1898): 933–35.

———. "Case of Absent Uterus: With Considerations on the Significance of Hermaphroditism." *American Journal of Obstetrics and Diseases of Women and Children* 32 (1895): 510–44.

———. "Case of Facial and Palatine Paralysis, and Loss of Equilibrium, Produced by a Fall on the Head." *Independent Practitioner* 2 (1881): 69. Reprinted in *Pathfinder*, 329–33.

———. "Case of Post-Epileptic Hysteria. Effect of Inhalation of Compressed Air. Phenomena of Transfer." *Journal of Nervous and Mental Diseases* 15 (1888): 442–45.

———. "Case of Probable Tumor of the Pons." *Journal of Nervous and Mental Diseases* 16 (1889): 115. Reprinted in *Pathfinder*, 446–57.

———. "Case of Tubercular Meningitis with Measurements of Cranial Temperatures." *Journal of Nervous and Mental Diseases* 7 (1880): 51–56.

———. "Case of Uterine Fibroid Treated by Apostoli's Method. Enucleation of the Tumor." *American Journal of Obstetrics and Diseases of Women and Children* 21 (1889): 806–15.

———. "Cerebro-Spinal Meningitis — Pseudo-Membranous Croup." *Medical Record* 12 (1877): 237–38.

———. *"Common Sense" Applied to Woman Suffrage*. New York: G. P. Putnam's Sons, 1894 (2nd edition, 1915).

———. "Considerations on Flechsig's 'Gehirn und Seele.'" *Journal of Nervous and Mental Disease* 24 (1897): 747–68.

———. "Contribution to Sphygmography: The Influence of Pain Upon the Pulse-Trace." *Archives of Medicine* 2 (1879): 51. Reprinted in *Pathfinder*, 326–28.

———. "Croup and Diphtheria." *Medical Record* 12 (1877): 125.

———. "Curious Congenital Deformities of Upper and Lower Extremities." *Medical Record* 13 (1878): 115.

———. "Cystic Ovaries — Battey's Operation." *Medical Record* 25 (1884): 705.

———. "The Discoveries of Pasteur, Koch, and Others: A Brief Review to Date." *The Century* 41 (April 1891): 954–57.

———. "Does Vivisection Help?" *The Century* 42 (March 1891): 157–58.

———. "Dr. Putnam-Jacobi on Prohibition." *The Woman's Journal*, 18 May 1889, 160.

———. "Dr. Putnam Jacobi on the 'Antis.'" *The Woman's Journal*, 23 June 1894, 198–99.

———. "Educational Needs." *North American Review* 136 (1883): 299–304.

———. *Essays on Hysteria, Brain-Tumor, and Some Other Cases of Nervous Disease*. New York: G. P. Putnam's Sons, 1888.

———. "Faradic Electricity in Rigidity of Os Uteri During Labor." *American Journal of Obstetrics and Diseases of Women and Children* 19 (1886): 36.

———. "Fatty Degeneration of the Placenta." *Medical Record* 16 (1879): 162.

———. "Female Physicians for Insane Women." *Medical Record* 37 (1890): 543.

———. "From Massachusetts to Turkey: A Paper Read before the League for Political Education, November 14th, 1896." New York: League for Political Education, 1896.

———. "General Miliary Tuberculosis and Endometritis." *Medical Record* 10 (1875): 27.

———. "Generalized Tuberculosis." *Medical Record* 16 (1879): 570.

———. "Hemorrhage into the Ovisacs during Pneumonia." *Medical Record* 9 (1874): 410–11.

———. "Hysterical Fever." *Journal of Nervous and Mental Disease* 17 (1890): 373. Reprinted in *Pathfinder*, 463–77.

———. "Inaugural Address at the Opening of the Woman's Medical College of the New York Infirmary, October 1, 1880." *Chicago Medical Journal and Examiner* 42 (1881): 561. Reprinted in *Pathfinder*, 334–56.

———. "The Indication for Quinine in Pneumonia." *New York Medical Journal* 45 (1887): 589, 620. Reprinted in *Pathfinder*, 419–45.

———. "Intestinal Obstruction." *Medical Record* 7 (1872): 208–9.

———. "Intra-uterine Therapeutics." *American Journal of Obstetrics and Diseases of Women and Children* 22 (1889): 449–57, 598–620.

———. "Letter from Dr. Mary Putnam Jacobi: Plato for Woman Suffrage." *The Woman's Journal*, 7 February 1885, 44.

———. "Limitations and Dangers of Intra-uterine Medication." *American Journal of Obstetrics and Diseases of Women and Children* 22 (1889): 589–620.

———. "Married Women's Right to Compensation." *The Woman's Journal*, 26 February 1887, 66.

———. *Mary Putnam Jacobi, M.D.: A Pathfinder in Medicine, with Selections from Her Writings and a Complete Bibliography.* Edited by Women's Medical Association of New York City. New York: G. P. Putnam's Sons, 1925.

———. "Mary Putnam Jacobi's Letter of Protest to S. Weir Mitchell." In *Transactions and Studies of the College of Physicians, Philadelphia*, edited by Nancy Cervetti, 110–14, Philadelphia, Pa.: The College, 1997.

———. "Mental Action and Physical Health." In Brackett, *Education of American Girls*, 257–306.

———. "Modern Female Invalidism." *Boston Medical and Surgical Journal* 133 (1895): 174. Reprinted in *Pathfinder*, 478–82.

———. "Monthly Abortions." *Medical Record* 11 (1876): 481–82.

———. "The Nature and Dangers of Intra-uterine Medication." *Medical Record* 33 (1888): 23–26.

———. "The Needs and Shortcomings of Women Physicians." *Boston Medical and Surgical Journal* 133 (1895): 146.

———. "Nitrite of Amyl and Belladonna in Dysmenorrhœa." *Medical Record* 10 (1875): 11–12.

———. "Notes on Uterine Versions and Flexions." *American Journal of Obstetrics and Diseases of Women and Children* 21 (1888): 225–38.

———. "Obituary of the Author: Susan Dimock." *Medical Record* 10 (1875): 357–58.

———. "On Atropine: A Lecture Delivered at the Woman's Medical College of the New York Infirmary." *Medical Record* 8 (1873): 249, 273. Reprinted in *Pathfinder*, 204–39.

———. "On the Opening of the Johns Hopkins Medical School to Women." *The Century* 41 (1891): 633–34.

———. "Opening Lecture on Diseases of Children, At the Post-Graduate Medical School, New York." *Boston Medical and Surgical Journal* 108 (1883): 121, 145. Reprinted in *Pathfinder*, 403–18.

———. "Ovarian Tumor." *Medical Record* 8 (1873): 342.

———. "Pathogeny of Infantile Paralysis." *American Journal of Obstetrics and Diseases of Women and Children* 7 (1874): 1. Reprinted in *Pathfinder*, 240–83.

———. *Physiological Notes on Primary Education and the Study of Language.* New York: G. P. Putnam's Sons, 1889.

———. "A Plea for Medical Women." *Medical Record* 37 (1890): 107.

———. "The Practical Study of Biology." *Boston Medical and Surgical Journal* 120 (1889): 631. Reprinted in *Pathfinder*, 458–62.

———. "Progress in Medical Education — The Women Taking the Lead." *Medical Record* 28 (1885): 584.

———. "Puerperal Fever, Infection from Ovary through Retro-peritoneal Glands." *Medical Record* 11 (1876): 307.

———. *The Question of Rest for Women during Menstruation.* New York: G. P. Putnam's Sons, 1877.

———. "Remarks Upon the Action of Nitrate of Silver on Epithelial and Gland Cells." Reprinted in *Pathfinder*, 284–98.

———. "Report of an Address to the Graduating Class of the Women's Medical College of the New York Infirmary." *Medical Record* 7 (1872): 215. Reprinted in *Pathfinder*, 201–3.

———. "Review of Dr. W. C. Wood's Book, *Fever: A Study in Morbid and Normal Physiology*." *Archives of Medicine* 5 (1881): 302–18.

———. "The Rights of Majorities." *The Woman's Journal*, 22 June 1889, 194.

———. "Salpingo-oöphorectomy." *New York Medical Journal* 39 (1884): 673.

———. "The School of Medicine for Women of the New York Infirmary." Edited by Woman's Medical College of the New York Infirmary. Laurel House, Lakewood, 3 March 1884.

———. "Shall Women Practice Medicine?" *North American Review* 134 (1882): 52. Reprinted in *Pathfinder*, 367–90.

———. "Social Aspects of the Readmission of Women into the Medical Profession." In *Papers Presented at the First Woman's Congress of the Association for the Advancement of Women*. New York, 1874.

———. "Some Considerations on Endometritis." *Boston Medical and Surgical Journal* 110 (1884): 468–70.

———. "Some Considerations on Hysteria." In *Essays on Hysteria, Brain-Tumor, and Some Other Cases of Nervous Disease*, 1–80. New York: G. P. Putnam's Sons, 1888.

———. "Specialism in Medicine." *Archives of Medicine* 7 (1882): 87. Reprinted in *Pathfinder*, 357–66.

———. "Sphygmographic Experiments Upon a Human Brain, Exposed by an Opening in the Cranium." *American Journal of Medical Sciences* 76 (1878): 10. Reprinted in *Pathfinder*, 299–310.

———. "The Stephenson Wave." *American Journal of Obstetrics and Diseases of Women and Children* 32 (1895): 90–92.

———. "Stomach Washing." *Reports and Transactions of the Annual Meetings of the Alumnae Association of the Woman's Medical College of Pennsylvania* (1889): 50–53.

———. *Stories and Sketches*. New York: G. P. Putnam's Sons, 1907.

———. "Studies in Endometritis." *American Journal of Obstetrics and Diseases of Women and Children* 18 (1885): 36–50, 113–28, 262–83, 376–86, 519–31, 596–606, 802–46, 915–32; 19 (1886): 352–86.

———. "Sudden Death without Apparent Cause." *Medical Record* 12 (1877): 476.

———. "A Suggestion in Regard to Suggestive Therapeutics." *New York Medical Journal* 67 (1898): 485. Reprinted in *Pathfinder*, 483–93.

———. "The 'Temptation of Johns Hopkins.'" *Medical Record* 38 (1890): 588–89.

———. "Thrombosis of Ovarian Veins." *Medical Record* 7 (1872): 305.

———. "The Treatment of Hydrophobia by Woorara." *Transactions of the Medical Society of the State of New York* (1877): 23–24.

———. "Treatment of Incipient Insanity" (aka "Some Considerations on the Moral, and on the Non-Asylum Treatment of Insanity"). *Journal of Social Science* 15 (1882): 77–96.

————. "Two Cases of Convulsive Disease without Convulsions." *Transactions of the Medical Society of the State of New York* (1877): 147–58.

————. "Two Peculiar Cases of Typhoid Fever — One at the Age of Six Months; One Beginning with Pneumonia, and with Heart Failure Conspicuous — Effect of Digitalis." *Archives of Medicine* 11 (1884): 30–72.

————. "Two Representative Women." *The Woman's Journal*, 23 December and 30 December 1893, 406–7, 410.

————. "The Use of Electricity in Gynaecology." *Report of the Proceedings of the Annual Meeting of the Alumnae Association of the Woman's Medical College of Pennsylvania* (1889): 60–73.

————. *The Value of Life: A Reply to Mr. Mallock's Essay, "Is Life Worth Living?"* New York: G. P. Putnam's Sons, 1879.

————. "Varieties of Nephritis." *Woman's Medical Journal* 7 (1898): 191.

————. "The Woman Suffrage Question: The Present Demand." *Outlook*, 12 May 1894, 820–21.

————. "Woman in Medicine." In *Woman's Work in America*, edited by Annie Nathan Meyer, 139–205. New York: Henry Holt & Co., 1891.

Jacobi, Mary Putnam, and Victoria A. White. *On the Use of the Cold Pack Followed by Massage in the Treatment of Anemia*. New York: G. P. Putnam's Sons, 1880.

Jex-Blake, Sophia. *Medical Women: A Thesis and a History*. Edinburgh: Oliphant, Anderson, and Ferrier, 1886.

Karl Marx, Frederick Engels: Collected Works. Translated by Richard Dixon et al. Vol. 39, 1852–55. New York: International Publishers, 1983.

Kimball, John C. "Woman's Medical College and Vivisection." *The Woman's Journal*, 15 May 1897, 153.

Knight, Denise D., ed., *The Abridged Diaries of Charlotte Perkins Gilman*. Charlottesville: University Press of Virginia, 1998.

Kölliker, Rudolph Albert von. *Manual of Human Microscopical Anatomy*. Translated by George Busk and Thomas Huxley. Edited by J. da Costa. Philadelphia: Lippincott, Grambo, 1854.

Leffingwell, Albert. "Does Vivisection Pay?" *Scribner's Monthly* 20 (1880): 391–99.

————. "On Vivisection in America." In Salt, ed., *Animals' Rights*, 133–68.

Lewis, Dio. *Our Girls*. New York: Harper and Brothers, 1871.

"Literature: The Question of Woman Suffrage." *The Critic* 25 (1894): 151–52.

"The Magazines for August." *The Nation*, 3 August 1871.

Mallock, William Hurrell. *Is Life Worth Living?* Chicago: Belfords, Clarke and Co., 1879.

————. *Memoirs of Life and Literature*. New York: Harper and Brothers, 1920.

————. *The New Paul and Virginia; or, Positivism on an Island*. Edited by John D. Margolis. Lincoln: University of Nebraska Press, 1970.

Marshall, Clara. *The Woman's Medical College of Pennsylvania: An Historical Outline*. Philadelphia: P. Blakiston, Son & Co., 1897.

Meigs, J. Forsyth, and William Pepper. *A Practical Treatise on the Diseases of Children*. 7th ed. London: Henry King Lewis, 1883.

"Methods of Sanitarians." *New York Times*, 11 July 1882, 8.

Mitchell, S. Weir. *Characteristics*. New York: The Century Co., 1900.

———. *Fat and Blood: And How to Make Them*. Philadelphia: J. B. Lippincott and Co., 1878.

———. *Lectures on Diseases of the Nervous System, Especially in Women*. Philadelphia: Henry C. Lea's Son & Co., 1881.

———. *Wear and Tear; or, Hints for the Overworked*. Philadelphia: J. B. Lippincott and Co., 1887.

Montanier, Henri. "La femme médecin." *Gazette des Hôpitaux* 34 (1868).

Moreau (de Tours), Jacques-Joseph. *Hashish and Mental Illness*. Edited by Hélèn Peters and Gabriel G. Nahas. Translated by Gordon J. Barnett. New York: Raven Press, 1973.

Mosher, Clelia Duel. *Health and the Woman Movement*. New York: Young Women's Christian Associations, 1916.

———. "Normal Menstruation and Some of the Factors Modifying to It." *Johns Hopkins Hospital Bulletin* (May–June 1901): 178–79.

Mundé, Paul F. "Report on the Progress of Gynecology during the Year 1875." *American Journal of Obstetrics and Gynecology* 9 (1876): 127–73.

Nathan, Maud. *The Story of an Epoch-Making Movement*. Garden City: Doubleday, Page, and Company, 1926.

New York State Woman Suffrage Association. *1894, Constitutional-Amendment Campaign Year: Report of the New York State Woman Suffrage Association* (aka "Record of the Campaign: Woman Suffrage and the Constitutional Convention, 1894"). Rochester, N.Y.: Charles Mann, Printer, 1895.

"No Compromise with 'Antis': Dr. Jacobi Gives the Woman Suffragists a War Cry." *New York Times*, 29 April 1894, 8.

Nott, Richard M. *Memoir of Abner Kingman Nott, Formerly Pastor of the First Baptist Church in the City of New York, with Copious Extracts from His Correspondence*. New York: Charles T. Evans, 1882.

Novak, Emil. *Menstruation and Its Disorders*. New York: D. Appleton and Company, 1921.

"On the Ballot for Women." *New York Times*, 8 June 1894, 8.

"Opponents of the Old Code." *New York Medical Journal* 37 (1883): 474.

Osler, William. "On the Opening of the Johns Hopkins Medical School to Women." *The Century* 41 (1891): 635.

Paine, Thomas. *Common Sense*. New York: Bantam Dell, 2004.

P. C. M. [Mary C. Putnam]. "Letters to the *Medical Record*, 1867–1870." Reprinted in *Pathfinder*, 1–170.

Peabody, Philip G. and Robert Green Ingersoll. *Personal Experiences of Two American Anti-Vivisectionists in Various Countries*. Boston: New England Anti-Vivisection Society, 1895.

"A Positivist Celebration." *Springfield Daily Republican*, 8 April 1872, 6.

Preston, Ann, M.D. *Valedictory Address to the Graduating Class of the Female Medical College of Pennsylvania, 12th Annual Commencement*. Philadelphia: William S. Young, 1864.

Putnam, George Haven. *George Palmer Putnam: A Memoir, Together with a Record of the Earlier Years of the Publishing House Founded by Him*. New York: G. P. Putnam's Sons, 1912.

———. *Memories of My Youth, 1844–1865*. New York: G. P. Putnam's Sons, 1914.

————. *A Prisoner of War in Virginia, 1864–65.* New York: G. P. Putnam's Sons, 1914.

Putnam, George Palmer. "Before and After the Battle: A Day and Night in 'Dixie.'" *Knickerbocker* 58 (1861): 231–50.

Putnam, Mary C. "The Clubs of Paris." *Scribner's Monthly* 3 (November 1871): 105–9.

————. "Concerning Charlotte." *Putnam's Monthly,* January–March 1870. Reprinted in *Stories and Sketches,* 262–389.

————. "De la graisse neutre et des acides gras [on neutral fat and fatty acids]: Thèse pour la doctorat en médecine présentée et soutenue le 23 juillet 1871." Medical thesis, École de Médecine. Paris: A. Parent, 1871. Translated by Andrew J. Cain.

————. "Found and Lost." *Atlantic Monthly,* April 1860. Reprinted in *Stories and Sketches,* 1–49.

————. "Hair Chains." *Atlantic Monthly,* November 1861. Reprinted in *Stories and Sketches,* 50–96.

————. "Imagination and Language." *Putnam's Monthly,* March 1868. Reprinted in *Stories and Sketches,* 97–125.

————. "A Martyr to Science." *Putnam's Monthly,* August 1869. Reprinted in *Stories and Sketches,* 212–61.

————. "Note on a Case of Human Nosencephalian Monster Who Lived Twenty-Nine Hours." *Archives of Scientific and Practical Medicine* 1 (1873): 342–50, 446–52.

————. "Phenomena Attending Section of the Right Restiform Body." *Medical Record* 8 (1873): 17–18.

————. "Sermon at Notre Dame." *Putnam's Monthly,* December 1868 and January 1869. Reprinted in *Stories and Sketches,* 166–211.

————. "Some Details in the Pathogeny of Pyæmia and Septicæmia." *Medical Record* 7 (1872): 73. Reprinted in *Pathfinder,* 171–200.

————. "Some of the French Leaders." *Scribner's Monthly,* August 1871. Reprinted in *Stories and Sketches,* 390–443.

————. "A Study of Still-Life (Paris)." *Putnam's Monthly,* December 1868. Reprinted in *Stories and Sketches,* 126–65.

————. "Woman's Right to Labor." In *Graduates' Reunion,* 62–71.

Putnam, Ruth. *Life and Letters of Mary Putnam Jacobi.* New York: G. P. Putnam's Sons, 1925.

Quain, Richard, ed. *A Dictionary of Medicine, Including General Pathology, General Therapeutics, Hygiene, and the Diseases Peculiar to Women and Children.* New York: D. Appleton & Co., 1883.

"Recent Fiction: Tales of an Earlier Time." *New York Times,* 2 September 1894, 23.

Reclus, Élie. *La Commune de Paris au jour le jour, 19 mars–28 mai 1871.* Edited by Roger Gonot. Paris: Atlancica, 2000.

Reilly, Frank W. *One Hundred Views of the Health-Lift.* Chicago: J. P. Marsh & Co., 1877.

Report of the Association for Preventing the Re-Enactment in the State of New York of the Present Code of Ethics of the American Medical Association. New York, 1883.

Report of the Association for the Advancement of the Medical Education of Women, with Addresses Delivered at Union League Hall, Tuesday, March 26th, 1878. New York: G. P. Putnam's Sons, 1878.

Reports and Transactions of the Annual Meetings of the Alumnae Association of the Woman's Medical College of Pennsylvania. 1875–1900. Drexel University College of Medicine,

Archives and Special Collections on Women in Medicine and Homeopathy. Philadelphia, Pa.

"Reviews and Book Notices." *Philadelphia Medical and Surgical Reporter* 36 (1877): 511.

Robinson, William J. "The Malice and Vindictiveness of the Anti-vivisectionists." *Medical Record* 51 (1897): 791.

Salt, Henry S., ed. *Animals' Rights Considered in Relation to Social Progress*. New York: Macmillan, 1894.

Schultze, Caroline. *Die Ärztin im XIX. Jahrhundert*. Leipzig: Hobbing, 1889.

———. "La femme-médecin au XIXe siècle." Paris: Librarie Ollier-Henry, 1888.

Stanton, Elizabeth Cady. *Eighty Years and More (1815–1897): Reminiscences of Elizabeth Cady Stanton*. London: T. Fisher Unwin, 1898.

———. "Has Christianity Benefited Woman?" *North American Review* 140 (1885): 389–99.

———. "Our Young Girls; An Essay Read Before the Seneca Falls Conversational, 12 February 1853." *The Lily*, 1 March 1853.

Stephenson, William. "On the Menstrual Wave." *American Journal of Obstetrics and Diseases of Women and Children* 15 (1882): 287–94.

Stewart, William Rhinelander. *The Philanthropic Work of Josephine Shaw Lowell*. New York: Macmillan, 1911.

"Suffragists on the Warpath." *New York Times*, 3 May 1894, 9.

"The Temptation of Johns Hopkins." *Medical Record* 38 (November 1890): 550.

Thomson, William. *A Practical Treatise on the Diseases of the Liver and Biliary Passages with Clinical Illustrations of Diseases of the Liver and Spleen*. Illustrations by William Twining. Philadelphia: Ed. Barrington & Geo. D. Haswell, 1842.

Tiemann, George, and Co. *American Armamentarium Chirurgicum*. New York: George Tiemann and Co., 1889.

Transactions of the New York Academy of Medicine. 1880–1900.

"Two Views of Woman Suffrage." *New York Daily Tribune*, 4 October 1894, 8.

Uffelmann, Julius. *Manual of the Domestic Hygiene of the Child: For the Use of Students, Physicians, Sanitary Officials, Teachers, and Mothers*. Translated by Harriot Ransom Milinowski. Edited by Mary Putnam Jacobi. New York: G. P. Putnam's Sons, 1891.

U.S. Census Bureau. *Ninth Census of the United States, 1870*. Washington, D.C.

———. *Tenth Census of the United States, 1880*. Washington, D.C.

———. *Eleventh Census of the United States, 1890*. Washington, D.C.

———. *Twelfth Census of the United States, 1900*. Washington, D.C.

———. *Thirteenth Census of the United States, 1910*. Washington, D.C.

Van Hoosen, Bertha. *Petticoat Surgeon*. Chicago: Pellegrini & Cudahy, 1947.

Virchow, Rudolf. *Cellular Pathology as Based Upon Physiological and Pathological Histology*. Translated by Frank Chance. New York: Dover Publications, 1971.

Vivisection: Hearing Before the Senate Committee on the District of Columbia, February 21, 1900, on the Bill S. 34, For the Further Prevention of Cruelty to Animals in the District Columbia. Washington, D.C.: Government Printing Office, 1900.

"'Vivisection': A Statement in Behalf of Science" (pamphlet). New York Academy of Medicine Library, 1896.

Warner, Anna B. *Susan Warner ("Elizabeth Wetherell")*. New York: G. P. Putnam's Sons, 1909.

Warner, Susan. *The Wide, Wide World*. With an Afterword by Jane Tompkins. New York: The Feminist Press, 1987.

White, Frances Emily. "Woman's Place in Nature." *Popular Science Monthly* 6 (1875): 292–301.

Wilson, Edmund B. *The Cell in Development and Inheritance*. New York: Macmillan, 1896.

The Woman's Journal. 1880–98.

Woman's Medical College of the New York Infirmary, Annual Catalogue and Announcement, 1870–71 (New York: S. Angell Printer, 1870).

Woman's Medical College of the New York Infirmary, Annual Catalogue and Announcement, 1869–97. In Woman's Medical College of the New York Infirmary Collection of Publications, National Library of Medicine, History of Medicine Division, Microfilm no. 2701065oR.

"Woman's Political Work: Dr. Mary Putnam Jacobi Delivers an Address to the League for Political Education." *New York Times*, 7 November 1897, 21.

"Women Against the Tiger: Social Leaders Express Their Opposition to Corruption." *New York Times*, 3 November 1894, 5.

"Women Are at Work." *New York Times*, 23 October 1890, 5.

"Women Pleading at Albany." *New York Times*, 1 June 1894, 2.

Women's Medical Association of New York City, ed. *In Memory of Mary Putnam Jacobi*. New York: Knickerbocker Press, 1907.

SECONDARY SOURCES

Abram, Ruth J. *"Send Us a Lady Physician": Women Doctors in America, 1835–1920*. New York: W. W. Norton & Co., 1985.

Ackerknecht, Erwin H. *Rudolf Virchow: Doctor, Statesman, Anthropologist*. Madison: University of Wisconsin Press, 1953.

Alan Mason Chesney Archives. *The Women's Medical Fund and the Opening of the Johns Hopkins School of Medicine*. Baltimore: Johns Hopkins Medical Institutions, 1979.

Alpern, Sara, ed. *The Challenge of Feminist Biography: Writing the Lives of Modern American Women*. Urbana: University of Illinois Press, 1992.

Anderson, Eric D. "Black Responses to Darwinism, 1859–1915." In Numbers and Stenhouse, eds., *Disseminating Darwinism*, 247–66.

Apple, Rima D. *Mothers and Medicine: A Social History of Infant Feeding, 1890–1950*. Madison: University of Wisconsin Press, 1987.

———. *Perfect Motherhood: Science and Childrearing in America*. New Brunswick, N.J.: Rutgers University Press, 2006.

Apple, Rima D., ed. *Women, Health, and Medicine in America: A Historical Handbook*. New York: Garland, 1990.

Attie, Jeanie. "Warwork and the Crisis of Domesticity in the North." In *Divided Houses: Gender and the Civil War*, edited by Catherine Clinton and Nina Silber, 247–59. New York: Oxford University Press, 1992.

Aufses, Arthur H., Jr., and Barbara Niss. *This House of Noble Deeds: The Mount Sinai Hospital, 1852–2002*. New York: New York University Press, 2002.

Ballard, Charles W. *A History of the College of Pharmacy, Columbia University*. New York: Columbia University Press, 1954.

Baym, Nina. *American Women of Letters and the Nineteenth-Century Sciences: Styles of Affiliation*. New Brunswick, N.J.: Rutgers University Press, 2002.

Bender, Thomas. *New York Intellect: A History of Intellectual Life in New York City From 1750 to the Beginnings of Our Own Time*. Baltimore: Johns Hopkins University Press, 1988.

Benson, Susan Porter. *Counter Cultures: Saleswomen, Managers, and Customers in American Department Stores, 1890–1940*. Urbana: University of Illinois Press, 1986.

Bidelman, Patrick Kay. *Pariahs Stand Up!: The Founding of the Liberal Feminist Movement in France, 1858–1889*. Westport, Conn.: Greenwood Press, 1982.

Bittel, Carla. "Mary Putnam Jacobi and the Nineteenth-Century Politics of Women's Health Research." In *Women Physicians and the Cultures of Medicine*, edited by Ellen S. More, Elizabeth Fee, and Manon Parry, 23–51. Baltimore: Johns Hopkins University Press, 2009.

———. "The Science of Women's Rights: The Medical and Political Worlds of Mary Putnam Jacobi." Ph.D. diss., Cornell University, 2003.

———. "Science, Suffrage, and Experimentation: Mary Putnam Jacobi and the Controversy Over Vivisection in Late Nineteenth-Century America." *Bulletin of the History of Medicine* 79 (2005): 664–94.

Bloor, David. *Knowledge and Social Imagery*. Chicago: University of Chicago Press, 1991.

Blum, Deborah., *Sex on the Brain: The Biological Differences Between Men and Women*. New York: Viking, 1997.

Blustein, Bonnie E. *Preserve Your Love for Science: Life of William A. Hammond, American Neurologist*. Cambridge: Cambridge University Press, 1991.

Boas, Norman Francis, and Barbara Linton Meyer. *Alma Farm: An Adirondack Meeting Place*. Bolton Landing, N.Y.: Boas and Meyer Publishers, 1999.

Bonner, Thomas Neville. *Becoming a Physician: Medical Education in Britain, France, Germany, and the United States, 1750–1945*. New York: Oxford University Press, 1995.

———. *To the Ends of the Earth: Women's Search for Education in Medicine*. Cambridge, Mass.: Harvard University Press, 1992.

Bordin, Ruth. *Woman and Temperance: The Quest for Power and Liberty, 1873–1900*. Philadelphia: Temple University Press, 1981.

Boyer, Paul S., and Stephen Nissenbaum. *Salem Possessed: The Social Origins of Witchcraft*. Cambridge, Mass.: Harvard University Press, 1974.

Brancaforte, Charlotte L., ed. *The German Forty-Eighters in the United States*. New York: Peter Lang, 1989.

Brandt, Allan M. *No Magic Bullet: A Social History of Venereal Disease in the United States since 1880*. New York: Oxford University Press, 1987.

Brizendine, Louann. *The Female Brain*. New York: Morgan Road Books, 2006.

Bruce, Robert V. *The Launching of Modern American Science, 1846–1876*. Ithaca, N.Y.: Cornell University Press, 1987.

Brumberg, Joan Jacobs. *The Body Project: An Intimate History of American Girls*. New York: Random House, 1997.

———. "Chlorotic Girls, 1870–1920: A Historical Perspective on Female Adolescence." *Child Development* 53 (1982): 1468–77.

———. *Fasting Girls: The Emergence of Anorexia Nervosa as a Modern Disease*. Cambridge, Mass.: Harvard University Press, 1988.

———. *Kansas Charley: The Story of a Nineteenth-Century Boy Murderer*. New York: Viking Press, 2003.

———. *Mission for Life: The Story of the Family of Adoniram Judson, the Dramatic Events of the First American Foreign Mission, and the Course of Evangelical Religion in the Nineteenth Century*. New York: Free Press, 1980.

Brumberg, Joan Jacobs, and Nancy Tomes. "Women in the Professions: A Research Agenda for American Historians." *Reviews in American History* (1982): 275–96.

Buettinger, Craig. "Women and Antivivisection in Late Nineteenth-Century America." *Journal of Social History* 30 (1997): 857–72.

Bullough, Vern, and Martha Voght. "Women, Menstruation, and Nineteenth-Century Medicine." In Leavitt, ed., *Women and Health in America*, 28–37.

Burrows, Edmin G., and Mike Wallace. *Gotham: A History of New York City to 1898*. New York: Oxford University Press, 1999.

Burstyn, Joan N. "Education and Sex: The Medical Case Against Higher Education for Women in England, 1870–1900." *Proceedings of the American Philosophical Society* 117 (1973): 79–89.

Butler, Judith. *Gender Trouble: Feminism and the Subversion of Identity*. New York: Routledge, 1999.

Carter, K. Codell. "Koch's Postulates in Relation to the Work of Jacob Henle and Edwin Klebs." *Medical History* 29 (1985): 353–74.

Carter, Paul A. *The Spiritual Crisis of the Gilded Age*. DeKalb: Northern Illinois University Press, 1971.

Cervetti, Nancy. "S. Weir Mitchell and His Snakes: Unraveling the 'United Web and Woof of Popular and Scientific Beliefs.'" *Journal of Medical Humanities* 28 (2007): 119–33.

———. "S. Weir Mitchell Representing 'a hell of pain': From Civil War to Rest Cure." *Arizona Quarterly* 59 (2003): 69–96.

Charlton, D. G. *Positivist Thought in France during the Second Empire, 1852–1870*. Oxford: Clarendon Press, 1959.

Cole, Douglas. *Franz Boas: The Early Years, 1858–1906*. Vancouver: Douglas and McIntyre, 1999.

Coleman, William C., and Frederic L. Holmes, eds. *The Investigative Enterprise: Experimental Physiology in Nineteenth-Century Medicine*. Berkeley: University of California Press, 1988.

Collins, Harry M. *Changing Order: Replication and Induction in Scientific Practice*. Beverly Hills: Sage Publications, 1985.

Collins, Harry M., and Robert Evans. *Rethinking Expertise*. Chicago: University of Chicago Press, 2007.

Cott, Nancy. "Young Women in the Second Great Awakening in New England." *Feminist Studies* 3 (Fall 1975): 15–29.

Cozzens, Susan E., and Edward J. Woodhouse. "Science, Government, and the Politics of Knowledge." In Jasanoff et al., eds., *Handbook of Science and Technology Studies*, 533–53.

Crosby, William H., M.D. "An Historical Sketch of Splenic Function and Splenectomy." *Lymphology* 16, no. 2 (1983): 52–55.

Cross, Gary S. *The Cute and the Cool: Wondrous Innocence and Modern American Children's Culture*. New York: Oxford University Press, 2004.

Cross, Whitney R. *The Burned-Over District: The Social and Intellectual History of Enthusiastic Religion in Western New York, 1800–1850*. New York: Harper and Row, 1965.

Cunningham, Andrew, and Perry Williams, eds. *The Laboratory Revolution in Medicine*. Cambridge: Cambridge University Press, 1992.

Curti, Merle E. *Human Nature in American Thought: A History*. Madison: University of Wisconsin Press, 1980.

Daston, Lorraine. "Objectivity and the Escape from Perspective." In *The Science Studies Reader*, edited by Mario Biagioli, 110–23. New York: Routledge, 1999.

Daston, Lorraine, and Peter Galison. *Objectivity*. New York: Zone Books, 2007.

Dear, Peter. "Mysteries of State, Mysteries of Nature: Authority, Knowledge, and Expertise in the Seventeenth Century." In Jasanoff, ed., *States of Knowledge*, 206–24.

Derrick, Peter. *Tunneling to the Future: The Story of the Great Subway Expansion That Saved New York*. New York: New York University Press, 2001.

Dictionary of American Medical Biography. Vol. 2. Edited by Martin Kaufman, Stuart Galishoff, and Todd L. Savitt. Westport, Conn.: Greenwood Press, 1984.

Dictionnaire de biographie française. Edited by Roman d'Amat, M. Prevost, H. Tribout de Morembert, and J. P. Loies et al. Paris: Librairie Letouzey et Ané, 1964, 1994.

Douglas, Ann. *The Feminization of American Culture*. New York: Alfred A. Knopf, 1977.

Drachman, Virginia G. *Hospital with a Heart: Women Doctors and the Paradox of Separatism at the New England Hospital, 1862–1969*. Ithaca, N.Y.: Cornell University Press, 1984.

Dreger, Alice Domurat. *Hermaphrodites and the Medical Invention of Sex*. Cambridge, Mass.: Harvard University Press, 1998.

DuBois, Ellen Carol. *Feminism and Suffrage: The Emergence of an Independent Women's Movement in America, 1848–1869*. Ithaca, N.Y.: Cornell University Press, 1978.

———. *Harriot Stanton Blatch and the Winning of Woman Suffrage*. New Haven, Conn.: Yale University Press, 1997.

———. "Working Women, Class Relations, and Suffrage Militance: Harriot Stanton Blatch and the New York Woman Suffrage Movement, 1894–1909." *Journal of American History* 74 (1987): 34–58.

Dunbar, Gary S. *Élisée Reclus: Historian of Nature*. Hamden, Conn.: Archon Books, 1978.

Ehrenreich, Barbara, and Deirdre English. *For Her Own Good: 150 Years of Experts' Advice to Women*. Garden City, N.Y.: Anchor Press, 1978.

Eichner, Carolyn J. *Surmounting the Barricades: Women in the Paris Commune*. Bloomington: Indiana University Press, 2004.

Elston, Mary Ann. "Women and Anti-Vivisection in Victorian England, 1870–1900." In Rupke, *Vivisection in Historical Perspective*, 259–94.

Epstein, Steven. *Impure Science: AIDS, Activism, and the Politics of Knowledge*. Berkeley: University of California Press, 1996.

Farley, Frances. "The New York Infirmary for Women and Children, 1870–1899: Women Doctors in Transition." Thesis, Duke University, 1983.

Faust, Drew Gilpin. *Mothers of Invention: Women of the Slaveholding South in the American Civil War*. Chapel Hill: University of North Carolina Press, 1996.

Fausto-Sterling, Anne. *Sexing the Body: Gender Politics and the Construction of Sexuality*. New York: Basic Books, 2000.

Fee, Elizabeth. "Nineteenth-Century Craniology: The Study of the Female Skull." *Bulletin of the History of Medicine* 53 (1979): 415–33.

Ferguson, Moira. *Animal Advocacy and Englishwomen, 1780–1900: Patriots, Nation, and Empire*. Ann Arbor: University of Michigan Press, 1998.

Fleming, Marie. *The Anarchist Way to Socialism: Elisée Reclus and Nineteenth-Century European Anarchism*. London: Croom Helm, 1979.

———. *The Geography of Freedom: The Odyssey of Elisée Reclus*. New York: Black Rose Books, 1988.

Frank, Robert G., Jr. "The Telltale Heart: Physiological Instruments, Graphic Methods, and Clinical Hopes, 1854–1914." In Coleman and Holmes, eds. *Investigative Enterprise*, 211–90.

French, Richard D. *Antivivisection and Medical Science in Victorian Society*. Princeton, N.J.: Princeton University Press, 1975.

Gallagher, Teresa Catherine. "From Family Helpmeet to Independent Professional: Women in American Pharmacy, 1870–1940." *Pharmacy in History* 31 (1989): 60–77.

Ganobcsik-Williams, Lisa. "The Intellectualism of Charlotte Perkins Gilman: Evolutionary Perspectives on Race, Ethnicity, and Class." In Rudd and Gough, eds., *Charlotte Perkins Gilman*, 16–41.

Gartner, Carol B. "Fussell's Folly: Academic Standards and the Case of Mary Putnam Jacobi." *Academic Medicine* 71 (May 1996): 470–77.

Geison, Gerald L. "Divided We Stand: Physiologists and Clinicians in the American Context." In Vogel and Rosenberg, eds., *Therapeutic Revolution*, 67–90.

Gieryn, Thomas F. "Boundaries of Science." In Jasanoff et al., eds., *Handbook of Science and Technology Studies*, 393–443.

———. "Boundary-Work and the Demarcation of Science from Non-Science: Strains and Interests in Professional Ideologies of Scientists." *American Sociological Review* 48 (1983): 781–95.

Gilbert, Scott F., and Karen A Rader. "Revisiting Women, Gender, and Feminism in Developmental Biology." In *Feminism in Twentieth-Century Science, Technology, and Medicine*, edited by Elizabeth Lunbeck, Angela N. H. Creager, and Londa Schiebinger, 73–97. Chicago: University of Chicago Press, 2001.

Golden, Janet, Richard A. Meckel, and Heather Munro Prescott, eds. *Children and Youth in Sickness and in Health: A Historical Handbook and Guide*. Westport, Conn.: Greenwood Press, 2004.

Goldstein, Jan. *Console and Classify: The French Psychiatric Profession in the Nineteenth Century*. New York: Cambridge University Press, 1987.

Gossel, Patricia Peck. "William Henry Welch and the Antivivisection Legislation in the District of Columbia, 1896–1900." *Journal of the History of Medicine and Allied Sciences* 40 (1985): 397–419.

Graham, Sara Hunter. "The Suffrage Renaissance: A New Image for a New Century, 1896–

1910." In *One Woman, One Vote: Rediscovering the Woman Suffrage Movement*, edited by Marjorie Spruill Wheeler, 157–78. Troutdale, Oreg.: NewSage Press, 1995.

Greenspan, Ezra. *George Palmer Putnam: Representative American Publisher*. University Park: Pennsylvania State University Press, 2000.

Guarneri, Carl. *The Utopian Alternative: Fourierism in Nineteenth-Century America*. Ithaca, N.Y.: Cornell University Press, 1991.

Guerrini, Anita. *Experimenting with Humans and Animals: From Galen to Animal Rights*. Baltimore: Johns Hopkins University Press, 2003.

Gullickson, Gay L. *Unruly Women of Paris: Images of the Commune*. Ithaca, N.Y.: Cornell University Press, 1996.

Halttunen, Karen. *Confidence Men and Painted Women: A Study of Middle-Class Culture in America, 1830–1870*. New Haven, Conn.: Yale University Press, 1982.

———. "Humanitarianism and the Pornography of Pain in Anglo-American Culture." *American Historical Review* 100 (1995): 303–34.

Hamlin, Kimberly A. "Beyond Adam's Rib: How Darwinian Evolutionary Theory Redefined Gender and Influenced American Feminist Thought, 1870–1920." Ph.D. diss., University of Texas at Austin, 2008.

Hammonds, Evelynn Maxine. *Childhood's Deadly Scourge: The Campaign to Control Diphtheria in New York City, 1880–1930*. Baltimore: Johns Hopkins University Press, 1999.

Haraway, Donna J. *Modest_Witness@Second_Millennium. FemaleMan©Meets_OncoMouse™: Feminism and Technoscience*. New York: Routledge, 1997.

———. "Situated Knowledges: The Science Question in Feminism and the Privilege of Partial Perspective." In Keller and Longino, eds., *Feminism and Science*, 249–63.

Hardesty, Nancy A. *Women Called to Witness: Evangelical Feminism in the Nineteenth Century*. Nashville, Tenn.: Abingdon Press, 1984.

Harding, Sandra G. "Rethinking Standpoint Epistemology: What Is 'Strong Objectivity'?" In Keller and Longino, eds., *Feminism and Science*, 235–48.

———. *The Science Question in Feminism*. Ithaca, N.Y.: Cornell University Press, 1986.

Harp, Gillis J. *Positivist Republic: Auguste Comte and the Reconstruction of American Liberalism, 1865–1920*. University Park: Pennsylvania State University Press, 1995.

Harth, Erica. *Cartesian Women: Versions and Subversions of Rational Discourse in the Old Regime*. Ithaca, N.Y.: Cornell University Press, 1992.

Harvey, Joy. "Clanging Eagles: The Marriage and Collaboration Between Two Nineteenth-Century Physicians, Mary Putman Jacobi and Abraham Jacobi." In *Creative Couples in the Sciences*, edited by Helena M. Pycior, Nancy G. Slack, and Pnina G. Abir-Am, 185–95. New Brunswick, N.J.: Rutgers University Press, 1996.

———. "'Faithful to Its Old Traditions'? Paris Clinical Medicine from the Second Empire to the Third Republic (1848–1872)." *Clio Medica* 50 (1998): 313–35.

———. "La Visite: Mary Putnam Jacobi and the Paris Medical Clinics." *Clio Medica* 25 (1994): 350–71.

———. "Medicine and Politics: Dr. Mary Putnam Jacobi and the Paris Commune." *Dialectical Anthropology* 15 (1990): 107–17.

Hedrick, Joan. *Harriet Beecher Stowe: A Life*. New York: Oxford University Press, 1994.

Herzig, Arno. *Abraham Jacobi: Die Entwicklung zum sozialistischen und revolutionären*

Demokraten: Briefe, Dokumente, Presseartikel, 1848–1853. Minden, Germany: Mindener Geschichtsverein, 1980.

Hines, Melissa. *Brain Gender.* New York: Oxford University Press, 2004.

Hirsh, Joseph, and Beka Doherty. *The First Hundred Years of the Mount Sinai Hospital of New York, 1852–1952.* New York: Random House, 1952.

Hoffman, Nancy. *Woman's "True" Profession: Voices from the History of Teaching.* New York: McGraw-Hill, 1981.

Holmes, Frederic Lawrence. *Claude Bernard and Animal Chemistry: The Emergence of a Scientist.* Cambridge, Mass.: Harvard University Press, 1974.

———. "Claude Bernard, the *Milieu Intérieur*, and Regulatory Physiology." *History and Philosophy of Life Sciences* 8 (1986): 3–25.

Hood, Clifton. *722 Miles: The Building of the Subways and How They Transformed New York.* New York: Simon & Schuster, 1993.

Horowitz, Helen Lefkowitz. *The Power and Passion of M. Carey Thomas.* New York: Alfred A. Knopf, 1994.

Horvath-Peterson, Sandra. *Victor Duruy and French Education: Liberal Reform in the Second Empire.* Baton Rouge: Louisiana State University Press, 1984.

Hunter, Jane H. *How Young Ladies Became Girls: The Victorian Origins of American Girlhood.* New Haven, Conn.: Yale University Press, 2002.

Jasanoff, Sheila, ed. *States of Knowledge: The Co-production of Science and Social Order.* New York: Routledge, 2004.

Jasanoff, Sheila, Gerald E. Markle, James C. Petersen, and Trevor Pinch, eds. *Handbook of Science and Technology Studies.* Thousand Oaks, Calif.: Sage Publications, 1995.

Jones, Susan D. *Valuing Animals: Veterinarians and Their Patients in Modern America.* Baltimore: Johns Hopkins University Press, 2003.

Kamminga, Harmke, and Andrew Cunningham. "The Science and Culture of Nutrition, 1840–1940." *Clio Medica* 32 (1995): 1–14.

Katz, Philip M. *From Appomattox to Montmarte: Americans and the Paris Commune.* Cambridge, Mass.: Harvard University Press, 1998.

Kaufman, Martin. *American Medical Education: The Formative Years, 1765–1910.* Westport, Conn.: Greenwood Press, 1976.

Keller, Evelyn Fox. "Developmental Biology as a Feminist Cause?" *Osiris* 12 (1997): 16–28.

———. *A Feeling for the Organism: The Life and Work of Barbara McClintock.* New York: W. H. Freeman Press, 1983.

———. *Reflections on Gender and Science.* New Haven, Conn.: Yale University Press, 1985.

———. *Secrets of Life, Secrets of Death: Essays on Language, Gender, and Science.* New York: Routledge Press, 1992.

Keller, Evelyn Fox, and Helen E. Longino, eds. *Feminism and Science.* New York: Oxford University Press, 1996.

Kelley, Mary. *Private Woman, Public Stage: Literary Domesticity in Nineteenth-Century America.* New York: Oxford University Press, 1984.

Kimura, Doreen. *Sex and Cognition.* Cambridge, Mass.: MIT Press, 1999.

King, Charles R. *Children's Health in America: A History.* New York: Twayne Publishers, 1993.

Kirschmann, Anne Taylor. *A Vital Force: Women in American Homeopathy.* New Brunswick, N.J.: Rutgers University Press, 2003.

Knight, Denise D. "'All the Facts of the Case': Gilman's Lost Letter to Dr. S. Weir Mitchell." *American Literary Realism* 37 (2005): 259–77.

Kohlstedt, Sally Gregory. *History of Women in the Sciences: Readings from Isis.* Chicago: University of Chicago Press, 1999.

Kohlstedt, Sally Gregory, and Mark R. Jorgensen. "'The Irrepressible Woman Question': Women's Responses to Evolutionary Ideology." In Numbers and Stenhouse, eds., *Disseminating Darwinism,* 267–93.

Kohlstedt, Sally Gregory, and Helen Longino. "The Women, Gender, and Science Question: What Do Research on Women in Science and Research on Gender and Science Have to Do with One Another?" *Osiris* 12 (1997): 3–15.

Kraditor, Aileen S. *The Ideas of the Woman Suffrage Movement, 1890–1920.* New York: Columbia University Press, 1965.

Kraut, Alan M. *Silent Travelers: Germs, Genes, and the "Immigrant Menace."* Baltimore: Johns Hopkins University Press, 1995.

Kremers, Edward. *Kremers and Urdang's History of Pharmacy.* Edited by Glenn Sonnedecker. Philadelphia: J. B. Lippincott Company, 1963.

Krug, Kate. "Women Ovulate, Men Spermate: Elizabeth Blackwell as a Feminist Physiologist." *Journal of the History of Sexuality* 7 (1996): 51–72.

Kuhn, Thomas S. *The Structure of Scientific Revolutions.* Chicago: University of Chicago Press, 1962.

Kunzel, Regina G. *Fallen Women, Problem Girls: Unmarried Mothers and the Professionalization of Social Work, 1890–1945.* New Haven, Conn.: Yale University Press, 1993.

Lane, Ann J. *To Herland and Beyond: The Life and Work of Charlotte Perkins Gilman.* New York: Pantheon Books, 1990.

Laqueur, Thomas. *Making Sex: Body and Gender from the Greeks to Freud.* Cambridge, Mass.: Harvard University Press, 1990.

Laslett, Barbara, Sally Gregory Kohlstedt, Helen Longino, and Evelyn Hammonds, eds. *Gender and Scientific Authority.* Chicago: University of Chicago Press, 1996.

Latour, Bruno. *The Pasteurization of France.* Translated by Alan Sheridan and John Law. Cambridge, Mass.: Harvard University Press, 1988.

———. *Science in Action: How to Follow Scientists and Engineers Through Society.* Cambridge, Mass.: Harvard University Press, 1987.

Latour, Bruno, and Steve Woolgar. *Laboratory Life: The Construction of Scientific Facts.* Beverly Hills: Sage Publications, 1979.

Leach, William. *True Love and Perfect Union: The Feminist Reform of Sex and Society.* Middletown, Conn.: Wesleyan University Press, 1989.

Leavitt, Judith Walzer. *Brought to Bed: Childbearing in America, 1750–1950.* New York: Oxford University Press, 1986.

———. "'A Worrying Profession': The Domestic Environment of Medical Practice in Nineteenth-Century America." *Bulletin of the History of Medicine* 69 (1995): 1–29.

———, ed. *Women and Health in America.* Madison: University of Wisconsin Press, 1984.

Leavitt, Judith Walzer, and Ronald L. Numbers, eds. *Sickness and Health in America: Readings in the History of Medicine and Public Health.* 3rd ed. Madison: University of Wisconsin Press, 1997.

Lederer, Susan E. "Moral Sensibility and Medical Science: Gender, Animal Experimentation, and the Doctor-Patient Relationship." In More and Milligan, eds. *Empathic Practitioner,* 59–73.

———. *Subjected to Science: Human Experimentation in America Before the Second World War.* Baltimore: Johns Hopkins University Press, 1995.

Lesch, John E. *Science and Medicine in France: The Emergence of Experimental Physiology, 1790–1855.* Cambridge, Mass.: Harvard University Press, 1984.

Leslie J. Reagan, Nancy Tomes, and Paula A. Treichler, eds. *Medicine's Moving Pictures: Medicine, Health, and Bodies in American Film and Television.* Rochester, NY: University of Rochester Press, 2007.

Levine, Bruce. *The Spirit of 1848: German Immigrants, Labor Conflict, and the Coming of the Civil War.* Urbana: University of Illinois Press, 1992.

Long, Diana Elizabeth, and Janet Golden, eds. *The American General Hospital: Communities and Social Contexts.* Ithaca, N.Y.: Cornell University Press, 1989.

Long, Kathryn Teresa. *The Revival of 1857–58: Interpreting an American Religious Awakening.* New York: Oxford University Press, 1998.

Longo, Lawrence D. "Electrotherapy in Gynecology: The American Experience." *Bulletin of the History of Medicine* 60 (1986): 343–66.

Ludmerer, Kenneth M. *Learning to Heal: The Development of American Medical Education.* New York: Basic Books, 1985.

Lutz, Tom. *American Nervousness, 1903: An Anecdotal History.* Ithaca, N.Y.: Cornell University Press, 1991.

Maines, Rachel P. *The Technology of Orgasm: "Hysteria," the Vibrator, and Women's Sexual Satisfaction.* Baltimore: Johns Hopkins University Press, 1999.

Margadant, Jo Burr, ed. *The New Biography: Performing Femininity in Nineteenth-Century France.* Berkeley: University of California Press, 2000.

Marrett, Cora Bagley. "On the Evolution of Women's Medical Societies." *Bulletin of the History of Medicine* 53 (1979): 434–48.

Marsh, Margaret, and Wanda Ronner. *The Empty Cradle: Infertility in America from Colonial Times to the Present.* Baltimore: Johns Hopkins University Press, 1996.

Marshall, Megan. *The Peabody Sisters: Three Women Who Ignited American Romanticism.* Boston: Houghton Mifflin Co., 2005.

McClusky, David A., III, Lee J. Skandalakis, Gene L. Colborn, and John E. Skandalakis. "Tribute to a Triad: History of Splenic Anatomy, Physiology, and Surgery, Parts I and II." *World Journal of Surgery* 23, nos. 3, 5 (1999): 311–25, 514–26.

McCollum, Elmer Verner. *A History of Nutrition: The Sequence of Ideas in Nutrition Investigations.* Boston: Houghton Mifflin Co., 1957.

McCormick, Richard L. *From Realignment to Reform: Political Change in New York State, 1893–1910.* Ithaca, N.Y.: Cornell University Press, 1981.

McDonald, David Kevin. "Organizing Womanhood: Women's Culture and the Politics of Woman Suffrage in New York State, 1865–1917." Ph.D. diss., State University of New York, Stony Brook, 1989.

McGregor, Deborah Kuhn. *From Midwives to Medicine: The Birth of American Gynecology.* New Brunswick, N.J.: Rutgers University Press, 1998.

McMillan, James F. *France and Women, 1789–1914: Gender, Society, and Politics.* New York: Routledge, 2000.

Merchant, Carolyn. *The Death of Nature: Women, Ecology, and the Scientific Revolution.* San Francisco: Harper and Row, 1980.

Moir, Anne, and David Jessel. *Brain Sex: The Real Difference between Men and Women.* New York: Carol Publishers, 1991.

Morantz, Regina Markell. "Feminism, Professionalism, and Germs: The Thought of Mary Putnam Jacobi and Elizabeth Blackwell." *American Quarterly* 34 (1982): 459–78.

———. "The Perils of Feminist History." *Journal of Interdisciplinary History* 4 (1973): 649–60.

Morantz-Sanchez, Regina. *Conduct Unbecoming a Woman: Medicine on Trial in Turn-of-the-Century Brooklyn.* New York: Oxford University Press, 1999.

———. "Female Patient Agency and the 1892 Trial of Dr. Mary Dixon Jones in Late Nineteenth-Century Brooklyn." In *Women Physicians and the Cultures of Medicine*, edited by Ellen S. More, Elizabeth Fee, and Manon Parry, 69–88. Baltimore: Johns Hopkins University Press, 2009.

———. "Feminist Theory and Historical Practice: Rereading Elizabeth Blackwell." *History and Theory* 31 (1992): 51–69.

———. *Sympathy and Science: Women Physicians in American Medicine*, 2nd ed. Chapel Hill: University of North Carolina Press, 2000.

———. *Sympathy and Science: Women Physicians in American Medicine.* New York: Oxford University Press, 1985.

More, Ellen S. *Restoring the Balance: Women Physicians and the Profession of Medicine, 1850–1995.* Cambridge, Mass.: Harvard University Press, 1999.

More, Ellen S., Elizabeth Fee, and Manon Parry, eds. *Women Physicians and the Cultures of Medicine.* Baltimore: Johns Hopkins University Press, 2009.

More, Ellen Singer, and Maureen A. Milligan, eds. *The Empathic Practitioner: Empathy, Gender, and Medicine.* New Brunswick, N.J.: Rutgers University Press, 1994.

Moses, Claire Goldberg. *French Feminism in the Nineteenth Century.* Albany: State University of New York Press, 1984.

Muncy, Robyn. *Creating a Female Dominion in American Reform, 1890–1935.* New York: Oxford University Press, 1991.

Nadel, Stanley. *Little Germany: Ethnicity, Religion, and Class in New York City, 1845–1880.* Urbana: University of Illinois Press, 1990.

Newman, Louise Michele. *White Women's Rights: The Racial Origins of Feminism in the United States.* New York: Oxford University Press, 1999.

Niven, John. *Connecticut Hero: Israel Putnam.* Hartford: The American Revolution Bicentennial Commission of Connecticut, 1977.

Noble, David F. *A World Without Women: The Christian Clerical Culture of Western Science.* New York: Oxford University Press, 1993.

Normandin, Sebastian. "Claude Bernard and *An Introduction to the Study of Experimental Medicine*: 'Physical Vitalism,' Dialectic, and Epistemology." *Journal of the History of Medicine and Allied Sciences* 62 (2007): 495–528.

Notable American Women, 1607–1950: A Biographical Dictionary. 3 vols. Edited by Edward T. James, Janet Wilson Jones, and Paul S. Boyer. Cambridge, Mass.: Belknap Press of Harvard University Press, 1971.

Numbers, Ronald L., and John Stenhouse, eds. *Disseminating Darwinism: The Role of Place, Race, Religion, and Gender.* Cambridge: Cambridge University Press, 1999.

O'Brien, Kathryn E. *The Great and the Gracious on Millionaires' Row: Lake George in Its Glory.* Sylvan Beach, N.Y.: North Country Books, 1978.

Odem, Mary E. *Delinquent Daughters: Protecting and Policing Adolescent Female Sexuality in the United States, 1885–1920.* Chapel Hill: University of North Carolina Press, 1995.

Offen, Karen. *European Feminisms, 1700–1950: A Political History.* Stanford, Calif.: Stanford University Press, 2000.

Oreskes, Naomi. "Objectivity or Heroism?: On the Invisibility of Women in Science." *Osiris* 11 (1996): 87–113.

The Oxford Medical Companion. Edited by Jeremiah A. Barondess, John Walton, and Stephen Lock. New York: Oxford University Press, 1994.

Patterson, James T. *The Dread Disease: Cancer and Modern American Culture.* Cambridge, Mass.: Harvard University Press, 1987.

Paxton, Nancy L. *George Eliot and Herbert Spencer: Feminism, Evolutionism, and the Reconstruction of Gender.* Princeton, N.J.: Princeton University Press, 1991.

Peiss, Kathy. *Cheap Amusements: Working Women and Leisure in Turn-of-the-Century New York.* Philadelphia: Temple University Press, 1986.

Peitzman, Steven J., M.D. *A New and Untried Course: Woman's Medical College and Medical College of Pennsylvania, 1850–1998.* New Brunswick, N.J.: Rutgers University Press, 2000.

———. "Why Support a Women's Medical College? Philadelphia's Early Male Medical Pro-Feminists." *Bulletin of the History of Medicine* 77 (2003): 576–99.

Pernick, Martin S. *A Calculus of Suffering: Pain, Professionalism, and Anesthesia in Nineteenth-Century America.* New York: Columbia University Press, 1985.

Pickering, Mary. *Auguste Comte: An Intellectual Biography.* Vol. 1. Cambridge: Cambridge University Press, 1993.

Pickstone, John V. *Ways of Knowing: A New History of Science, Technology, and Medicine.* Chicago: University of Chicago Press, 2001.

Pittenger, Mark. *American Socialists and Evolutionary Thought, 1870–1920.* Madison: University of Wisconsin Press, 1993.

Porter, Dorothy, and Roy Porter. *Patient's Progress: Doctors and Doctoring in Eighteenth-Century England.* Stanford, Calif.: Stanford University Press, 1989.

Porter, Roy. *The Greatest Benefit to Mankind: A Medical History of Humanity.* New York: W. W. Norton & Company, 1997.

Porter, Theodore M. *The Rise of Statistical Thinking, 1820–1900.* Princeton, N.J.: Princeton University Press, 1986.

———. *Trust in Numbers: The Pursuit of Objectivity in Science and Public Life.* Princeton, N.J.: Princeton University Press, 1995.

Preston, Jo Anne. "Domestic Ideology, School Reformers, and Female Teachers: Schoolteaching Becomes Women's Work in Nineteenth-Century New England." *New England Quarterly* 66 (1993): 531–51.

Reis, Elizabeth. "Impossible Hermaphrodites: Intersex in America, 1620–1960." *Journal of American History* 92 (2005): 411–41.

Rhoads, Steven E. *Taking Sex Differences Seriously*. San Francisco: Encounter Books, 2004.

Rippley, La Vern J. *The German-Americans*. Boston: Twayne Publishers, 1976.

Rischin, Moses. *The Promised City: New York's Jews, 1870–1914*. Cambridge, Mass.: Harvard University Press, 1962.

Risdon, Wilfred. *Robert Lawson Tait*. London: National Anti-Vivisection Society, 1967.

Rodgers, Daniel T. *Atlantic Crossings: Social Politics in a Progressive Age*. Cambridge, Mass.: Belknap Press of Harvard University Press, 1998.

Rogers, Naomi. *An Alternative Path: The Making and Remaking of Hahnemann Medical College and Hospital of Philadelphia*. New Brunswick, N.J.: Rutgers University Press, 1998.

———. "American Medicine and the Politics of Filmmaking: Sister Kenny (RKO, 1946)." In Reagan, Tomes, and Treichler, eds., *Medicine's Moving Pictures*, 199–238.

Romano, Terrie M. *Making Medicine Scientific: John Burdon Sanderson and the Culture of Victorian Science*. Baltimore: Johns Hopkins University Press, 2002.

Rosenberg, Charles E. *The Care of Strangers: The Rise of America's Hospital System*. New York: Basic Books, 1987.

———. *The Cholera Years: The United States in 1832, 1849, and 1866*. Chicago: University of Chicago Press, 1962.

———. *No Other Gods: On Science and American Social Thought*. Baltimore: Johns Hopkins University Press, 1997.

———. "The Therapeutic Revolution: Medicine, Meaning, and Social Change in Nineteenth-Century America." In Vogel and Rosenberg, eds., *Therapeutic Revolution*, 3–25.

———. *The Trial of the Assassin Guiteau: Psychiatry and Law in the Gilded Age*. Chicago: University of Chicago Press, 1968.

Rosenberg, Charles E., and Janet Golden, eds. *Framing Disease: Studies in Cultural History*. New Brunswick, N.J.: Rutgers University Press, 1992.

Rosenberg, Rosalind. *Beyond Separate Spheres: Intellectual Roots of Modern Feminism*. New Haven, Conn.: Yale University Press, 1982.

Rosenkrantz, Barbara Gutman. "The Search for Professional Order in Nineteenth-Century American Medicine." In Leavitt and Numbers, eds., *Sickness and Health in America* (1985), 219–32.

Rosner, Lisa. "The Professional Context of Electrotherapeutics." *Journal of the History of Medicine and Allied Sciences* 43 (1988): 64–82.

Rossiter, Margaret W. *Women Scientists in America: Before Affirmative Action, 1940–1972*. Baltimore: Johns Hopkins University Press, 1995.

———. *Women Scientists in America: Struggles and Strategies to 1940*. Baltimore: Johns Hopkins University Press, 1982.

Rothman, David J. *The Discovery of the Asylum: Social Order and Disorder in the New Republic*. Boston: Little, Brown and Company, 1971.

Rothstein, William G. *American Medical Schools and the Practice of Medicine: A History*. New York: Oxford University Press, 1987.

Rudd, Jill, and Val Gough, eds. *Charlotte Perkins Gilman: Optimist Reformer*. Iowa City: University of Iowa Press, 1999.

Rupke, Nicolaas A. *Vivisection in Historical Perspective*. London: Croom Helm, 1987.

Rusby, Henry H. *The College of Pharmacy of the City of New York*. New York: New York College of Pharmacy Faculty, 1895.

Russett, Cynthia Eagle. *Sexual Science: The Victorian Construction of Womanhood*. Cambridge, Mass.: Harvard University Press, 1989.

Sahli, Nancy Ann. *Elizabeth Blackwell, M.D., 1821–1910: A Biography*. New York: Arno Press, 1982.

Sappol, Michael. *A Traffic of Dead Bodies: Anatomy and Embodied Social Identity in Nineteenth-Century America*. Princeton, N.J.: Princeton University Press, 2002.

Sax, Leonard. *Why Gender Matters: What Parents and Teachers Need to Know About the Emerging Science of Sex Differences*. New York: Double Day, 2005.

Schiebinger, Londa. *The Mind Has No Sex? Women in the Origins of Modern Science*. Cambridge, Mass.: Harvard University Press, 1989.

———. *Nature's Body: Gender in the Making of Modern Science*. Boston: Beacon Press, 1993.

Schultz, Jane E. *Women at the Front: Hospital Workers in Civil War America*. Chapel Hill: University of North Carolina Press, 2004.

Schuster, David G. "Personalizing Illness and Modernity: S. Weir Mitchell, Literary Women, and Neurasthenia, 1870–1914." *Bulletin of the History of Medicine* 79 (2005): 695–722.

Scott, Joan Wallach. *Gender and the Politics of History*. New York: Columbia University Press, 1988.

Shafer, David A. *The Paris Commune: French Politics, Culture, and Society at the Crossroads of the Revolutionary Tradition and Revolutionary Socialism*. New York: Palgrave Macmillan, 2005.

Shapin, Steven. "Cordelia's Love: Credibility and the Social Studies of Science." *Perspectives on Science* 3 (1995): 255–75.

———. *A Social History of Truth: Civility and Science in Seventeenth-Century England*. Chicago: University of Chicago Press, 1994.

Shapin, Steven, and Simon Schaffer. *Leviathan and the Air-Pump: Hobbes, Boyle, and the Experimental Life*. Princeton, N.J.: Princeton University Press, 1985.

Shorter, Edward. *From Paralysis to Fatigue: A History of Psychosomatic Illness in the Modern Era*. New York: Free Press, 1992.

Showalter, Elaine. *The Female Malady: Women, Madness, and English Culture, 1830–1980*. New York: Pantheon Books, 1985.

Sicherman, Barbara. *Alice Hamilton: A Life in Letters*. Cambridge, Mass.: Harvard University Press, 1984.

———. "The Paradox of Prudence: Mental Health in the Gilded Age." *Journal of American History* 62 (1976): 890–912.

———. "The Uses of a Diagnosis: Doctors, Patients, and Neurasthenia." *Journal of the History of Medicine and Allied Sciences* 32 (1977): 33–54.

Simon, Walter Michael. *European Positivism in the Nineteenth Century: An Essay in Intellectual History*. Ithaca, N.Y.: Cornell University Press, 1963.

Sklar, Kathryn Kish. *Catharine Beecher: A Study in American Domesticity.* New York: W. W. Norton and Company, 1976.

―――. *Florence Kelley and the Nation's Work: The Rise of Women's Political Culture, 1830–1900.* New Haven, Conn.: Yale University Press, 1995.

Smith-Rosenberg, Carroll. *Disorderly Conduct: Visions of Gender in Victorian America.* New York: Alfred A. Knopf, 1985.

―――. "The Female World of Love and Ritual: Relations between Women in Nineteenth-Century America." *Signs* 1 (1975): 1–29.

Smith-Rosenberg, Carroll, and Charles E. Rosenberg. "The Female Animal: Medical and Biological Views of Woman and Her Role in Nineteenth-Century America." In Leavitt, ed., *Women and Health in America,* 12–27.

Sperber, Jonathan. *Rhineland Radicals: The Democratic Movement and the Revolution of 1848–1849.* Princeton, N.J.: Princeton University Press, 1991.

Spiegel, Allen D. "New York Medical College: An Early Center of Excellence in American Medical Education." *Journal of Community Health* 18 (1993): 293–315.

Stage, Sarah, and Virginia B. Vincenti, eds. *Rethinking Home Economics: Women and the History of a Profession.* Ithaca, N.Y.: Cornell University Press, 1997.

Stampp, Kenneth M. *America in 1857: A Nation on the Brink.* New York: Oxford University Press, 1990.

Starr, Paul. *The Social Transformation of American Medicine: The Rise of a Sovereign Profession and the Making of a Vast Industry.* New York: Basic Books, 1982.

Stepan, Nancy Leys, and Sander L. Gilman. "Appropriating the Idioms of Science: The Rejection of Scientific Racism." In *The Bounds of Race: Perspectives on Hegemony and Resistance,* edited by Dominick LaCapra, 72–103. Ithaca, N.Y.: Cornell University Press, 1991.

Stern, Alexandra Minna, and Howard Markel, eds. *Formative Years: Children's Health in the United States, 1880–2000.* Ann Arbor: University of Michigan Press, 2002.

Swetlitz, Marc. "American Jewish Responses to Darwin and Evolutionary Theory, 1860–1890." In Numbers and Stenhouse, eds., *Disseminating Darwinism,* 209–45.

Taylor, Keith. *The Political Ideas of the Utopian Socialists.* Totowa, N.J.: Frank Cass, 1982.

Theriot, Nancy M. "Women's Voices in Nineteenth-Century Medical Discourse: A Step toward Deconstructing Science." *Signs* 19 (Autumn 1993): 1–31.

Todd, Jan. *Physical Culture and the Body Beautiful: Purposive Exercise in the Lives of American Women, 1800–1870.* Macon, Ga.: Mercer University Press, 1998.

Tombs, Robert. *The Paris Commune, 1871.* New York: Longman Press, 1999.

Tomes, Nancy. *The Gospel of Germs: Men, Women, and the Microbe in American Life.* Cambridge, Mass.: Harvard University Press, 1998.

Tomlinson, Stephen. "From Rousseau to Evolutionism: Herbert Spencer on the Science of Education." *History of Education* 25 (1996): 235–54.

Truax, Rhoda. *The Doctors Jacobi.* Boston: Little, Brown and Company, 1952.

Tuchman, Arleen Marcia. "'Only in a Republic Can It be Proved that Science Has No Sex': Marie Elizabeth Zakrzewska (1829–1902) and the Multiple Meanings of Science in the Nineteenth-Century United States." *Journal of Women's History* 11 (1999): 121–42.

————. *Science Has No Sex: The Life of Marie Zakrzewska, M.D.* Chapel Hill: University of North Carolina Press, 2006.

————. *Science, Medicine, and the State in Germany: The Case of Baden, 1815–1871.* New York: Oxford University Press, 1993.

————. "Situating Gender: Marie E. Zakrzewska and the Place of Science in Women's Medical Education." *Isis* 95 (2004): 34–57.

Turner, James. *Reckoning with the Beast: Animals, Pain, and Humanity in the Victorian Mind.* Baltimore: Johns Hopkins University Press, 1980.

Tuttle, Jennifer S. "Letters from Elizabeth Stuart Phelps (Ward) to S. Weir Mitchell, M.D., 1884–1897." *Legacy* 17 (2000): 83–94.

Verbrugge, Martha H. *Able-Bodied Womanhood: Personal Health and Social Change in Nineteenth-Century Boston.* New York: Oxford University Press, 1988.

Viner, Russell. "Abraham Jacobi and German Medical Radicalism in Antebellum New York." *Bulletin of the History of Medicine* 72 (1998): 434–63.

————. "Abraham Jacobi and the Origins of Scientific Pediatrics in America." In Stern and Markel, eds., *Formative Years*, 23–46.

————. "Healthy Children for a New World: Abraham Jacobi and the Making of American Pediatrics." Ph.D. diss., University of Cambridge, 1997.

Vogel, Morris J., and Charles E. Rosenberg, eds. *The Therapeutic Revolution: Essays in the Social History of American Medicine.* Philadelphia: University of Pennsylvania Press, 1979.

Vostral, Sharra L. *Under Wraps: A History of Menstrual Hygiene Technology.* Lanham, Md.: Lexington Books, 2008.

Wailoo, Keith. *Drawing Blood: Technology and Disease Identity in Twentieth-Century America.* Baltimore: Johns Hopkins University Press, 1997.

Walsh, James J. *History of Medicine in New York: Three Centuries of Medical Progress.* Vol. 1–5. New York: National Americana Society, 1919.

Walsh, Mary Roth. *"Doctors Wanted; No Women Need Apply": Sexual Barriers in the Medical Profession, 1835–1975.* New Haven, Conn.: Yale University Press, 1977.

Ward, Patricia Spain. "Hygeia's Sisters: A History of Women in Pharmacy." *Caduceus* 4 (Autumn/Winter 1988): 1–54.

Warner, John Harley. *Against the Spirit of System: The French Impulse in Nineteenth-Century American Medicine.* Princeton, N.J.: Princeton University Press, 1998.

————. "The Fall and Rise of Professional Mystery: Epistemology, Authority, and the Emergence of Laboratory Medicine in Nineteenth-Century America." In Cunningham and Williams, eds., *Laboratory Revolution in Medicine*, 110–41.

————. "Ideals of Science and Their Discontents in Late-Nineteenth-Century American Medicine." *Isis* 82 (1991): 454–78.

————. *The Therapeutic Perspective: Medical Practice, Knowledge, and Identity in America, 1820–1885.* Cambridge, Mass.: Harvard University Press, 1986.

Waugh, Joan. *Unsentimental Reformer: The Life of Josephine Shaw Lowell.* Cambridge, Mass.: Harvard University Press, 1997.

Weber, A. S. *Nineteenth-Century Science: A Selection of Original Texts.* Peterborough, Ont.: Broadview Press, 2000.

Wegener, Frederick. "'What a Comfort a Woman Doctor Is!': Medical Women in the Life and Writing of Charlotte Perkins Gilman." In Rudd and Gough, eds., *Charlotte Perkins Gilman*, 45–73.

Wells, Susan. *Out of the Dead House: Nineteenth-Century Women Physicians and the Writing of Medicine.* Madison: University of Wisconsin Press, 2001.

Whorton, James C. *Crusaders for Fitness: The History of American Health Reformers.* Princeton, N.J.: Princeton University Press, 1982.

Wilson, Dorothy Clarke. *Lone Woman: The Story of Elizabeth Blackwell, the First Woman Doctor.* Boston: Little, Brown and Company, 1970.

Wimmer, Curt P. *The College of Pharmacy of the City of New York, Included in Columbia University in 1904.* Baltimore: Read-Taylor, 1929.

Wood, Ann Douglas. "'The Fashionable Diseases': Women's Complaints and Their Treatment in Nineteenth-Century America." *Journal of Interdisciplinary History* 4 (1973): 25–52.

Woolsey, Thomas A., and Robert E. Burke. "The Playwright, the Practitioner, the Politician, the President, and the Pathologist: A Guide to the 1900 Senate Document Titled 'Vivisection.'" *Perspectives in Biology and Medicine* 30 (1987): 235–58.

Zelizer, Viviana A. Rotman. *Pricing the Priceless Child: The Changing Social Value of Children.* New York: Basic Books, 1985.

Zschoche, Sue. "Dr. Clarke Revisited: Science, True Womanhood, and Female Collegiate Education." *History of Education Quarterly* 29 (1989): 545–69.

Index

Adler, Isaac, 164
Adolescence, 125, 136, 142
African Americans, 93, 94, 204, 215
Agassiz, Alexander, 135
Agassiz, Mrs. Louis, 222
"Aims and Ends" (M. Putnam), 28
Alexina B. (Herculine Barbin), 150
Algeria, 68
Allyson, June, 230
Alma Farm (Lake George, N.Y.), 166
Alumnae Association of the Woman's
  Medical College of Pennsylvania, 47,
  221–22, 230
AMA. *See* American Medical Association
American Anti-Vivisection Society, 198–99
American Humane Association, 198–99
*American Journal of Obstetrics and Diseases
  of Women and Children*, 134, 147
American Medical Association, 33, 104,
  203; Code of Ethics, 181–82
American Society for the Regulation
  of Vivisection, 197
American Woman Suffrage Association, 199
Anarchism, 71, 72, 73
Anderson, Thomas D., 31, 32
Anemia, 136, 142–43, 147
Anesthetics, 197
Angel, Anne A., 100, 181
Animal experimentation. *See* Vivisection

Animal welfare movement, 114, 196, 197, 201
Anthony, Susan B., 208, 209, 210
Anticlericalism, 157
Antis (woman suffrage opponents), 209
Anti-Vivisection (journal), 199
Antivivisection movement, 196–204
Apostoli, Georges, 141
Archives de Médecine (journal), 84
Association for Preventing the Re-
  Enactment in the State of New York
  of the Present Code of Ethics of the
  American Medical Association, 182
Association for the Advancement of the
  Medical Education of Women, 100, 221
Association for the Advancement
  of Women, 96
Atelectasis pulmonum, 164
Atlantic Monthly (magazine), 30
Atropine, 110, 111
Autopsy, 112

Bacteriology, 13, 201; physician resistance
  to theory of, 13, 184–88
Baker, C. Alice, 126–27
Bakunin, Michael, 72
Baldwin, Helen, 226, 227
Ball, Benjamin, 58
Baptist church, 19–20, 21, 22, 23, 31
Barnard College, 145, 190

Barringer, Emily Dunning, 230–31

Battey, Robert, 142

Battey's Operation, 142

Beaujon, the (Paris), 59

Beecher, Henry Ward, 27

Behier, Dr., 63

Bellevue Hospital (N.Y.C.), 104

Bennett, J. H., 42

Bernard, Claude, 53–54, 60, 83–84, 91, 101, 113, 177

Bethune, George, 27

Bibliothèque Nationale (Paris), 71

Bigelow, Henry Jacob, 126, 198

Biological determinism, 1–2, 54, 115, 116–26, 233; Clarke's emphasis on, 1, 122–23, 126–27, 128; male bias and, 116–17; Mary Jacobi's version of, 117, 119–20, 152–53; hysteria debate and, 136. See also Sex differences

Biology. See Cell theory; Cellular pathology; Evolution theory; Physiology; Science; Scientific medicine; other specific aspects

Biology of sex. See Biological determinism; Sex differences

Birth control, 121–22

Blackwell, Alice Stone, 199–200, 206

Blackwell, Elizabeth, 45, 62, 66, 210, 231; New York Infirmary and, 5, 33, 102–3; sympathetic model of medicine and, 10, 101, 231; medical studies in Paris of, 57–58; religion and, 99; Woman's Medical College of the New York Infirmary and, 101, 104–5, 107–8; male physicians' support for, 104; as vivisection opponent, 107–8; ovarian surgery concerns of, 120; on sex differences, 120; bacteriology and, 184

Blackwell, Emily, 9, 102, 107, 108–9, 135, 164, 222

Blackwell, Henry, 204

Blake, Lillie Devereux, 207

Blatch, Harriot Stanton, 207

Bleecker, George W., 17

B. M. (Mary Jacobi patient), 147–50, 153

Boas, Franz, 163, 166

Boas, Sophie Meyer, 156, 158, 163, 170

Boas, Toni, 170

Boston Medical and Surgical Journal, 114

Bourgeois culture, 74, 155

Bowditch, Henry Pickering, 133, 201

Bowery to Bellevue: The Story of New York's First Woman Ambulance Surgeon (Barringer), 230

Boylston Prize, 8, 126–28, 133, 134, 135, 232

Brackett, Anna C., 123, 127

Brain: emotions and, 125; male vs. female, 152. See also Mental activity

Brain tumors, 8, 227–29; progression of symptoms of, 228

Breast milk, 154, 179, 180

Bremer, Fredrika, 25, 26, 241 (n. 43)

Bres, Madeleine, 63, 67

Bright's disease, 62

Brizendine, Louann, 233

Browning, Robert, 50

Brown-Séquard, Charles Édouard, 111

Bryn Mawr College, 222

Butler Health Lift, 141

Cancer. See Tumors

"Case" (M. P. Jacobi), 227, 229

"Case of Absent Uterus" (M. P. Jacobi), 147

Catholicism, 54, 74, 88–89, 90, 157

Catt, Carrie Chapman, 208

Celibacy, 121

Cell, The (Wilson), 145, 146

Cell theory, 32, 33, 41–43, 91–92

Cellular pathology, 5, 7, 41, 42, 60, 157, 159, 177; tumors and, 8, 227–29

Century (publication), 196, 200

"Characteristics" (Mitchell), 143–44

Charcot, Jean-Martin, 58, 111

Chemistry, 105, 106, 117; Mary Jacobi's study of, 48, 58, 60, 83; physiology and, 83; menstruation research and, 130

Childbearing, 94, 99; professional women and, 95; family size limit and, 121–22. *See also* Reproductive health

Child health. *See* Pediatrics

Childhood mortality, 163, 164, 178–79

Chloroform, 197

Chlorosis. *See* Anemia

Cholera infantum, 154, 178, 179

Christianity, 88; Mary Jacobi's critique of, 89–90. *See also* Catholicism; Evangelicalism

Civil service reform, 191, 214

Civil Service Reform Association, 214

Civil War, 4, 35–39, 80

Clarke, Edward H., 1, 6, 8, 122–28, 132, 232, 233

Class: Mary Jacobi's views on, 8, 12, 146; hierarchies and, 8, 93–94, 146, 213, 215, 234; hysteria and, 137; as Abraham Jacobi concern, 156, 173, 180; woman suffrage and, 207, 208, 213, 214. *See also* Working class

Cleveland, Emeline Horton, 47

Clinical Society of the New York Post-Graduate Medical School, 188

Code of Ethics (AMA), 181–82

Coeducation, 124–29, 135, 176, 210; seen as women's health threat, 1, 122–26; women's campaign for at Johns Hopkins, 222–25

Cogitationes de vita rerum naturalium (A. Jacobi), 157

Cole, Isabella, 22

Collectivism, 73, 92, 216

Cologne Communist Trial, 158

Columbia University College of Physicians and Surgeons, 160–61

"Common Sense" (Paine), 212

"Common Sense" Applied to Woman Suffrage (M. P. Jacobi), 212–14, 216

Commune de Paris au jour le jour, La: 19 mars–28 mai, 1871 (Reclus), 71

Communist League of Karl Marx and Friedrich Engels, 156

Comte, Auguste, 8, 51, 73, 87, 88, 90, 91, 93. *See also* Positivism

Congress, U.S., 201

Consumerism, 159

Consumers' League, 176, 190, 215, 216, 217–20, 230

Contraband, Sarah (servant), 37

Cooperative movement, 72

Cooper Institute (N.Y.C.), 208

Co-production, idiom of, 12

Cornell University, 106, 210, 224

Cornil, André-Victor, 60, 62, 69

Corps Législatif (France), 66, 78

Corruption reform, 195, 211, 214

Critic, The (publication), 214

Croly, David G., 88

Curtis, Edward, 188

Curtis, George William, 27

Cushier, Elizabeth, 229

"Cyclical Theory of Menstruation, The" (Goodman), 133

Cytogenesis, 41

Dana, Charles L., 9, 227, 229

Danton, Joseph-Arsène, 65

Danville Prison (Va.), 38

Darwin, Charles, 88, 148, 197

Darwinism. *See* Evolution theory

Deacks, Mary, 187

Declaration of Independence, 174, 175

"De la graisse neutre et des acides gras" (M. Putnam thesis), 83, 84–85

Democracy, 173

Democratic Party, 214

Democratic socialism, 173–74

Denonvilliers, Charles-Pierre, 63

Department store workers, 217–18, 219

"Dialysis" (M. Putnam thesis), 34

Digestion, 124–25

Dimock, Susan, 47–48, 127

Diphtheria: Jacobi children and, 167, 170–73; bacteria theory and, 184–88

Disease: somatic manifestations of, 7, 136; tenement life and, 102; electrical

therapy treatment and, 141–42, 145; nutrition factor and, 180; bacteriology and, 184–88. *See also specific conditions*
Dissection, 6, 106–7, 110–11. *See also* Vivisection
Doctors. *See* Medical profession; Women physicians
Doctors Jacobi, The (Truax), 230
Domesticity, 93, 96, 137, 217
Drugs: pharmacy studies and, 3, 33–34; medical training in, 105, 106; Mary Jacobi's research on, 110, 111, 183; for pain relief, 197, 202
DuBois, Ellen Carol, 207
Dumesnil, Alfred, 69, 74
Duruy, Victor, 65, 66, 67, 68
Dynamometer, 130

École de Médecine (Paris), 3, 5, 50, 54, 56, 57, 58, 59, 60, 62–69, 82–85, 99
École Pratique (Paris), 57, 62
Economic crisis of 1857, 17–19
Education: hygiene and, 125; women's progress in, 129, 210, 214; vivisection and, 201. *See also* Coeducation; Medical schools; Women's higher education
Education of American Girls, The (Brackett), 123
"Effeminacy" (M. Putnam), 29
Electrical therapy, 141–42, 145
Embryonic development, 148, 149, 151
Emotions, 98, 125, 138
Endocrinology, 149
Endometritis, 134–35
Engelmann, George J., 133, 141
Engels, Friedrich, 158, 159
Enlightenment, 73, 156, 159
Episcopal church, 20
Essays on Hysteria (M. P. Jacobi), 139, 227
Estrus, 132
Ether, 197
Eugenie, empress of France, 67, 68
Eulenberg, Albert, 139

Evangelicalism, 19, 21, 90; women and, 4, 16, 89, 199
Evolutionary biology. *See* Evolution theory
Evolutionary socialism, 92
Evolution of Sex (Geddes and Thomson), 151
Evolution theory, 13, 118, 123, 197; sex differences argument and, 8, 54, 148, 194, 195; social/racial hierarchy and, 8, 93–94, 146, 213, 234; social progress and, 73, 145–46, 210; woman suffrage argument and, 194, 210, 213, 225; gendered division of labor and, 216–17
Exercise. *See* Physical activity
Experimentalism and laboratory science, 105–14; dissection and, 6, 106–7, 110–11; medical practice and, 6, 182–85; Mary Jacobi's belief in, 6–7, 10, 12, 54, 60, 83, 87, 91, 109–14, 122, 135, 183–84, 195, 196, 203, 221; bacteriology and, 13, 184–86; French medical studies and, 53; positivism and, 91; Elizabeth Blackwell's view of, 101, 107–88; women medical students and, 106–7, 221–22, 225; human subjects and, 111–14, 197, 203–4; nutrition studies and, 122, 130; anemia studies and, 142–43. *See also* Vivisection
Experimental psychology, 232

Faradization, 141–42
Fat and Blood (Mitchell), 136, 143
Female (later Woman's) Medical College of Pennsylvania, 224; Mary Jacobi's studies at, 3, 15, 16, 39, 41, 43–47, 48, 66; alumnae association of, 47, 221–22, 230
Female body. *See* Biological determinism; Female maladies; Reproductive health; Women's health
Female Brain, The (Brizendine), 233
Female maladies, 7, 13, 123–24, 129, 134–35, 141, 205; invalidism and, 11, 99, 115, 118; cultural obsession with, 118. *See also* Hysteria
Female physicians. *See* Women physicians

Femininity, 29, 234; women physicians and, 6, 10, 56, 65, 67, 99, 109–10; Victorian view of, 10, 28, 48–49, 109–10, 136, 138; true womanhood and, 28, 32; active model of, 118; vivisection debate and, 198–200, 203. *See also* Gender roles

Feminism. *See* Women's rights movement

Field, Adele M., 207

Figaro, Le (Paris newspaper), 68, 84

Films, 230–31

First Baptist Church (N.Y.C.), 19, 21, 22, 23, 31

Force: sex differences and, 148, 151. *See also* Nerve force

Forget, Monsieur, 66

Forty-Eighters, 158, 166

"Found and Lost" (M. Putnam), 30–31

Fourier, Charles, 74, 92–93

France, 8, 50–56, 66–85; radical thought and, 5, 71–73, 77; Second Empire climate in, 50, 51, 53, 54, 55, 66–68, 78; women's status in, 50, 53, 54–56, 73, 82, 85; republicanism and, 51, 73, 80–82, 85, 87; positivism and, 51, 150; laboratory science and, 53; medical profession and, 53–56; feminism and, 55, 67, 68, 69, 73, 82, 85. *See also* Paris

Franco-Prussian War, 5, 51, 69, 72–73, 77–80

Freedmen, 36, 37, 38

Freedmen's Bureau, 35, 38

Freemasonry, 72

Free Thinkers, 72

Frémont, John C., 27

Fussell, Edwin, 45–46, 246 (nn. 137, 142)

Galen, 41

Galvanization, 141

Ganglionic system, 124–25

Garrett, Elizabeth, 66, 67

Garrett, Mary, 121, 222, 223

Garrison, William Lloyd, 172

Geddes, Patrick, 151, 152

Gender equality. *See* Women's rights movement

Gender politics, 1–2, 12, 100, 215, 231–32, 234; Jacobis' marriage and, 174–75, 193; women's rational capacity and, 195. *See also* Biological determinism; Sex differences

Gender roles, 84, 132, 144, 174–76; Victorian-era norms and, 1–2, 6, 10, 13, 24, 28, 48–49, 109–10, 115, 116, 118, 148, 153; biological argument for, 1–2, 11–14, 54, 114–26, 152–53, 233; scientific study and, 5, 11–12, 94, 96–99, 114–15, 117, 146, 148, 152, 195, 231–34; medical practice and, 6, 155; Jacobis' differing perspectives on, 9, 10–11, 169, 174, 175–76; New Woman icon and, 24, 232, 234; True womanhood image and, 28, 32; Civil War's effect on, 39; France and, 50, 53, 54–56, 73, 82, 85; Fourier utopianism and, 74, 92–93; Comte's positivism and, 93; domesticity and, 93, 96, 137, 217; women's reproductive function and, 94; hysteria and, 136–37; in Near East, 215; division of labor and, 216–17. *See also* Femininity; Masculinity; Women; Women's rights movement

Geneva Medical College, 210

Geography, 72

German Dispensary of the City of New York, 159–60, 163, 185

German Hospital (N.Y.C.), 161

Germany, 7, 155–58; scientific medicine and, 182, 185–86

Germ-layer theory, 149

Germ theory. *See* Bacteriology

Gilded Age, 5, 88, 216

Gilder, Richard Watson, 230

Gilman, Charlotte Perkins, 144–46, 216–17, 230

Gilman, Daniel C., 224

Girl in White (film), 230–31

Goncharova, Ekaterina, 67

Goodman, John, 133

Göttingen University (Germany), 156

G. P. Putnam (publisher), 17–19, 25, 26

G. P. Putnam's Sons (publisher), 123, 128, 212, 236 (n. 12)
Grace Church (N.Y.C.), 191
Gray, Henry, 42
Great Britain, 17, 55, 114, 158
Greeley, Horace, 26
Greenspan, Ezra, 36
Green-Wood Cemetery (Brooklyn), 171, 192, 229
Gregory, Samuel, 44–45
Gynecology, 7, 8, 103. *See also* Reproductive health

"Hair Chains" (M. Putnam), 29
Hale, Edward Everett, 27
Hall, G. Stanley, 148
Hammond, William A., 143
Hammonds, Evelynn, 184
Harpers (publisher), 26
Harvard Medical School, 127, 135
Harvard University, 1, 101, 224; sex differences controversies and, 126–28, 232–33. *See also* Boylston Prize
Harvey, William, 41
Havemeyer, William Frederick, 154
Health reform movement, 44, 141
Hemoglobin, 122, 142
Hérard, Hippolyte-Victor, 58, 61
Heredity, 145–46
Hermaphroditism, 117, 147–53; as metaphor for society, 153
Hewitt, Graily, 119
Hiawatha Island (Lake George, N.Y.), 165, 166; shrine to Ernst Jacobi at, 171
Higher education. *See* Medical schools; Women's higher education
Hippocrates, 88, 132
Histology, 5, 6–7, 41, 42, 60, 69, 91; tumor formation and, 228
Hodges, Richard M., 128
Holabird, Samuel B., 37, 38
Hollingworth, Leta Stetter, 232
Home Journal (magazine), 213
Homeopathy, 44, 181–82

Homes of the New World (Bremer), 26
Hôpital de la Maternité (Paris), 57–58
Hopkins, Nancy, 233
Hospital of the Women's Medical College of Pennsylvania, 230
Hôtel Dieu (Paris), 77
Hovey, Marion, 127, 135
Human experimentation, 111–14, 197, 203–4
Humanitarianism, 109
Human Work (Gilman), 145
Hunt, Harriot, 127
Hunter, Jane, 24
Hygiene, 39, 103, 125, 154, 178, 187
Hysteria, 8, 54, 58, 59, 119, 135–42; male labeling of, 11; Mary Jacobi's treatment of, 117, 138–42, 144–46; disagreement on causes of, 138

Illness. *See* Disease; Female maladies; Women's health; *specific conditions*
Immigrants, 93, 102, 113, 158–59, 187, 215
Indigestion, 125
Industrialization, 158, 159, 173, 177, 216
Infant Diet (A. Jacobi), 154, 179–81
Infant mortality, 163, 164, 178
Infant nutrition, 154, 178–81
Infections, 178, 187
Innervation sensation (Meynert theory), 139
Insanity, 59, 144
Intelligence training. *See* Mental activity
Intercourse, 121
International Working Men's Association, 72
Introduction to the Study of Experimental Medicine, An (Bernard), 53
Invalidism, 11, 99, 115, 117, 118; hysteria and, 137, 138
Irving, Washington, 17
Is Life Worth Living? (Mallock), 90

Jacobi, Abraham, 104, 154–93; pediatrics and, 3, 7, 100, 159–61, 177–83; personal losses of, 7, 9, 163, 164, 166, 170–73,

192; courtship and marriage to Mary Putnam, 7, 13, 86–87, 111, 154; political/social activism and, 7, 154–55, 156–59, 173–77; background of, 7, 155–59; previous marriages of, 7, 162–63, 192; marital/professional relationship of, 13, 121, 154–55, 169–70, 172–73, 192–93, 206; medical societies and, 86, 154, 175, 181, 186; education of, 156–58; German Dispensary and, 159–60, 163, 185; Schurz close friendship with, 166, 169, 229; as father, 166–73, 184, 188, 189, 190–92; diphtheria theories of, 170, 172, 184–88; effect of death of son on, 170–73, 192; gender politics and, 174–75; scientific medicine and, 182–88; as grandfather, 192; grave site of, 192; wife Mary's fatal illness and, 226, 229

Jacobi, Eleasar (A. Jacobi's father), 155

Jacobi, Ernst (son), 166–73; death of, 7, 170, 173, 184, 187, 188, 189, 190, 229; birth of, 166–67; burial site of, 171, 192, 229

Jacobi, Julie Abel (A. Jacobi's mother), 155

Jacobi, Kate Rosalie (A. Jacobi's second wife), 163

Jacobi, Marjorie ("Grete") (daughter), 7, 9, 10, 167–69, 187; birth of, 167; death of brother and, 170; education of, 189–90; marriage to McAneny of, 190–92

Jacobi, Mary Putnam: menstruation studies of, 1, 8, 11, 112, 117, 118–19, 122–35, 232; Clarke rebuttal of, 1, 8, 122, 123–30, 132, 232; social/political activism and, 2, 3, 5, 7, 8, 13, 50, 51, 53, 69, 71, 73–77, 85, 94, 146, 176–77, 194–95, 204–25; women's rights and, 2, 7–8, 9, 73–74, 87, 89, 94, 146, 231, 232, 234; medical reputation of, 2–3, 5, 7–8, 9–10, 11, 13, 114, 195–96, 220–24, 229–30; accomplishments of, 2–3, 225, 231–34; education of, 3, 4, 5, 23–24, 29–30; medical education of, 3, 5, 16, 32–35, 39–51, 53–60, 62–67, 69, 77, 79, 82–85; courtship and marriage of, 3, 7, 9, 10, 13, 86–87, 111, 121, 154, 154–55, 161–62;

pharmacy studies of, 3, 16, 33–35; medical society membership of, 3, 86, 114, 175, 181, 195, 220, 221; birth of, 3–4; family background of, 3–4, 155; early interests of, 3–4, 229; childhood and youth of, 4, 17–31; religion and, 4–5, 15–16, 19–23, 31–32, 33, 74–77, 89–90, 99; scientific conversion of, 4–5, 15–17, 31–34; Paris experience of, 5, 8, 13, 50–85; New York Infirmary and, 5, 86, 100, 103, 112, 129, 195; medical school faculty and, 5, 86, 100–101, 103, 104–9, 114, 195; pediatrics and, 7, 100, 112, 177, 179–81, 183; children of, 7, 164–73, 189–92; effect of death of son on, 7, 170–73, 184, 188, 189, 192, 206; hysteria studies of, 8, 11, 117, 135–46; positivism's influence on, 8, 12, 13, 51, 73, 87–94, 99, 109, 114, 124, 135, 136, 153, 213, 231; Boylston Prize and, 8, 126–28, 133, 134, 135, 232; woman suffrage advocacy and, 8, 146, 194, 195, 204–15, 225; complexity of, 8–9; Lake George retreat of, 9, 154, 164–66, 171, 190, 226; personal intensity of, 9–10, 169; Civil War activities of, 35–39, 80; engagement to Mayer of, 48, 161; engagement to Monsieur M. of, 71, 82, 161; rejection of bourgeois culture by, 74, 155; New York City medical office of, 86; vivisection defense of, 107, 108, 109–11, 113, 183, 195, 196, 197, 199, 200–204, 225, 226; goals achieved by, 114; career focus shifts of, 117; hermaphroditism studies of, 117, 147–53; marital/professional relationship of, 121, 154–55, 161–62, 169–70, 172–73, 177–89, 192–93, 206; Gilman association with, 144–46; Progressive Era causes of, 146, 177, 195, 225; infant nutrition work of, 179–81; as grandmother, 192, 226; grave site of, 192, 229; brain tumor of, 226–29; death of, 229; memorialization of, 229–31; film/literary/radio representations of, 230–31 —writings of: unpublished autobiography, 4; *Medical Record* articles, 5, 58, 60–62,

86, 105, 111, 134, 223; *Question of Rest for Women during Menstruation*, 8, 126, 128–33, 134, 216, 232; "Theorae ad lienis officium," 15, 39–43, 45; early stories, 25–31; "Dialysis," 34; "Martyr to Science," 61; "Sermon at Notre Dame," 75–77; "De la graisse neutre et des acides gras," 83, 84–85; *Value of Life, The: A Reply to Mallock's Essay*, 90–91; "Mental Action and Physical Health," 123; "Studies on Endometritis," 134–35; *Essays on Hysteria*, 139, 227; *Physiological Notes on Primary Education and the Study of Language*, 145, 189; "Case of Absent Uterus," 147; *"Common Sense" Applied to Woman Suffrage*, 212–14, 216; "Case," 227, 229
Jacobi Point (Lake George, N.Y.), 166
Jarjavay, Jean-François, 59
Jasanoff, Sheila, 12
Jews, 7, 94, 155–56
Jex-Blake, Sophia, 127
Johns Hopkins University, 222–24
Jones, Mary Dixon, 11–12, 120, 142, 231

Keen, William Williams, 201, 202
Kelley, Florence, 219–20, 230
Kimball, John C., 198, 200
Kinkel, Gottfried, 156
Kleindeutschland ("Little Germany" N.Y.C. neighborhood), 158, 159, 163
Koch, Robert, 186
Kölliker, Rudolf Albert von, 42
Krackowizer, Ernst, 159, 166

Laboratory studies. *See* Experimentalism and laboratory science
Labor movement, 8, 190, 194–95, 215–20, 225; women's health and, 176, 216–17, 220; woman suffrage and, 207. *See also* Working women
Lake George, N.Y., 9, 154, 164–66, 171, 190, 226
Language acquisition, 145

Lariboisière (Paris hospital), 58, 59
Lavoisier, Antoine, 83
Leach, William, 89
League for Political Education, 214–15
League of Peace and Freedom, 72
Leavitt, Jonathan, 17
Lederer, Susan, 197
Leffingwell, Albert T., 197–98, 202, 203
Le Gendre, Paul, 151
Leslie, John, 19, 22
Leukemia, 42, 245 (n. 124)
L'Herminez, Fanny, 75
Liebig's volumetric method, 130
"Life in the Country" (M. Putnam), 28
Lincoln, Abraham, 36
Löffler, Friedrich, 186, 188
Longfellow, Henry Wadsworth, 26, 165
Lowell, Josephine Shaw, 207, 217, 218
Loyal National League, 36

M., Monsieur (Mary Putnam fiancé), 71, 161
Madame Curie (film), 231
Maines, Rachel, 141
Mallock, William Hurrell, 90
Malnutrition, 178
Manchester (England), 158
Manhattan Borough presidency, 191
Mann, Horace, 168
Mann, Mary Tyler Peabody, 168
Manual of Pathological Histology (Ranvier and Cornil), 60
Manual of the Domestic Hygiene of the Child (Uffelmann), 181
Marriage: Mary Jacobi's view of, 75, 121, 161–62; women's economic autonomy and, 95, 144, 216–17; women physicians and, 99, 162; parental roles and, 153, 169
"Martyr to Science, A" (M. Putnam), 61
Marx, Karl, 158, 159
Masculinity: science and, 6, 11–12, 155; patriarchy and, 32, 54, 55, 215; experimentalism and, 110, 198. *See also* Gender roles
Massachusetts Medical Society, 113

Massage therapy, 142

Maternalism, 3, 117, 120

Mayer, Ferdinand F., 48, 161

McAneny, George, 172, 192, 214; marriage to Marjorie Jacobi of, 190–92

Medical journals, 5, 133, 134

Medical profession: Mary Jacobi as leader in, 2–3, 5, 7–8, 9–10, 11, 13, 114, 195–96, 220–24, 229–30; Paris as center for, 3, 53–54, 84; post–Civil War expanded influence of, 6; women physicians percentage (1900) of, 6; gender norms and, 6, 155; women's manipulation by, 11, 144; nursing and, 39, 98–99; homeopathy and, 44, 181–82; women's ability to work in, 152; Mary and Abraham Jacobis' professional relationship and, 155, 177–89; reform movement and, 157, 159; Abraham Jacobi's activism in, 173–77. See also Pediatrics; Scientific medicine; Women physicians

Medical Record (journal), 58, 60–62, 86, 105, 111, 133, 223

Medical schools, 3, 5, 43–48, 99–109; France and, 3, 5, 50, 54–60, 62–69, 82–85, 99; AMA guidelines for, 33, 104; barriers for women and, 54–56, 127, 135, 222–25; vivisection debate and, 107–9. See also specific institutions

Medical societies, 111, 112, 113; Mary Jacobi's membership in, 3, 86, 114, 175, 181, 195, 220, 221; women physicians and, 175, 220–22. See also specific groups

Medical Society of the County of New York, 86, 154, 175

Menstrual waves, 119, 133

Menstruation: Mary Jacobi's work on, 1, 8, 11, 112, 117, 118–19, 122–35, 232; Clarke's views on, 1, 122–28, 130, 232; normalization of, 125; plethoric theory of, 132

"Mental Action and Physical Health" (M. P. Jacobi), 123

Mental activity, 1, 2, 7; Mary Jacobi's training exercises in, 117, 144–46, 189; menstruation's compatibility with, 124–25; hysteria linked with, 136; sex differences and, 152

Mental health, 7, 118, 136; rest cure's effect on, 144. See also Hysteria

Mercantile Inspection Bill (1896), 219

Metabolism, 7, 148, 151

Metropolitan Fair Association, 36

Meyer, Fanny (A. Jacobi's first wife), 156, 158, 162–63

Meyer, Sophie. See Boas, Sophie Meyer

Meyer, Theodore, 166

Meyer, Willy, 166, 190

Meynert, Theodor, 139

Michelet, Jules, 55, 124

Microscopy, 60

Midwives, 16, 68

Milieu intérieur concept, 53, 83–84, 91

Ministry of Education, French, 55, 62, 66, 68

Minority groups, 93–94. See also Immigrants; Race

Mitchell, Mrs. S. Weir, 222

Mitchell, S. Weir, 113, 119, 121, 142, 143–44, 146; hysteria theories of, 136–38, 141

Montanier, Henri, 54

Morantz-Sanchez, Regina, 3, 101

Moreau de Tours, Jacques-Joseph, 59

Morphine, 197

Mosher, Clelia Duel, 232

Mother's Congress of the City of New York, 194

Motor hysteria, 136

Mount Sinai Hospital (N.Y.C.), 100, 104, 161, 181; Pediatric Clinic, 5, 112

Municipal reform, 195

Muscle mass, 119, 130–31

Napoléon III, emperor of the French, 51, 55, 66–67, 77, 78

"Napoleon Bonaparte" (M. Putnam), 28

Napoleonic Code, 54

Nation (magazine), 81, 133

National Academy of Sciences, 233

National American Woman Suffrage Association, 208, 226

National Bureau of Economic Research Conference on Diversifying the Science and Engineering Workforce, 232

National Consumers' League, 220

National Freedmen's Relief Association, 38

Nationalism, 72–73

Native Americans, 27

Natural law, 73, 94

NAWSA. *See* National American Woman Suffrage Association

Neighbors, The (Bremer), 26

Nerve force, 138, 139, 141–42

Nervous disorders, 59, 136, 138–39; tumor symptoms vs., 228. *See also* Hysteria

Nervous system, 124–25, 138

Neurasthenia, 138

Neurology, 7, 117, 195–96; brain tumor research and, 8, 227–29; hysteria and, 136, 139, 143

New England Female Medical College, 44–45

New England Hospital for Women and Children, 44–45, 47

New Orleans Times (newspaper), 38

New Woman icon, 24, 232, 234

New York Academy of Medicine, 86, 114, 139, 143, 175, 186, 229

New York Board of Health, 179

New York City: Mary Jacobi's medical career initiation in, 86; as academic and medical center, 87, 104; as cultural center, 87–88; German neighborhood in, 158, 159, 163; McAneny's political role in, 191, 214; woman suffrage campaign in, 204–11

New York College of Pharmacy, 3, 16, 33–34, 45, 66, 243 (n. 92)

New York Dispensary for Poor Women and Children, 102

New York Evening Post (newspaper), 61, 84

New York Eye and Ear Infirmary, 104

New York Herald (newspaper), 61

New York Infirmary for Indigent Women and Children, 102–3

New York Infirmary for Women and Children, 5, 33, 86, 100, 102–3, 112, 129, 195. *See also* Woman's Medical College of the New York Infirmary

New York Kommunisten Klub, 159

New York Medical College, 32–33, 45, 160

New York Medical Journal, 183

New York Neurological Society, 143, 175

New York Obstetrical Society, 175

New York Pathological Society, 175

New York Positivist Society, 87–89

New York Post-Graduate Medical School, 5, 114

New York State Constitutional Convention (1894), 207, 211–12, 214

New York Times (newspaper), 209, 214

New York Tribune (newspaper), 84, 214

New York University, 34

Nitrate of silver, 110

Noeggerath, Emil, 159

Nolan, Josie, 113

Nott, Abner Kingman, 19–20, 21–23, 240 (n. 28)

Nouvelle Géographie Universelle, La (Reclus), 72

Nursery and Child's Hospital (N.Y.C.), 104, 161

Nursing (lactation). *See* Breast milk

Nursing (profession), 39, 98–99

Nutrition, 6–7, 83, 91–92; women's health and, 6–7, 91, 118–22, 129–32, 134, 136, 138; pulse rate and, 111; hysteria and, 136, 138, 139, 145; anemia and, 142–43; sex differences and, 148, 151; pediatrics and, 154, 178–81; breast milk and, 154, 179, 180

Nutritional waves, 133

Obstetrics, 7, 177

Olympic Games (1896), 215

Original sin, 32, 33

Osler, William, 201, 202, 224, 229–30
Osler, Mrs. William, 222
Ovarian determinism, 119–20, 123
Ovarian disease. *See* Utero-ovarian disease
Ovariotomy, 120, 142, 200–201
Ovulation theory, 131–32, 133

Pain: menstruation and, 125; vivisection debate and, 197, 202
Paine, Thomas, 212
Parenthood: scientific motherhood and, 96; gender roles and, 153, 169; Jacobis' values and, 168–70
Paris, 13, 50–85; medical profession and, 3, 53–54, 84; Mary Jacobi's medical studies in, 5, 8, 62–68, 84–85; political and social climate of, 51, 53, 55, 78–82. *See also* École de Médecine
Paris Commune (1871), 5, 51, 69, 71, 80–82, 85
Pathology, 7, 112. *See also* Cellular pathology
Patriarchy, 32, 54, 55, 215
Peabody, Elizabeth Palmer, 168
Pediatrics, 3, 5, 7, 100, 154, 159–61, 173, 177–88; pathological studies and, 112
Percy, Samuel, 32, 45
Periodicity, 131
Pharmacy studies, 3, 33–34. *See also* Drugs
Philadelphia Medical and Surgical Reporter, 133
Phillips, Wendell, 27
Physical activity: women's health and, 1, 125, 131, 141, 142, 145, 194; as hysteria treatment, 117, 141, 142, 145; breast milk and, 180
Physicians. *See* Medical profession; Women physicians; *specific specialties*
Physiological Notes on Primary Education and the Study of Language (M. P. Jacobi), 145, 189
Physiology, 83, 91, 117, 133; women's health and, 6–7, 87, 124, 126, 152, 153; medical training and, 106, 107, 111; reproduction

and, 121, 131; hysteria and, 136, 138; of learning and memory, 189
Plato, 88, 205–6
Plethoric theory of menstruation, 132
Pneumonia, 183
Politics, 7, 8, 13; women's participation in, 2, 95–96; France and, 5, 51, 71–73, 77, 80–82, 85, 87; woman suffrage and, 8, 146, 194, 195, 205–15, 225; science integrated with, 51, 73, 94, 96, 154–55, 157, 195. *See also* Gender politics; Progressive Era; Socialism; Social reform
Positivism, 12, 13, 51, 72, 87–94, 99, 109, 114, 135, 136, 213; Mary Jacobi's selective adoption of, 8, 73, 89, 90–91, 94; women and, 87, 89, 93, 94, 99, 124, 153, 195; New York intellectuals and, 87–89; beliefs of, 88, 93–94, 231; critics of, 90
Post-feminism, 231
Poverty, 178, 185
Pregnancy. *See* Childbearing
Presbyterian Hospital (N.Y.C.), 104
Professional work, women and, 2, 94, 95–96, 97, 117. *See also* Women physicians
Progress, belief in, 73, 93, 94, 145, 210
Progressive Era, 8, 146, 177, 234; major causes of, 93, 195; women's reform approach and, 96; intellectual strands of, 215, 225
Prohibition, 206–7, 225
Pseudomembranes, 184, 185, 186
Psychology, 139, 232
Puberty, 119, 125
Public health, 39. *See also* Sanitation
Publishing industry, 3–4, 17–19, 24–26, 77, 87
Pulse rates, 111, 112–13, 122, 130, 141
Putnam, Amy (M. P. Jacobi's sister), 121, 167, 226
Putnam, Bishop (M. P. Jacobi's brother), 164
Putnam, Catherine (M. P. Jacobi's grandmother), 19, 21, 23, 25

Putnam, Edith (M. P. Jacobi's sister), 4, 20, 36, 38, 57, 161

Putnam, George Haven (M. P. Jacobi's brother), 4, 20, 21, 73, 164; Civil War and, 35, 36–38

Putnam, George Palmer (M. P. Jacobi's father), 17–20, 24–27, 30, 48, 86, 239 (n. 7); publishing industry and, 3–4, 17–19, 24–26, 77, 78, 87; financial losses of, 19; religion and, 19–20, 22; daughter Mary's medical studies and, 34, 48–49; Civil War and, 36, 38

Putnam, Israel (ancestor), 3

Putnam, Mary Corinna (Minnie). See Jacobi, Mary Putnam

Putnam, Rufus (ancestor), 3

Putnam, Victorine Haven (M. P. Jacobi's mother), 3, 4, 17, 20, 24, 48, 167

"Putnam's Handy Book Series of Things Worth Knowing," 179

Putnam's Monthly (magazine), 17, 26, 61, 75, 78, 241 (n. 52)

"Queen Marie Antoinette" (M. Putnam), 28

Question of Rest for Women during Menstruation, The (M. P. Jacobi), 8, 126, 128–33, 134, 216, 232

"Questions of the Day" book series, 212

Quinine, 183

Race, 8, 12, 146, 204, 215; positivism and, 93–94; woman suffrage and, 213

Ranvier, Louis-Antoine, 60, 62

Rationality, 12, 32, 125, 195

Reclus, Élie, 69, 71–72, 78, 161

Reclus, Élisée, 51, 69–73, 75, 79, 82, 85, 87, 92, 161

Reclus, Noémi, 69, 71, 82

Reconstruction era, 204

Reflex theory, 124, 136, 138

Reform, Die (publication), 159

Reform movements. See Social reform; Women's rights movement

Relief workshops, 216

Religion: women and, 4, 16, 89; Mary Jacobi and, 4–5, 15–16, 19–23, 31–32, 33, 74–77, 89–90, 99, 169; science and, 5, 32, 33, 73, 76, 77, 155; secularization and, 5, 12, 88, 197; patriarchy and, 32, 54; positivism and, 73, 88–90; female portrayals in, 89; evolution theory and, 94; women physicians and, 99; Abraham Jacobi and, 157, 169

Reproduction. See Childbearing; Sexuality

Reproductive health, 117, 118–35, 138, 142; coeducation seen as threat to, 1; New York Infirmary and, 103; ovariotomy and, 120, 142, 200–201; physiology and, 121, 131; ovulation theory and, 131–32, 133. See also Menstruation

Republicanism, French, 51, 73, 78–82, 85, 87, 155

Republican Party (U.S.), 27, 36, 212

Rest cure: menstruation and, 123, 125, 129; hysteria and, 137–38, 141; anemia and, 142; Gilman's critique of, 144

Revivalism. See Evangelicalism

"Revolutions" (M. Putnam), 28

Revolutions of 1848, 7, 156, 157, 158

Rhinehart Commission (N.Y.S.), 219

Riis, Jacob, 187

Robin, Charles, 64, 65, 69

Roosevelt Hospital (N.Y.C.), 161

Rousseau, Jean-Jacques, 73, 79

"Rules for Feeding Babies" (A. Jacobi), 179

Russia, 68

Sage, Olivia Slocum, 207

St. Mark's Hospital (N.Y.C.), 5, 195

Saint-Simon, Claude-Henri de, 92

Salem witch trials, 3

Salpêtrière (Paris hospital), 58–59

Sanitary Commission, U.S., 36, 38, 39

Sanitation, 39, 178, 185, 186–87, 195

Sappey, Marie Philibert Constant, 69

Schleiden, Matthias, 41

Schurz, Agatha, 204, 218

Schurz, Carl, 156, 158, 166, 169, 190, 212, 229

Schwann, Theodor, 41

Science, 2–7; Mary Jacobi's belief in, 4–5, 15–17, 31–34, 39–41, 154–55; women's capacity for, 5, 11–12, 94, 96–99, 114–15, 117, 146, 148, 152, 195, 231–34; religion and, 5, 32, 33, 73, 76, 77, 155; education in, 6–7, 8, 201; politics integrated with, 51, 73, 94, 96, 154–55, 157, 195; positivism and, 90–91; women's domestic application of, 96; socialism and, 155. *See also specific disciplines*

Science of sex. *See* Sex differences

Scientific medicine, 182–88, 201; Mary Jacobi's emphasis on, 1–2, 3, 6–7, 10–12, 83–84, 114; debate about role of, 6; positivism and, 73; Mary Jacobi's expertise and, 117; Jacobis' differing views on, 158, 183–84; German model of, 182, 185–86. *See also* Experimentalism and laboratory science

Scientific motherhood, 96

Scientific racism, 93–94

Scott, Francis M., 212

Scribner's Monthly (magazine), 81

Second Empire (France), 50, 51, 53, 54, 55, 66–68, 78

Second Great Awakening, 4

Secularization, 5, 12, 88, 197

Sedgwick, Catharine Maria, 25

Senate Bill 34 for the Further Prevention of Cruelty to Animals in the District of Columbia, 201

Sentimentalism, 159, 200, 206

Separate spheres ideology, 6, 13, 116, 153

"Sermon at Notre Dame, A" (M. Putnam), 75–77

Sewall, Lucy, 47, 58, 66

Seward, William, 36

Sex differences, 1–2; Mary Jacobi's theories and, 2, 8, 13, 116–17, 126, 132, 147–48, 194, 195, 196, 215, 225, 231–33, 234; arguments supporting, 2, 8, 54, 148, 188, 194, 195; gender codes and, 12; continuing debate over, 14, 232–34; hermaphroditism

and, 117, 147–53; women physicians' various views on, 120–21; nutrition and, 148, 151; feelings and, 152; woman suffrage arguments and, 210–11; gender equality and, 234. *See also* Biological determinism; Gender roles; Women

Sex in Education; or, A Fair Chance for the Girls (Clarke), 1, 122–23, 126–27, 128

Sexual identity, 148

Sexuality, 121, 132, 136, 152

Shalala, Donna E., 233

Sherry's (N.Y.C. restaurant), 208

Shrady, George Frederick, 61

"Sketches of Character" (newspaper series), 38

Slavery, 27, 35, 37, 72

Smith, Duncan, 22

Smith, Elizabeth Putnam, 22

Smith, Isaac, 22

Social class. *See* Class

Social hierarchies, 8, 93–94, 146, 213, 215, 234

Socialism: as Mary Jacobi influence, 5, 50, 51, 55, 69, 71–77, 85, 87, 90, 94, 144–45, 194–95; feminism and, 73–74, 146; utopianism and, 74, 92–93; social body concept and, 92; as Gilman influence, 144–45, 146; science and, 155; Abraham Jacobi and, 159, 173–74, 176–77

Social justice, 7, 8

Social organism, 153, 155, 174, 177, 181, 196; natural law and, 73, 94; women and, 73, 94, 122, 173, 194, 205, 216; nutrition analogy and, 91–92, 117; popularity of concept, 92–93

"Social Organism, The" (Spencer), 92

Social progress. *See* Progress, belief in

Social reform, 8, 13, 93, 173; pediatrics and, 7, 178; women and, 8, 13, 16, 96, 97; Mary Jacobi's projects and, 8, 13, 194–95, 215–20; religion and, 16; evolutionary progress and, 73; Progressive Era and, 96, 195; in health and medicine, 141, 157, 159; science and, 154–55. *See also* Labor movement; Women's rights movement

Social Register, 218
Social science, 195, 220, 232
Social work, 96, 220
Société de la Revendication de Droits
   de la Femme, La, 69
Sociology, 232
"Some of the French Leaders"
   (M. Putnam), 81
Sorbonne (Paris), 66
Spencer, Herbert, 88, 92, 145, 148
Sphygmograph, 112–13, 130, 140, 141
Spleen, 15, 39–43, 245 (n. 119)
Stanton, Elizabeth Cady, 16, 89, 208
Stephenson, William, 133
Stephenson's Wave, 133
Stone, Lucy, 86, 199, 204, 208
Storer, David Humphreys, 126
Strength building, as hysteria treatment,
   138, 139
Stress, 138
"Studies in Endometritis" (M. Jacobi),
   134–35
Suffrage, universal, 204, 205, 211, 213.
   See also Woman suffrage
Summers, Lawrence, 232–33, 234
Surgery, 59, 200–201. See also
   Ovariotomy
Swift, Mary, 22
Sympathetic model of medicine, 3, 10, 11,
   98, 199, 200; Elizabeth Blackwell and, 10,
   101, 231; vivisection debate and, 199, 200
Sympathy and Science: Women Physicians in
   American Medicine (Morantz-Sanchez), 3

Tait, (Robert) Lawson, 198, 203
Tammany machine (N.Y.C.), 214
Teaching profession, 30
Temperance movement, 198–99, 206–7, 225
"Temptation of Johns Hopkins, The"
   (editorial), 223–24
Tenements, 102, 179, 181, 195
Terre, La (Reclus), 72
"Theorae ad lienis officium" (Putnam
   thesis), 15, 39–43, 45

Therapeutical Society of New York,
   175
Thiers, Adolphe, 80, 82
Thomas, M. Carey, 121, 222–23
Thomson, J. Arthur, 151, 152
Thoreau, Henry David, 26
"Three Paths of Life" (M. Putnam), 27
Treatise on Diphtheria (A. Jacobi), 184
Truax, Rhoda, 230
True womanhood, cult of, 28, 32
"Truth" (M. Putnam), 28
Tuchman, Arleen, 120, 184
Tumors, 8, 227–29; nervous disease
   symptoms vs., 228
Twain, Mark, 198
Twelfth Street School (N.Y.C.), 23–24,
   29–30, 226
Twining, William, 42

Uffelmann, Julius, 181
Union League Club of New York, 36
University of Greifswald (Germany), 156
University of the City of New York, 160
Urea, 122, 130, 142
Utero-ovarian disease, 118, 120, 129, 134, 138,
   141, 142
Utopian socialists, 74, 92–93

Value of Life, The: A Reply to Mallock's Essay
   (M. P. Jacobi), 90–91
Vascoeuil (Dumesnil country estate), 69,
   71, 74, 166
Vesalius, Andreas, 41
Victorian era: gender ideology and, 1–2, 6,
   10, 24, 28, 48–49, 109–10, 115, 118, 136, 138,
   148, 234; hysteria diagnosis and, 135–38;
   sentimental culture of, 159, 200;
   vivisection debate and, 196–98; pain
   perspective of, 197
Villard, Fanny Garrison, 172
Villard, Henry Hilgard, 172
Viner, Russell, 160
Virchow, Rudolf, 33, 41, 42, 60, 157, 159, 177,
   183, 185, 227–28

Vivisection, 107–11, 155; opposition to, 107–8, 114, 196–204; defense of, 108–9, 113, 183, 195, 196, 201, 225, 226

Voltaire, 73, 79, 88

Voting rights. *See* Suffrage, universal; Woman suffrage

Wadleigh, Lydia F., 23–24

Warner, John Harley, 182

Warner, Susan, 25–26, 27

Wave theory, 133

WCTU. *See* Woman's Christian Temperance Union

Wear and Tear (Mitchell), 136

Wedigan, Emma, 187

Welch, William, 201, 202, 224

Wellesley College, 141

Wells, Susan, 106

Wetherell, Elizabeth (pseudonym of Susan Warner), 25

White, Frances Emily, 120, 199

White, Victoria, 170

"White List" campaign, 218, 219

Wide, Wide World, The (Warner), 25–26, 27, 31

Wilder, Burt, 106

Wiley and Long (publisher), 17

Wilson, E. B., 145, 146

"Within Our Gates" (radio program), 230

Woman question. *See* Gender roles

Woman's Christian Temperance Union, 198–99

Woman's Journal (magazine), 108, 204, 205, 206, 208, 209, 214

Woman's Medical College of Pennsylvania. *See* Female (later Woman's) Medical College of Pennsylvania

Woman's Medical College of the New York Infirmary, 5, 33, 86, 99–109, 114, 195, 200, 221; laboratory instruction and, 108–9

Woman suffrage, 8, 55, 146, 194, 195; vivisection debate and, 196–97, 199–200; Mary Jacobi's arguments for, 204–15, 225; opponents of, 209

Women: weakness/inferiority attributed to, 1–2, 54, 114–19, 123–32, 135; professional work and, 2, 94, 95–96, 97, 117; evangelicalism and, 4, 16, 89, 199; reform movements and, 8, 13, 16, 96, 97; as nurses and midwives, 16, 39, 68, 98–99; writing careers and, 23, 25–26, 27, 28; pharmacy studies and, 33, 34; social organism concept and, 73, 94, 122, 173, 194, 205, 216; positivism and, 89, 93, 94, 99, 124, 153; financial independence and, 94–95, 144, 216–17; political power and, 95–96; antivivisection movement and, 198–200, 202, 203, 204. *See also* Femininity; Gender roles; Menstruation; Sex differences; Women's health; Women's rights movement; Working women

Women and Economics (Gilman), 216–17

Women physicians: gender issues and, 2, 10–12, 54–56, 95–99, 152; Morantz-Sanchez's work on, 3; sympathetic model of medicine and, 3, 10, 11, 98, 101, 199, 200, 231; medical schools and, 3, 43–48, 54–56, 99–109, 127, 135, 222–25; Mary Jacobi's eminence among, 5, 9, 220–24, 229–30; opposition to, 5–6, 43–44, 49, 54–56, 62–63, 84–85, 143–44; medical profession percentage (1900) of, 6; femininity and, 6, 10, 56, 65, 67, 99, 109–10; women's rights and, 12, 144, 195, 220, 231; French attitudes toward, 54–56, 63–65, 67–68, 84–85; political power and, 95–96; marriage and, 99, 162; varying views on sex difference among, 120–21; Abraham Jacobi's support for, 175; medical societies and, 175, 220–22; vivisection debate and, 199, 200; films and books about, 230–31

Women's clubs, 195, 214

Women's Conference of the Society for Ethical Culture, 216

Women's Fund Committee, 222, 223, 224

Women's health, 6–8, 9, 13, 83, 91, 117–46, 194, 216, 232; education seen as threat to, 1, 107, 122–26; physical activity and, 1, 125, 131, 141, 142, 145, 194; masculine bias concerning, 2, 6, 116–17, 122–23, 137; nutrition and, 6–7, 91, 118–22, 129–32, 134, 136, 138; work and, 94–95, 124; New York Infirmary and, 102–3; reproductive system and, 103, 117, 118–35, 138, 142; labor movement and, 176, 216–17, 220, 225; impact on infant's nutrition of, 180; suffrage's link with, 205. *See also* Biological determinism; Female maladies; Hysteria

Women's higher education: Clarke's arguments against, 1, 2, 122–23; Mary Jacobi's arguments for, 2, 8, 94, 95, 117, 123–29, 195, 210; in France, 55, 68. *See also* Coeducation; Medical schools

Women's Medical Association of New York City, 229, 230

Women's Municipal League, 214

Women's rights movement, 7–9, 27; Clarke theory refutation and, 1, 123, 124, 127; women physicians and, 12, 144, 220, 231; critique of religion and, 16; in France, 55, 67, 68, 69, 73, 82, 85; socialism and, 73–74, 146; Fourier's support for, 74, 92–93; positivism and, 87, 89, 93, 94, 135; Saint-Simon and, 92; science and, 94, 117, 135, 146, 148; marriage and, 161–62; Abraham Jacobi's view of, 174–75;

evolution theory and, 194; vivisection debate and, 195, 197, 199–200; political issues of, 206; women's progress and, 210; Mary Jacobi's significance to, 231–34

Women's suffrage. *See* Woman suffrage

Woodbridge, Alice, 217

Woods, Matthew C., 198, 202–3

Woolley, Helen Bradford Thompson, 232

Working class, 8; social reform and, 93; labor movement and, 95, 129, 215–16; child health and, 178; disease transmission and, 187; woman suffrage and, 207

Working women, 94–96, 124, 144, 152; economic independence and, 94–95, 144, 216–17; rest concerns and, 129; Abraham Jacobi's view of, 176; labor reform and, 194–95, 215–20; woman suffrage and, 207, 210. *See also* Nursing; Women physicians

Working Women's Society, 216, 217

Wulfert, Elizabeth, 150

Wurtz, Adolphe, 63, 65

Wyman, Morrill, 126, 127, 135

Yellow Wallpaper, The (Gilman), 144

Yonkers (N.Y.), 27

Young Women's Christian Association, 218

Zakrzewska, Marie, 11–12, 44–45, 47, 102, 120, 135, 184, 231

Zymotic hypothesis, 185

Studies in Social Medicine

Nancy M. P. King, Gail E. Henderson, and Jane Stein, eds., *Beyond Regulations: Ethics in Human Subjects Research* (1999).

Laurie Zoloth, *Health Care and the Ethics of Encounter: A Jewish Discussion of Social Justice* (1999).

Susan M. Reverby, ed., *Tuskegee's Truths: Rethinking the Tuskegee Syphilis Study* (2000).

Beatrix Hoffman, *The Wages of Sickness: The Politics of Health Insurance in Progressive America* (2000).

Margarete Sandelowski, *Devices and Desires: Gender, Technology, and American Nursing* (2000).

Keith Wailoo, *Dying in the City of the Blues: Sickle Cell Anemia and the Politics of Race and Health* (2001).

Judith Andre, *Bioethics as Practice* (2002).

Chris Feudtner, *Bittersweet: Diabetes, Insulin, and the Transformation of Illness* (2003).

Ann Folwell Stanford, *Bodies in a Broken World: Women Novelists of Color and the Politics of Medicine* (2003).

Lawrence O. Gostin, *The AIDS Pandemic: Complacency, Injustice, and Unfulfilled Expectations* (2004).

Arthur A. Daemmrich, *Pharmacopolitics: Drug Regulation in the United States and Germany* (2004).

Carl Elliott and Tod Chambers, eds., *Prozac as a Way of Life* (2004).

Steven M. Stowe, *Doctoring the South: Southern Physicians and Everyday Medicine in the Mid-Nineteenth Century* (2004).

Arleen Marcia Tuchman, *Science Has No Sex: The Life of Marie Zakrzewska, M.D.* (2006).

Michael H. Cohen, *Healing at the Borderland of Medicine and Religion* (2006).

Keith Wailoo, Julie Livingston, and Peter Guarnaccia, eds., *A Death Retold: Jesica Santillan, the Bungled Transplant, and Paradoxes of Medical Citizenship* (2006).

Michelle T. Moran, *Colonizing Leprosy: Imperialism and the Politics of Public Health in the United States* (2007).

Karey Harwood, *The Infertility Treadmill: Feminist Ethics, Personal Choice, and the Use of Reproductive Technologies* (2007).

Carla Bittel, *Mary Putnam Jacobi and the Politics of Medicine in Nineteenth-Century America* (2009)